Mental Well-Being

Corey L.M. Keyes
Editor

Mental Well-Being

International Contributions to the Study of Positive Mental Health

Springer

Editor
Corey L.M. Keyes
Department of Sociology
Emory University
Atlanta, GA, USA

ISBN 978-94-007-5194-1 ISBN 978-94-007-5195-8 (eBook)
DOI 10.1007/978-94-007-5195-8
Springer Dordrecht Heidelberg New York London

Library of Congress Control Number: 2012953135

Printed on acid-free paper

Springer is part of Springer Science+Business Media (www.springer.com)

Prologue

There is a new generation of research in which scholars are investigating mental health and human development as not merely the absence of mental illness but also the presence of subjective well-being. Subjective well-being is a fundamental facet of the quality of life that can be assessed externally and objectively or internally and subjectively. From an objective standpoint, other people measure and judge another's life according to criteria such as income or educational attainment. Individuals who are wealthier, have more education, or live longer are considered to have higher quality of life or personal well-being. The subjective standpoint emerged shortly after World War II as an important alternative to the objective approach to measuring individual's well-being. Subjectively, individuals evaluate their own lives as evaluations made, in theory, after reviewing, summing, and weighing the substance of their lives in social context. In short, subjective well-being is an evaluation or declaration that individuals make about the quality of their lives in terms of how they feel about their lives and how well they see themselves functioning in life.

Research has clearly shown that measures of subjective well-being, which are conceptualized as indicators of mental health (or "mental well-being"), are factorially distinct from but correlated with measures of symptoms of common mental disorders such as depression. Despite countless proclamations that health is not merely the absence of illness, there had been little or no empirical research to verify this assumption. Research now supports the hypothesis that health is not merely the absence of illness but also the presence of higher levels of subjective well-being.

In turn, there is growing recognition of the personal and social utility of subjective well-being, both higher levels of hedonic and eudaimonic well-being. Increased subjective well-being has been linked with higher personal and social "goods": higher business profits, more worker productivity, and greater employee retention; increased protection against mortality; increased protection against the onset and increase of physical disability with aging; improved cognitive and immune system functioning; and increased levels of social capital such as civic responsibility, generativity, community involvement, and volunteering.

This edited volume is my humble attempt to bring together for the first time the growing scientific literature on positive mental health that is now being conducted in many countries around the world. My hope is that this volume will provide students and scholars with an invaluable source for teaching and for generating new ideas for furthering this important line of research so that the promotion and protection of good mental health becomes a truly international endeavor.

Atlanta, GA, USA Corey L.M. Keyes

Contents

Part I
Toward an International Epidemiology of Positive Mental Health

Chapter 1
Promoting and Protecting Positive Mental Health: Early and Often Throughout the Lifespan

Corey L.M. Keyes

Ancient civilizations conceived of well-being—synonymous with "good health"—as one of the highest goods in life (Sigerist 1941). Well-being was not merely an end, but it also was a means to creating and sustaining a good society. Today, mental as well as physical health are considered forms of human capital because studies consistently link the presence of mental illness and chronic physical disease to high levels of social and economic burden to society (i.e., disability, premature death, and direct and indirect costs). Health—not solely industriousness—is now viewed among the greatest sources of the "wealth" of a nation, for it is tied to the growth and development of nations (Berger et al. 2003; Bloom and Canning 2000; Sullivan 2004).

Mental illness has always been seen as problematic but not as a public health issue or impediment to the development of nations until 1996, when the World Health Organization published the results of the first Global Burden of Disease study. This study estimated the total contribution of 107 acute and chronic medical conditions and illnesses by including disability in the equation to calculate disability life-adjusted years (DALYs). The DALY reflects the total number of years in a population that were either lived with disability or abbreviated prematurely due to specific physical or mental conditions. Depression was the fourth leading cause of disease burden, accounting for 3.7% of DALYs in 1990, 4.4% in 2000, and projected to be 15% of DALYs by 2020 and to be the leading cause of burden to all nations by 2030 (Ustun 1999; Ustun et al. 2004). As such, the debate is over as whether mental illness is a serious public health issue—it is.

The biggest issue facing governments around the world is what can and should be done to reduce the number of cases of mental illness and those suffering from it. Most governments choose the de facto approach of providing treatment to more individuals (Chisholm et al. 2004). All evidence points to the fact that the de facto

C.L.M. Keyes (✉)
Department of Sociology, Emory University, Atlanta, GA, USA
e-mail: ckeyes@emory.edu

C.L.M. Keyes (ed.), *Mental Well-Being: International Contributions to the Study of Positive Mental Health*, DOI 10.1007/978-94-007-5195-8_1,

approach of talk or drug therapies is not reducing the prevalence, burden, or early age of onset for mental disorders (Kessler et al. 2005; Insel and Scolnick 2006). Albee (2006) reiterated that "public health teaches us that no mass disease or disorder has ever been controlled or eliminated through individual treatment" (p. 449), a point he delivered to the US Congress in his 1959 (Albee 1959) book on behalf of the Joint Commission on Mental Health and Illness which informed the creation of the National Institute of Mental Health.

A viable alternative is mental health promotion, which seeks to elevate levels of positive mental health and protect against its loss (Davis 2002; Jané-Llopis et al. 2005; Keyes 2007; Secker 1998). Whereas treatment targets those with mental illness and risk reduction prevention targets those vulnerable to mental illness, mental health promotion targets those with good mental health and those with less than optimal mental health—i.e., all members of a population.

To make the shift toward mental health promotion requires overcoming the bias to focus exclusively on the presence and absence of mental illness rather than also the presence and absence of mental well-being. This is an unfortunate bias in the scientific and policy community, which is the assumption that individuals who are not ill are therefore healthy. This assumption is false according research on the two- (or "dual"-) continua model of health as applied to mental illness and mental health (Keyes 2005a, b). The study of the two-continua model has led to advances in understanding how to best measure the presence and absence of good (or "positive") mental health (hereafter referred to only as "mental health") that is comparable to the measurement of mental illnesses. It has also confirmed the long-standing notion that mental health is a complete state, not merely the absence of mental illness but also the presence of sufficiently high levels of well-being that constitutes the condition Keyes (2002) calls "flourishing" mental health.

Subjective Well-Being: Mental Health as "Something Positive"

The quality of an individual's life can be assessed externally and objectively or internally and subjectively. From an objective standpoint, other people measure and judge another's life according to criteria such as wealth or income, educational attainment, occupational prestige, and health status or longevity. Nations, communities, or individuals who are wealthier, have more education, and live longer are considered to have higher quality of life or personal well-being. The subjective standpoint emerged during the 1950s as an important alternative to the objective approach to measuring individual's well-being. Subjectively, individuals evaluate their own lives as evaluations made, in theory, after reviewing, summing, and weighing the substance of their lives. In short, subjective well-being is an evaluation or declaration that individuals make about the quality of their lives (Diener et al. 1999; Keyes et al. 2002).

Well-being has been a paramount concern of thinkers since ancient times as witnessed in much of Greek philosophical writings. It became a topic of scientific inquiry during the 1950s when interest in fostering a better life was facilitated by the Zeitgeist following World War II. The world's recovery from the manifold devastation—physical, psychological, social, and moral—of the world war encouraged a commitment to social welfare, the diversity of people and viewpoints, and a greater appreciation of the individual. This atmosphere manifested itself in philosophical (e.g., phenomenology and existentialism), sociological (e.g., symbolic interactionism), and psychological (e.g., cognitive psychology) movements that focused on the centrality of the individual's perceptions and viewpoints and the importance of personal meaning and concerns about life. Subjective well-being therefore emerged as a scientific field in the late 1950s when social scientists developed indicators of quality of life to monitor social change and to improve social policy as well as pursue a humanistic scientific agenda.

Humanistic writings emphasized several concerns and constructs that buttressed the study of subjective well-being. In reaction to Orthodox psychoanalysis, humanistic scholars scientifically catalogued the individual's capacity for positive adjustment through the development of positive characteristics such as maturity, ego strength, generativity, and virtues (see, e.g., Erik Erikson's writings). In reaction to behaviorism, humanistic writers welcomed introspection and subjective appraisal as meaningful data. Humanistic social scientists also sought to understand whole lives by asking people how their lives looked to them and how they felt about their own lives. The humanism exemplified through the study of subjective well-being was distilled by Gordon Allport (cited in Severin 1965), who pronounced that "it is not enough to know how man reacts: we must know how he feels, how he sees his world, ... why he lives, what he fears, for what he would be willing to die. Such questions of existence must be put to man directly" (p. 42).

During this same historical period, the US Congress passed the "Mental Health Act" that earmarked future funds for the creation of a "National Institute of Mental Health" (NIMH), which came into being at the end of the 1940s. It is almost ironic that the Joint Commission on Mental Health and Illness, which served as the advisory board for the creation of the future NIMH, may have planted the intellectual seeds of the two dominant streams of research on subjective well-being today. This commission, chaired and dominated by psychiatrists, requested several topical reports ranging from the state of mental health services to epidemiology of mental illness. Though clearly in the minority, several Ph.D.s, including M. Brewster Smith (1959), were responsible for two separate reports on mental health, both of which reported on the status of theory and research on subjective well-being.

The first publication was Marie Jahoda's (1958) now seminal volume on positive mental health. This volume reviewed the personality and clinical psychology literatures regarding dimensions of psychological well-being (e.g., purpose in life, personal growth, and self-acceptance). The second volume, in terms of its publication, was Gurin, Veroff, and Feld's (1960) book on the state of American's mental health. This volume featured subjective well-being as through individuals' assessments of their satisfaction and happiness with life and domains of life.

The overwhelming odds of psychiatry pitted against mainstream social psychologists in the mid-1940s played history's ironic cards: The Mental Health Act of 1946 gave way in title only to the National Institute of Mental ***Health***. In practice and programs, the NIMH remains committed to the promotion of America's mental health through the study of the etiology and treatment of mental ***illness***. Although subjective well-being did not become part of this nation's mental health agenda, the impetus to launch the NIMH may have been responsible for planting the seeds of the study of subjective well-being as it appears today (Keyes et al. 2002).

Since Jahoda's (1958) and Gurin et al.'s (1960) now seminal reviews of elements of "mental health," social scientific scholars have spent the past 40 years moving forward the nascent agenda of mental health via the study of subjective well-being. In the 1980s, two seminal journal articles brought the study of subjective well-being and its two traditions into the mainstream of social science. The first was Ed Diener's (1984) review article of the state of the first generation of research and theory on subjective well-being, which had focused squarely on hedonic (i.e., happiness, life satisfaction, or affect balance) well-being. The third was Carol Ryff's (1989) article that operationalized the theory of psychological well-being outlined in Jahoda's (1958) volume.

Feeling Good About, and Functioning Well in, Life

The study of subjective well-being has been divided into two streams of research, one that equates well-being with happiness as feeling good and the other with happiness as human potential that, when pursued and developed, results in positive functioning in life. The streams of subjective well-being research grew from two distinct ancient philosophical viewpoints on happiness—one reflecting the Epicurean view that believed happiness was about feeling positive emotions (i.e., hedonic) and another reflecting the Aristotelian (and Socratic) view that happiness was about striving toward excellence and positive functioning (i.e., eudaimonia—pronounced "you-day-monia") as an individual and as a member of society (i.e., as a citizen).

The hedonic tradition that embodies human concerns with maximizing the amount or duration of positive, pleasant feelings while minimizing the amount or duration of negative, unpleasant feelings. The hedonic tradition is reflected in the stream of research on subjective *emotional* well-being (i.e., happiness, satisfaction, and affect balance). The second is the tradition of eudaimonia that animates human concerns with developing nascent abilities and capacities toward becoming a more fully functioning person and citizen. This tradition is reflected in the stream of research on subjective *psychological* (Ryff 1989) and *social* (Keyes 1998) well-being that reflect how well individuals see themselves functioning in life, striving to achieve secular standards of excellence such as purpose, contribution, integration, intimacy, acceptance, and mastery.

Social scientists have devised self-report measures to unveil people's views of the quality of their lives. Although research shows that people use multiple criteria to evaluate their subjective experiences, there are two general lines of research that have evolved. According to one line of well-being research, evaluations of the degree of positive feelings (e.g., happiness) experienced and perceptions (e.g., satisfaction) toward one's life overall constitute subjective well-being (Gurin et al. 1960). A second stream of well-being research specifies dimensions of positive functioning in terms of psychological well-being (Jahoda 1958; Keyes 1998; Ryff 1989; Ryff and Keyes 1995) and social well-being (Keyes 1998). Overall, subjective well-being consists of two broad domains—emotional well-being and positive functioning. These domains, their conceptions, and the quality of their measures will be reviewed in this section.

The Hedonic Tradition: Feeling Good About Life

Emotional well-being is a specific dimension of subjective well-being that consists of perceptions of avowed happiness and satisfaction with life and the balancing of positive and negative affects. Whereas happiness is based upon spontaneous reflections of pleasant and unpleasant affects in one's immediate experience, life satisfaction represents a long-term assessment of one's life.

Single-item measures of life satisfaction are adaptations of Cantril's (1965) self-anchoring scale, which asks respondents to "rate their life overall these days" on a scale from 0 to 10, where 0 meant the "worst possible life overall" and 10 meant "the best possible life overall." Variants of Cantril's measure have been used extensively and have been applied to the measurement of avowed happiness with life (Andrews and Withey 1976). Multi-item scales of life satisfaction and happiness also have been developed and used extensively (Campbell et al. 1976; Larsen et al. 1985). Most positive and negative affect measures tap the frequency with which a respondent reports experiencing the symptoms of these affects. For example, individuals often are asked to indicate how much of the time during the past 30 days they have felt six types of negative and six types of positive indicators of affect: "all," "most," "some," "a little," or "none of the time." Symptoms of negative affect usually include feeling (1) so sad nothing could cheer you up, (2) nervous, (3) restless or fidgety, (4) hopeless, (5) that everything was an effort, and (6) worthless. Symptoms of positive affect usually involve feeling (1) cheerful, (2) in good spirits, (3) extremely happy, (4) calm and peaceful, (5) satisfied, and (6) full of life (Mroczek and Kolarz 1998).[1]

The Eudaimonic Tradition: Functioning Well in Life

A variety of concepts from personality, developmental, and clinical psychology have been synthesized by Ryff (1989) to operationalize psychological well-being. In contrast to hedonic measures of subjective well-being, psychological well-being

[1] In my own research, I have not included the measure of negative affect to assess emotional well-being, because my research seeks to connect positive mental health with mental illnesses like depression, where negative affect (e.g., depressed mood) is part of its assessment.

requires individuals to self-report about the quality with which they are functioning in their lives (not feelings or emotions toward or about life). Each of the six dimensions of psychological well-being indicates the challenges that individuals encounter as they strive to function fully and realize their unique talents (Ryff 1989; Ryff and Keyes 1995). The six dimensions encompass a breadth of well-being: a positive evaluation of oneself and one's past life, a sense of continued growth and development as a person, the belief that one's life is purposeful and meaningful, the possession of quality relations with others, the capacity to manage effectively one's life and surrounding world, and a sense of self-determination (Ryff and Keyes 1995).

Self-acceptance is the criterion toward which individuals must strive in order to feel good about themselves. Such self-acceptance is characterized by a positive attitude toward the self and acknowledging and accepting multiple aspects of self, including unpleasant personal aspects. In addition, self-acceptance includes positive feelings about past life. *Positive relations with others* is the possession of, or the ability to cultivate, warm, trusting, intimate relationships with others. A concern for the welfare of others and the ability to empathize, to cooperate, and to compromise are all implied aspects of the ability to develop warm and trusting interpersonal relationships. *Autonomy* reflects the seeking of self-determination and personal authority or independence in a society that sometimes compels obedience and compliance. The abilities to resist social pressures so as to think or behave in certain ways, and to guide and evaluate behavior based on internalized standards and values, are crucial in this domain.

Environmental mastery includes the ability to manage everyday affairs, to control a complex array of external activities, to make effective use of surrounding opportunities, and to choose or create contexts suitable to personal needs. A sense of mastery results when individuals recognize personal needs and desires and also feel capable, and permitted, to take an active role in getting what they need from their environments. *Purpose in life* consists of one's aims and objectives for living, including the presence of life goals and a sense of directedness. Those with high purpose in life see their daily lives as fulfilling a direction and purpose and therefore view their present and past life as meaningful. Finally, *personal growth* reflects the continuous pursuit of existing skills, talents, and opportunities for personal development and for realizing one's potential. In addition, personal growth includes the capacity to remain open to experience and to identify challenges in a variety of circumstances.

Whereas psychological well-being is conceptualized as a primarily private phenomenon that is focused on the challenges encountered by individuals in their personal lives, social well-being represents a more public experience that is focused on the social tasks encountered by individuals in their social structures and communities. Social well-being consists of five elements that indicate whether and to what degree individuals are functioning well in their social world (e.g., as neighbors, as coworkers, and as citizens) (Keyes 1998). Social well-being originates in the sociological interest in individuals' anomie and alienation in society, which were classic themes in the writings of Emile Durkheim and Karl Marx. Drawing on these theoretical roots, Keyes (1998) developed multiple operational dimensions of social well-being that represent the challenges individuals face as members of society, groups, institutions, and communities.

Social integration is the evaluation of the quality of one's relationship to society and community. Integration is therefore the extent to which people feel they have something in common with others who constitute their social reality (e.g., their neighborhood), as well as the degree to which they feel that they belong to their communities and society. *Social contribution* is the evaluation of one's value to society. It includes the belief that one is a vital member of society, with something of value to give to the world. Social coherence is the perception of the quality, organization, and operation of the social world, and it includes a concern for knowing about the world. *Social coherence* is analogous to meaningfulness in life that involves appraisals that society is discernable, sensible, and predictable.

Social actualization is the evaluation of the potential and the trajectory of society. This is the belief in the evolution of society and the sense that society has a potential that is being realized through its institutions and citizens. *Social acceptance* is the construal of society through the character and qualities of other people as a generalized category. Individuals must function in a public arena that consists primarily of strangers. Individuals who illustrate social acceptance trust others, think that others are capable of kindness, and believe that people can be industrious. Socially accepting people hold favorable views of human nature and feel comfortable with others.

In the eudaimonic stream of research, confirmatory factor analysis models have revealed strong support for the proposed five-factor theory of social well-being (Keyes 1998), and the proposed six-factor theory of psychological well-being is the best-fitting model in representative sampled of US adults (Ryff and Keyes 1995). Moreover, the constructs of social well-being and psychological well-being are correlated but empirically distinct, as reported in my doctoral dissertation. That is, the scales of social and psychological well-being correlated as high as .44, and exploratory factor analysis revealed two correlated ($r = .34$) factors with the scales of social well-being loading on a separate factor from the items measuring happiness, satisfaction, and the overall scale of psychological well-being.

Measures of social well-being also represent distinct latent factors from traditional measures (happiness and satisfaction) of emotional well-being. Measures of emotional well-being (positive and negative affect, life satisfaction) are factorially distinct from the measures of psychological well-being (Keyes et al. 2002). In fact, McGregor and Little's (1998) factor analysis also yielded two distinct factors that reveal an underlying emotional factor (including depression, positive affect, and life satisfaction) and an underlying psychological functioning factor (including four of the psychological well-being scales: personal growth, purpose in life, positive relations with others, and autonomy).

Subjective Well-Being: Is It More Complex Than Feeling Good?

The description of the traditions, or streams, of research on well-being suggests that there is more to well-being than happiness or feeling good. This question was investigated in adolescents in 2002 by administering a more comprehensive assessment of subjective well-being that included emotional (items 1–3 below), social (items 4–8 below), and psychological (items 9–14 below) well-being:

1. Happy
2. Interested in life
3. Satisfied
4. That you had something important to contribute to society
5. That you belonged to a community (like a social group, your school,[2] or your neighborhood)
6. That our society is becoming a better place for people like you
7. That people are basically good
8. That the way our society works made sense to you
9. That you liked most parts of your personality
10. Good at managing the responsibilities of your daily life
11. That you had warm and trusting relationships with others
12. That you had experiences that challenged you to grow and become a better person
13. Confident to think or express your own ideas and opinions
14. That your life has a sense of direction or meaning to it

The above set of items was included in the 2002 Child Development Supplement (CDS) of the Panel Study of Income Dynamics (PSID). All families participating in the PSID in 1997 with children between the ages of 0 and 12 years old were asked to complete the CDS, resulting in a sample of 3,563. Out of all CDS families interviewed in 1997, a total of 94% of the children had parents who had remained active in the PSID as of 2001 ($n=3{,}271$), and these children were reinterviewed during the fall of 2002 and spring of 2003, resulting in a sample of 2,907 children and youth ages 5–18. All youth ages 12 or older at that time were administered the comprehensive assessment of subjective well-being.

The measures of subjective well-being were administered by audio computer-assisted self-interview. Youth read each question and listened to each questioned read to them through headphones and responded directly into a computer laptop. Youth were asked when, in the past month, they had felt or experienced the following, either "never," "once or twice," "about once a week," "two or three times a week," "almost every day," or "every day."

With a sample size of just over 1,200 adolescents, confirmatory factor analyses were performed on the CDS subjective well-being items to test various theories about the latent structure of this measure. The best-fitting model to the data (i.e., the correlations among the well-being items) was a three-factor model. That is, items measuring emotional well-being, psychological well-being, and social well-being are reflections of three distinct, but correlated, latent factors (Keyes 2005b). The two-factor model in which the items of psychological and social well-being

[2] The difference between the adult and adolescent version of the MHC-SF is that the reference to "your school" in question 5 is omitted for the adult version.

belong to a separate (i.e., eudaimonic) latent factor from the items measuring emotional (i.e., hedonic) well-being was superior to the single-factor model. Thus, superiority of the three-factor model of the aforementioned two-factor model suggests that the domain of positive (i.e., eudaimonic) function consists of two sides: a psychological form of functioning well in life and a social form of functioning well in life.

The correlations between the three latent factors were similar to the observed bivariate correlations between the subjective well-being scales. There is a slight tendency for a stronger correlation between the scale of emotional well-being and psychological well-being than between either of these two scales with the scale of social well-being. However, all correlations—both latent and observed—are modestly strong (i.e., no lower than $r = .57$) but not extremely high (i.e., no higher than $r = .71$), as would be expected from the confirmatory factor analysis results that supported the three-factor model. The internal reliabilities of the scales ranged from .78 (psychological well-being), .80 (social well-being), to .84 (emotional well-being).

The scales of subjective well-being in youth exhibited good construct validity. All three scales of subjective well-being correlated most strongly and positively with the global self-concept scale by Marsh (1990). This scale measures how much time youth ("never," "rarely," "sometimes," "most of the time," or "always") feel (1) "I have a lot to be proud of," (2) "I can do things as well as most people," (3) "I'm as good as most other people," (4) "Other people think I am a good person," (5) "When I do something, I do it well," and (6) "A lot of things about me are good." The global self-concept scale, which can be construed as a measure of confidence, correlated between .44 (with social well-being) and a high of .54 (with psychological well-being). Thus, youth who report greater levels of each component of positive mental health also tend to report more self-confidence.

The scales of subjective well-being also correlated modestly with a multi-item measure of self-determination, which is a reflection of the positive developmental outcome of competence. To measure self-determination, the youth in the CDS indicated how much of the time—"never," "rarely," "sometimes," "most of the time," or "always"—the following described them: (1) "I stay with a task until I solve it," (2) "Even when a task is difficult, I want to solve it anyway," (3) "I keep my things orderly," (4) "I try to do my best on all my work," and (5) "When I start something, I follow it through to the end." The scale of self-determination, which can be construed as an indicator of competence, correlated between .35 (with social well-being) and a high of .46 (with psychological well-being). Thus, youth who report greater levels of each component of positive mental health also tend to report more competence in terms of more self-determination (i.e., efficacy).

The CDS study measured perceived closeness to significant others and a sense of school integration, both of which are proxies for the positive outcome of connection. Youth were asked how close they felt toward six individuals—mother (or stepmother), father (or stepfather), sibling, friends, teacher, or other adults outside of school. Youth indicated whether they felt "extremely," "quite," "fairly," or "not very" close to each of the six individuals. A total score was constructed by measuring the number of individuals of the six toward which a youth felt either "quite close" or "extremely close." A higher score on this variable means that youth felt closer to more significant others. The CDS study also measured school integration, asking youth to indicate how often ("never," "once or twice in the last month," "about once a week," "two or three times a week," "almost every day," or "every day") they felt (1) part of their school, (2) close to people at their school, (3) happy to be at their school, and (4) safe at their school. A higher score on the school integration scale means that youth felt more integrated in their school—i.e., more frequently happy, safe, connected to, and close to people at their school.

The measure of perceived closeness correlated .29 with emotional well-being and .31 with psychological well-being and with social well-being. The scale measuring school integration correlated .37 with both emotional and psychological well-being and .42 with social well-being. Compared with the measure of perceived closeness, the scale measuring school integration correlated more strongly with the subjective well-being outcomes. However, as expected, youth who felt higher levels of the components of positive mental health also were more likely to report feeling closer to more significant others, and they were more likely to report higher levels of feeling integrated into their school.

The final category of positive outcomes is character, which reflects the ability to engage in normative and prosocial behaviors and refrain from antisocial and non-normative behaviors. One measure of character is participation in conduct problems such as skipping school, being arrested, smoking cigarettes, smoking marijuana, drinking alcohol, or using inhalants. As reported in Keyes (2006), flourishing youth reported the lowest prevalence of any of the aforementioned conduct problems, followed by moderately mentally healthy youth, while languishing youth reported the highest prevalence on all indicators of conduct problems. Moreover, while 25% of languishing youth engaged in at least three or more of the conduct problems, compared with 13% of moderately mentally healthy youth, only 6.5% of flourishing youth had three or more conduct problems.

Another way to assess character would be to assess how much youth care for others, or engage in prosocial behavior. Toward that end, in the CDS study, youth were also asked how frequently they helped and gave support to friends, family, and siblings in the past 6 months, using a scale from 1 (almost never) to 7 (every day). Youth were asked how often they helped friends, and how often they helped their siblings, with things they had to get done, such as homework or chores, and how often they helped parents with things they had to get done, such as chores or running errands. Youth were also asked how often they provided emotional support to their friends (as well as to siblings), such as giving them advice on a problem or making them feel better when they were sad, and how often they provide emotional support to their parents, such as making them feel better when they were sad. The average of help provided to others across the six questions (i.e., help to friends, siblings, and parents; support to friends, siblings, and parents) correlated .30 ($p < .001$) with the continuous measure of overall positive mental health. As frequency of helping others increases, level of positive mental health also tends to increase. Using the

Tukey's honestly significant difference test for pairwise contrast (and a *p*-value of .05 or less), the flourishing youth provided more support (M = 4.1, SD = 1.2) than moderately mental healthy youth (M = 3.5, SD = 1.1), who in turn provided more help to others than languishing youth (M = 3.2, SD = 1.2). Based on the response scale for helping and supporting others, the findings suggest that the difference between languishing and flourishing youth is that the former helped others "one to three times a month" on average, while flourishing youth helped others on average "about once a week." Thus, while they exhibit the lowest level of conduct problems, flourishing youth also engage in more prosocial behavior, providing more help and emotional support to friends, siblings, and parents.

The Mental Health Continuum

Though each dimension of subjective well-being represents an important domain of study in itself, Keyes (2002, 2005b) has argued that these scales collectively measure the presence and absence of mental health. That is, mental health, like mental illness, is a syndrome of symptoms of subjective well-being.

The 14 items of subjective well-being shown above represent the Mental Health Continuum-Short Form (MHC-SF), which was created for more efficient integration into epidemiological and clinical research as well as public health surveillance. The MHC-SF is derived from the long form (MHC-LF), which consisted of seven items measuring emotional well-being, six 3-item scales (or 18 items total) that measured the six dimensions of Ryff's (1989) model of psychological well-being, and five 3-item scales (or 15 items total) that measure the five dimensions of Keyes' (1998) model of social well-being. The measure of emotional well-being in the MHC-LF included six items measuring the frequency of positive affect that was derived, in part, from Bradburn's (1969) affect balance scale and a single item of the quality of life overall based on Cantril's (1965) self-anchoring items. The estimates of internal consistency reliability for each of the three sets of measures—emotional, psychological, and social well-being—in the MHC short and long forms have all been high (>.80; see, e.g., Keyes 2005a). The MHC-LF form measures of social and psychological well-being have been validated (see Keyes 1998; Ryff 1989; Ryff and Keyes 1995) and used in hundreds of studies over the past two decades, and their use as a measure of overall positive mental health was first introduced by Keyes (2002) and recently summarized in Keyes (2007).

While the MHC-LF consisted of 40 items, the MHC-SF consists of 14 items that were chosen as the most prototypical items representing the construct definition for each facet of well-being. Three items were chosen (happy, interested in life, and satisfied) to represent emotional well-being, six items (one item from each of the six dimensions) were chosen to represent psychological well-being, and five items (one item from each of the five dimensions) were chosen to represent social well-being. The response option for the short form was changed to measure the frequency with which respondents experienced each symptom of positive mental health and thereby provided a clear standard for the assessment and a categorization of levels of positive mental health that was similar to the standard used to assess and diagnosis major depressive episode (see Keyes 2002, 2005a, 2007). To be diagnosed with *flourishing* mental health, individuals must experience "every day" or "almost every day" at least one of the 3 signs of hedonic well-being and at least 6 of the 11 signs of positive functioning during the past month. Individuals who exhibit low levels (i.e., "never" or "once or twice" during the past month) on at least one measure of hedonic well-being and low levels on at least six measures of positive functioning are diagnosed with *languishing* mental health. Individuals who are neither flourishing nor languishing are diagnosed with *moderate* mental health.

The short form of the MHC has shown excellent internal consistency (>.80) and discriminant validity in adolescents (ages 12–18) and adults in the USA, in the Netherlands, and in South Africa (Keyes 2005b, 2006; Keyes et al. 2008; Lamers et al. 2010; Westerhof and Keyes 2010). The 4-week test-retest reliability estimates for the long-form scales ranging from .57 for the overall psychological well-being domain, .64 for the overall emotional well-being domain, to .71 for the overall social well-being domain (Robitschek and Keyes 2006, 2009). The test-retest reliability of the MHC-SF over three successive 3-month periods averaged .68, and the 9-month test-retest was .65 (Lamers et al. 2010). The three-factor structure of the long and short forms of the MHC—emotional, psychological, and social well-being—has been confirmed in nationally representative samples of US adults (Gallagher et al. 2009) and college students (Robitschek and Keyes 2009) and in a nationally representative sample of adolescents between the ages of 12 and 18 (Keyes 2005b, 2009) as well as in South Africa (Keyes et al. 2008) and the Netherlands (Lamers et al. 2010).

The well-being dimensions of the MHC-SF are reflected in the recent definition of mental health offered by the World Health Organization (WHO). The WHO (2004) defined good mental health as "… a state of well–being in which the individual realizes his or her own abilities, can cope with the normal stresses of life, can work productively and fruitfully, and is able to make a contribution to his or her community" (p. 12). According to Westerhof and Keyes (2010), the WHO reference to a "state of well-being" is reflected in the measurement of emotional well-being, the reference to the ability of people to "realize their abilities and cope with normal stress" is reflected in the measurement of psychological well-being, while the reference to individuals' abilities to "work productively" and "make a contribution to community" is reflected in the measurement of social well-being.

Moreover, the merger of feeling good about a life in which individuals are functioning well, I have argued (Keyes 2002), constitutes the presence of good mental health. In the same way that depression requires symptoms of *an*hedonia, mental health consists of symptoms of hedonia. But, feeling good, in the same way as only feeling sad or losing interest in life, is not sufficient for the diagnosis of a clinical state. Rather, and in the same way that major depression consists of symptoms of *mal*functioning, mental health must also consist of symptoms of positive functioning. In turn, the mental health continuum (Keyes 2002) consists of three diagnostic categories, or levels, of positive mental health: flourishing,

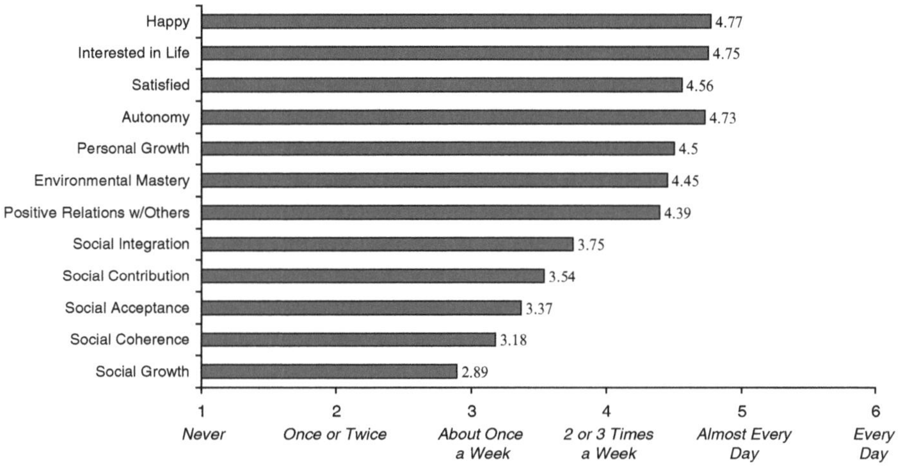

Fig. 1.1 Mean frequency of each component of mental health in the past month. U.S. adolescents, ages 12–18, in 2002 (Data from the child development supplement) ($n = 1{,}260$)

moderate, and languishing mental health. Individuals with flourishing mental health report feeling at least one measure of hedonic well-being plus six or more of the measures of positive functioning almost every day or every day during the past month. Individuals with languishing mental health, however, report feeling at least one measure of hedonic well-being with six or more measures of positive functioning never or maybe once or twice during the past month. Languishing is the absence of mental health—a state of being mentally ***un***healthy—which is tantamount to being stuck and stagnant or feeling empty or that life lacks interest and engagement. Individuals who are neither flourishing nor languishing are diagnosed with moderate mental health.

The categorical diagnosis and the continuous assessment yield very similar estimates of the prevalence of mental health in American adolescents. As such, I will report here only the categorical diagnosis, which revealed that 38% of youth between the ages of 12 and 18 are flourishing. Over half—about 56%—of adolescent are moderately mentally healthy, while 6% are languishing. Further analyses revealed a small and negative correlation of age with the continuous assessment of mental health ($r = -.07$; $p < .02$), revealing that level of mental health declines slightly between the ages of 12 and 18. Using the categorical diagnosis and grouping youth into middle school (ages 12–14) and high school (ages 15–18) revealed a 9% drop in prevalence of flourishing between middle school and high school. While the prevalence of languishing remained constant between middle school and high school, the prevalence of flourishing declined from a high of 49% in middle school to 40% in high school.

Figure 1.1 provides insight into the specific dimensions of positive mental health where youth are succeeding and where they are falling short. As reported in Keyes (2005a), mean level of overall emotional well-being was not different from the overall mean of psychological well-being. However, overall social well-being was lower than both overall emotional well-being and overall psychological well-being. Figure 1.1 reiterates these findings by revealing how all five dimensions of social well-being fall below the level at which youth are experiencing them even two or three times a week. Youth experience a sense of integration (i.e., that they belong to a community like a social group or their school) and a sense of social contribution (i.e., that they had something to contribute to society) about two or three times a week. Even worse, youth experience about once a week a sense of social growth (i.e., that our society is becoming a better place), social acceptance, (i.e., that people are basically good), and social coherence (i.e., that the way society works makes sense to them). In comparison, youth experience the dimensions of psychological and emotion well-being almost every day. In short, any attempts to improve the positive mental health of youth will clearly need to address the deficit of social well-being in the lives of US adolescents.

With Measurement We Can Test the Two-Continua Hypothesis

The importance of measuring mental health in the same way as mental illness cannot be overstated, because it allows scientists to finally adequately test the hypothesis that mental health and illness belong to two separate continua. Indeed, mental health promotion and protection is premised on the two-continua model because good mental health is presumed to belong to a separate continuum from mental illness (Health and Welfare Canada 1988). Yet, the studies that did exist on the subject only measured mental health emotionally in terms of life satisfaction or happiness (Greenspoon and Saklofske 2001; Headey et al. 1993; Huppert and Whittington 2003; Masse et al. 1998; Suldo and Shaffer 2008). Numerous studies in mainstream psychology of emotion have shown that positive and negative emotions belong to separate continua (e.g., Bradburn 1969; Watson and Clark 1997), but as mentioned earlier, emotional disturbance or emotional vitality does not, in themselves, constitute states of mental illness or mental health.

Findings based MHC-LF in the MIDUS study (Keyes 2005b) support the two-continua model: one continuum indicating the presence and absence of positive mental health and the other indicating the presence and absence of mental illness symptoms. For example, the latent factors of mental illness and mental health correlated ($r = -.53$), but only 28.1% of their variance is shared in the MIDUS data (Keyes 2005b). The two-continua model has been replicated in a nationally representative sample of US adolescents (ages 12–18) with data from the Panel Study of Income Dynamics' Child Development Supplement (Keyes 2009), in a national study of Dutch adults (Westerhof and Keyes 2008, 2010), and in Setswana-speaking South African adults using the MHC-SF (Keyes et al. 2008).

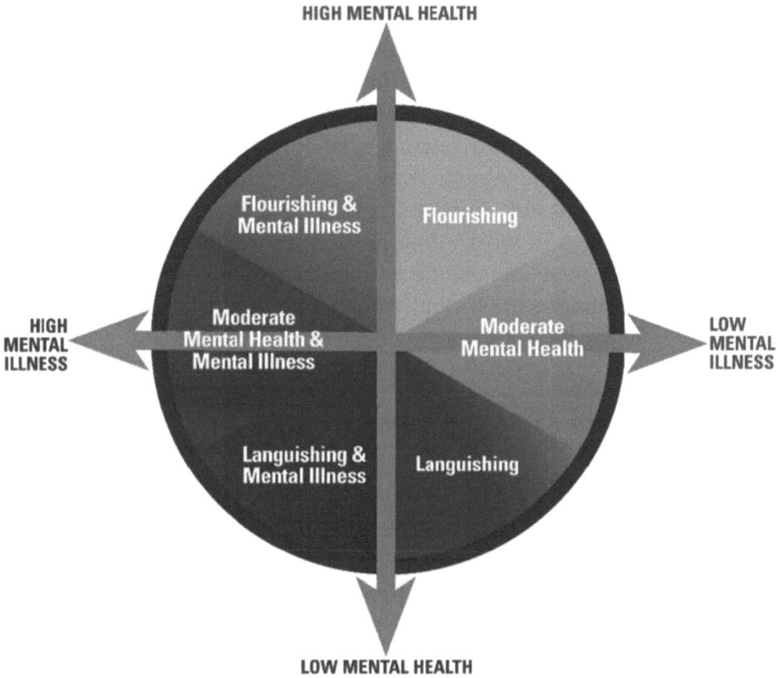

According to the dual-continua model[3] shown above, individuals can be categorized by their recent mental illness status and according to their level of mental health—whether they have languishing, moderate, or flourishing mental health. One implication of the dual-continua model is that the absence of mental illness does not imply the presence of mental health. In the American adult population between 25 and 74 years, just over 75% were free of three common mental disorders during the past year (i.e., major depressive episode [MDE], panic disorder [PD], and generalized anxiety [GAD]). However, while just over three-quarters were free of mental illness during the past year, only about 20% were flourishing. A second implication of the dual continua is that the presence of mental illness does not imply the absence of mental health. Of the 23% of adults with any mental illness, 14.5% had moderate, and 1.5% had flourishing mental health. Thus, almost seven of every ten adults with a recent mental illness (MDE, Panic or GAD) had moderate or flourishing mental health. While the absence of mental illness does not mean the presence of mental health (i.e., flourishing), the presence of mental illness does not imply the absence of some level of good mental health.

Another important implication of the dual-continua model is that level of mental health should differentiate level of functioning among individuals free of, and

[3] This graphic was commissioned by the Winnipeg Regional Health Authority's mental health promotion team and was created by the "That 2 Graphics" in Winnipeg, Manitoba, Canada. Copyright of Fig. 1.1 remains with the author (Corey L. M. Keyes), and permission to reprint it should be directed to Corey L. M. Keyes.

those with, a mental illness. Put differently, anything less than flourishing mental health is associated with impaired functioning both for those with a mental illness and individuals free of a mental illness. Findings consistently show that adults and adolescents who are diagnosed as anything less than flourishing are functioning worse in terms of physical health outcomes, health-care utilization, missed days of work, and psychosocial functioning (Keyes 2002, 2005b, 2006, 2007, 2009a, b). Over all outcomes to date, individuals who are flourishing function better (e.g., fewer missed days of work) than those with moderate mental health, who in turn function better than languishing individuals—and this is true for individuals with a recent mental illness and for individuals free of a recent mental illness.

The Dual-Continua Model in Youth

In the CDS study, the Children's Depression Inventory (Kovacs 1992) scale was the only measure of mental illness. As a screening tool, the CDI provides a threshold above which youth are expected to screen for depression under clinical assessment. The manual for the CDI recommends slightly different thresholds for boy (a score of 7 or higher) than girls (a score of 6 or higher). For our purposes here, the lower of the threshold, a score of 6 or higher, is used to suggest that an adolescent would screen for depression.

Only 4.9% of flourishing youth would screen for depression, compared with 17.3% of youth with moderate mental health. In sharp contrast, 51.5% of languishing youth would screen for depression. Thus, and compared with flourishing youth, moderately mentally healthy youth are about 3.5 times more likely to screen for depression, and languishing youth are 10.5 times more likely to screen for depression. Compared with moderately mental health youth, languishing youth are about three times more likely to screen for depression.

According to the dual-continua model, level of mental health is hypothesized to differentiate level of psychosocial functioning among individuals with and without a mental disorder. To that end, one-way ANOVAs were used to test whether level of mental health (i.e., languishing, moderate mental health, or flourishing) exerts a main effect in addition to (or interactively with) mental illness (in this case, whether or not youth are above the threshold of a score of 6 or higher on the CDI scale). The outcomes investigated included the four validation scales reported earlier (global self-concept, self-determination, perceived closeness to others, and school integration) as well as conduct problems and helping behavior. For all outcomes, level of mental health exerted a main effect (all F tests, $p < .001$), with level of conduct problems decreasing, while all other outcomes increased, as level of mental health increased. There was a main effect for the dichotomous variable of mental illness (i.e., whether or not youth had a score of 6 or higher on CDI) for the outcomes of global self-concept (F test, $p < .001$), school integration (F test, $p < .05$), and conduct problems (F test, $p < .001$), but not for the following measures: self-determination, perceived closeness to others, and helping behavior. There were no interaction effects between mental health and mental illness.

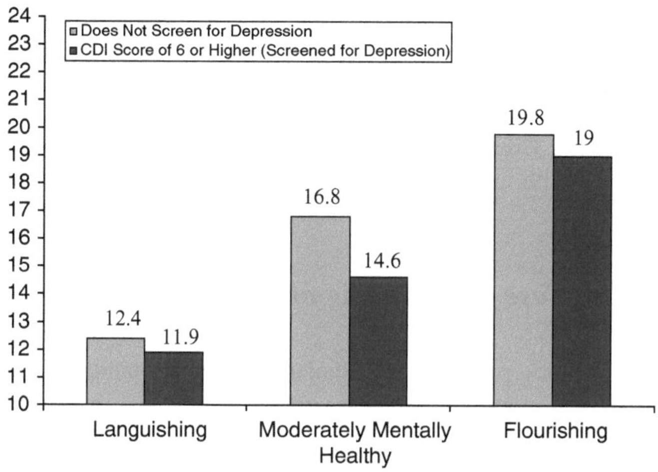

Fig. 1.2 Mean level of perceived school integration by level of mental health and whether youth screens for depression ($n = 1,260$)

Figure 1.2 presents as one example the mean level of perceived integration into school by level of mental health and by mental illness. The main effect for mental illness reveals that perceived integration into school is lower for youth who screen for depression than for youth who would screen as being free of depression, and this is true at all levels of mental health. The main effect for level of mental health reveals that level of perceived integration into school increases as level of mental health increases for youth who would screen as "depression-free" as well as for youth who would screen for depression. In other words, level of mental health matters whether youth have, or do not have, a mental disorder like depression.

How many youth in America are truly mentally healthy, i.e., flourishing in life rather than merely free of mental illness? The CDS study was not designed for the purpose of psychiatric epidemiology of youth; it therefore only provides a single screening measure of depression. Although 14% of youth were screened for depression, the estimate of overall mental illness would likely be higher if the CDS had included measures of anxiety and personality disorders. Yet studies reviewed earlier that used more comprehensive assessments of mental disorders suggest the upper limit of mental illness in youth is about 20%. As such, the findings reported here (14% screening for depression) may not be that far from the best estimate of 20% overall mental illness in youth. What is unique for the CDS is that it permits demarcating the population of youth with a mental illness (as well as without) by level of mental health.

Most youth who screened for depression had moderate mental health (9.7%), while only 1.9% was flourishing and 2.7% was languishing. The fact that the proportion of youth who are languishing with possible depression is good news because youth who screen for depression and are languishing function worse than those with moderate mental health (e.g., in terms of conduct problems). Of those who did not screen for depression, only 2.5% is languishing. Languishing in the absence of a mental disorder is rare in youth compared with adults, where languishing in the absence of mental disorders is 9.5% (Keyes 2007). Of those who do not screen for depression, just over 46% of youth are moderately mentally healthy and 37% are flourishing. By comparison, over half (50.8%) of adults otherwise free of an episode of mental disorder are moderately mentally healthy, and only 16.8% of adults are flourishing. Compared with their adult counterparts, youth in the USA are mentally healthier, with just over 20% more youth than adults flourishing.

Summary: The Case for Focusing on Youth

Despite a long-standing prejudice for scholars and the lay public to equate subjective well-being with emotional well-being (i.e., happiness), research clearly has shown that subjective well-being in US youth and adults is a multifaceted and multidimensional construct. One result of the nearly 50 years of research on this important concept is that researchers have proliferated upward of 13 facets of subjective well-being. In turn, theory and research has supported the metatheoretical models of hedonia and eudaimonia that reflect different kinds of well-being. That is, subjective well-being consists of a cluster of measures reflecting emotional, or hedonic, well-being and a cluster of measures reflecting positive functioning, or eudaimonic, well-being.

Research on the subjective well-being of youth, as with adults, has focused exclusively on the dimension of hedonia, or emotional well-being. However, the research reviewed here indicates that well-being in youth is more complex and whether its structure is equivalent to the structure of subjective well-being found among adults. Findings based on data from the nationally representative CDS sample of youth clearly supported the complex, comprehensive approach to the subjective well-being of youth. That is, among youth ages 12–18, subjective well-being is characterized in terms of distinct dimensions of emotional, psychological, and social well-being. These measures exhibit good construct validity, correlating highly with measures of the quality of one's self-concept, a youth's self-determination, as well as the degree to which youth felt integrated into their school. Moreover, the well-being measures also correlated modestly with the Kovacs (1992) Child Depression Inventory and a measure of self-rated overall health and weakly with perceived math and reading skill.

Findings also revealed that levels of emotional well-being are highest, followed closely by psychological well-being, and levels of social well-being are lowest in youth between the ages of 12 and 18. Roughly speaking, these findings suggest that American adolescents experience social well-being about once a week. What this means is that typical American adolescents felt they had something to contribute to the world about once a week; adolescents felt liked they belonged somewhere about once a week; they felt that the way our society works made sense to them about once a week; they felt that our society was becoming a better place about once a week; and our adolescents felt that people in our society were basically good about once a week. It appears more sober when put this way, making it clearer, I hope, that

America's youth sorely lack social well-being. In contrast, youth reported that they experienced psychological well-being (i.e., managing responsibilities, trusting relationships with kids, growth-producing experiences, and confidence to express ideas) about two or three times a week during the past month. However, youth reported that they experienced emotional well-being—i.e., interest in life, happiness, and satisfaction—about every day during the past month.

Is it sufficient to have youth who regularly feel happy, only rarely feel that they have experiences that challenge them to grow and become a better person, but infrequently feel that they have something important to contribute to society? Parents may hope they can raise children who become happy adults; parents probably also aspire to raise children who are and become psychological healthy and socially healthy human beings. Indeed, any nation that claims to prepare its youth to become democratically engaged citizens must have youth who know how to be, and feel, integrated into society, contributing to society, accepting of people not like them, working to improve and understand society, to have a purpose in life, self-accepting and autonomous, but also able to cultivate positive relations with others while exerting some mastery over their immediate environments and, above all, capable of continued personal growth throughout life. A comprehensive approach to the assessment of youth subjective well-being can provide a more detailed picture of the strengths and weakness of our youth, and such an approach will suggest directions for future programmatic initiatives.

Indeed, it must because less than four in every ten American adolescents are flourishing. Findings suggest that fewer adolescents are mentally healthy—nearly 40%—than would be implied by taking the obverse of the best estimate of any mental disorder in youth, which would imply that about 80% or youth are free of a mental illness and therefore mentally healthy. Just over one-half of adolescents fit the criteria for moderate mental health, while 6% were mentally unhealthy, as they fit the criteria for languishing. Moreover, findings here suggest that flourishing may decline, while moderate mental health increases, during adolescence. Nearly one-half of the middle school youth, ages 12–14, were flourishing. Flourishing was the most prevalent mental health status among adolescents aged 12–14; moderate mental health was the most prevalent mental health status among adolescents aged 15–18. These data suggest—although causality cannot be inferred from them—that there is approximately a 10% loss of flourishing between middle school and high school.

Findings support the descriptive hypotheses that flourishing youth function better than moderately mentally healthy youth, who in turn function better than languishing youth. Flourishing youth had the *fewest* depressive symptoms and conduct problems and the *highest levels* of global self-concept, self-determination, closeness to other people, and school integration. Languishing youth had the *highest number* of depressive symptoms and conduct problems and the *lowest levels* of global self-concept, self-determination, closeness to other people, and school integration. Conduct problems were higher in the older, than younger, adolescents. However, flourishing in both age groups was associated with the lowest level of conduct problems; languishing (i.e., the absence of mental health) was associated with the highest level of conduct problems in both age groups.

Continued research on the epidemiology of children's mental health in the CDS and other national studies of youth can point toward new directions for prevention of mental illness and for the study of resilience. Findings reviewed thus far in this report indicate that flourishing in adolescence is associated with developmentally desirable outcomes (e.g., low depression, few conduct problems, and high psychosocial functioning). Because these data are cross-sectional, future research is needed to determine the important question of whether positive mental health is a cause or consequence (or both) of conduct problems and psychosocial functioning. What youth are most likely to be flourishing and what factors (intrapersonal, familial, educational, and community) explain how youth come to flourishing over time could provide new insights for promoting positive development and resilience in youth and their transition into adulthood.

Ultimately, the research summarized here raises questions for (1) national public mental health goals and (2) creating effective techniques and interventions for promoting mental health in youth. Nations can no longer blithely announce that they seek to promote the mental health of their citizens while only investing in the study, treatment, and risk reduction and prevention of mental illness. The two-continua model clearly debunks this as a "wanting-doing gap" because we say we want mental ***health***, but we engage in activities directed solely toward mental ***illness***. We cannot promote mental health by solely reducing mental illness, and no amount of wishful political thinking will make this fact go away. We can, of course, politically ignore the fact of the two-continua model, and this will serve only to sacrifice more young lives to the recurrent, chronic, and incurable condition of mental illness. Indeed, I'm not convinced anymore that we, as a nation, can reduce mental illness without promoting mental health.

In turn, and in recognition that subjective well-being includes the hedonic and eudaimonic traditions, it may be necessary to better understand that feeling good and functioning well (or functioning better) may not always be compatible. Can individuals feel good about their lives at the same time they are attempting or being pushed to grow, to become better people, and to become fully contributing members of society? Studies suggest that in the short term when individuals make improvements in their functioning life, hedonic well-being may be sacrificed (Keyes 2002; Keyes and Ryff 2002). In the long run, striving to function better in life, and being supported by a nation that supports that endeavor, will clearly result in the revival of feeling good about a life in which our youth can also function well.

The Case for Mental Health Promotion

Progress has been slow in bringing mental health promotion and protection (MHPP) into the mainstream of debates about how to address the problem of mental illness. Admittedly, there has been a deficit of scientific evidence supporting the "promotion" and the "protection" axioms of MHPP. Central to the argument behind ***promotion*** is the hypothesis that gains in level of mental health should decrease the risk of mental illness over time. Central to the argument behind ***protection*** is the hypothesis that losses of mental health increase the risk of mental illness over time, and therefore efforts should be made to prevent, and to respond to, the loss of good mental health. Findings recently published (Keyes et al. 2010) using the 10-year follow-up of the MIDUS national sample strongly supported the protection and promotion hypotheses.

In 1995 and in the 2005 follow-up of the MIDUS sample, adults completed the long form of the Mental Health Continuum (MHC-LF; Keyes 2002, 2005b) and the Composite International Diagnostic Interview-Short Form (CIDI-SF; Kessler et al. 1998). Studies have shown that the CIDI-SF has excellent diagnostic sensitivity and diagnostic specificity as compared with diagnoses based on the full CIDI in the National Comorbidity Survey (Kessler et al. 1999). During the telephone interview, the CIDI-SF was used to assess whether respondents exhibited symptoms indicative of major depression episode (MDE), generalized anxiety disorder (GAD), and panic disorder (PD) during the past 12 months.

We found that the prevalence of levels of mental health and illness in 1995 and 2005 were similar, suggesting stability. The prevalence of mental illness was about the same in 1995 (18.5%) as in 2005 (17.5%); approximately eight out of every ten adults were free of any mental illness in 1995 and in 2005. The prevalence of any mental illness and the absence of mental illness appear to be stable over time. However, of the 17.5% with any mental illness in 2005, just over half (52%) were "new cases" of mental illness insofar as these adults did not have any of the three mental disorders in 1995. Thus, mental illness is dynamic over time, with about half recovering that is replaced by another half of new cases of mental illness.

The prevalence of flourishing is 3.2% higher in 2005, up from 19.2% in 1995. The prevalence of moderate mental health is 3.7% lower in 2005, which is down from 64.1% in 1995. The prevalence of languishing is 0.5% higher in 2005, slightly up from 16.7% in 1995. Compared with mental illness, levels of mental health—particularly moderate mental health and flourishing—appear slightly more dynamic at the level of the population. That is, there is a slight decline in moderate and slight increase in flourishing mental health at the level of the population. Overall, mental health appears to be relatively stable at the population level. However, only 45% of those languishing in 1995 are languishing in 2005; 51% improved to moderate, and 4% improved to flourishing mental health in 2005. Only 51% of those flourishing in 1995 are flourishing in 2005—46% declined to moderate, and 3% declined to languishing mental health in 2005. Two-thirds of those with moderate mental health in 1995 had moderate mental health in 2005. Of those with moderate mental health in 1995, about 19% improved to flourishing, and 14% declined to languishing mental health in 2005. Like mental illness, level of mental health is dynamic over time.

The Promotion and Protection Hypotheses

The changes in mental health level were strongly predictive of future mental illness. First, findings supported the protection hypothesis. Those who declined to moderate mental health were nearly four times (adjusted[4] odds ratio [OR] = 3.7) more likely to have a mental illness in 2005 as those who stayed flourishing. Thus, the first loss of good mental health—from flourishing to moderate mental health—results in a rise in the risk of future mental illness. Adults whose mental health stayed at moderate were over four times (OR = 4.4) as likely to have a 2005 mental illness as those who stayed flourishing. Compared to those who stayed at moderate mental health, those who declined to languishing—almost all of whom had moderate mental health in 1995—represented an 86% increase in the odds ratio of a 2005 mental illness (i.e., 8.2–4.4 = 3.2 ÷ 4.4 = .864). Thus, protection against the loss of moderate mental health can mitigate the risk of future mental illness.

Findings also supported the promotion hypothesis. Individuals who stayed languishing were over six times (OR = 6.6), and those who improved to moderate mental health were over three times (OR = 3.4), as likely as those who stayed flourishing to have a 2005 mental illness. Compared to staying languishing, improving to moderate mental health cuts the risk of future mental illness by nearly half (i.e., 6.6–3.4 = 3.2 ÷ 6.6 = .484). Individuals who improved to flourishing—most of whom had moderate mental health in 1995—had no more high risk of future mental illness than those who stayed flourishing.

Individuals who had any of the three mental illnesses in 1995 were five times (OR = 5.0) more likely than those who stayed flourishing to have one of the same mental illnesses in 2005. Our findings illustrate that the absence of flourishing mental health is as serious a risk factor for future mental illness as those who started with one of the mental illness. Almost half of the study sample who were free of any mental illness in 1995 but had moderate mental health in 2005 (i.e., 7.8% declined + 35.5% stayed + 4.7% improved = 48% with moderate mental health in 2005) had nearly as high an odds of mental illness in 2005 as the 18.5% who had a mental illness in 1995. Moreover, one in ten of the study sample who was free of any mental illness in 1995 but had languishing mental health in 2005 (i.e., 3.9% stayed + 6.5% declined = 10.4% with languishing in 2005) had a higher odds of mental illness in 2005 than the 18.5% who had a mental illness in 1995. In short, nearly six in every ten American adults (i.e., 48% with moderate + 10.4% with languishing mental health = 58.4%) otherwise free of MDE, GAD, or PD have about as high or even higher risk of a future mental illness than individuals who had one of those mental disorders to start.

Conclusion

Research supports the two fundamental axioms of MHPP for addressing the mental illness and mental health needs of the population. First, gains in mental health resulted in decreasing odds of mental illness over time, suggesting that promoting mental

[4] All models controlled for mental illness, age, sex, race, and education in 1995; marital status in 2005 and employment status in 2005; and whether respondents had any of 25 physical health conditions in 1995.

health could reduce the incidence and prevalence of mental illness. Second, losses of mental health resulted in increasing odds of mental illness over time, suggesting that protecting against loss of mental health could reduce the incidence and prevalence of mental illness. Third, mental health is dynamic over time, although the point prevalence estimates of any mental illness and level of mental health appear stable from 1995 to 2005. The reason for this apparent stability is that approximately half of the mental illness in 2005 represent new cases, while half of those flourishing in 2005 are new cases, and over half of those languishing in 2005 are new cases.

Further, research suggests that governments should invest in MHPP to keep pace with—i.e., prevent—the rise of new cases of mental illness. While having had a mental illness in the past is a good predictor of future mental illness, the absence of mental health is an equally good, and in some cases a better, predictor of future mental illness. Nearly 60% of the US adult population free of mental illness but with less than optimal mental health have as high, or higher, risk of a future mental illness as individuals who already have a mental illness. Failure to address the problem of the absence of positive mental health in populations means risking failure in attacking the problem of mental illness.

Ultimately, the research summarized here raises questions for (1) national public mental health goals and (2) creating effective techniques and interventions for MHPP. Government and public health officials can no longer blithely announce that they seek to promote the mental health of their population while investing mainly in treatment and the study of mental illness. The two-continua model debunks this as a "wanting-doing gap" in public health policy, where policies pronounce national efforts to seek ***health*** but engage in activities directed primarily or solely toward ***illness***. If a nation wants better mental health, it must focus on positive mental health—promoting flourishing and protecting against its loss. Governments cannot promote mental health by solely reducing mental illness, and no amount of wishful thinking will make this fact disappear. Nations can ignore the science supporting the two-continua model, but this will serve only to sacrifice more lives to the recurrent, chronic, and currently incurable condition of mental illness. The alternative and complementary approach to treatment is public mental health promotion and protection.

The question is no longer whether mental illness is a public health issue—it is. The question is no longer whether we have any alternative to treatment for reducing mental illness—we do. Research has clarified where citizens and governments should want to be; the debate, then, is not where we want to be—it is flourishing.

The most important next step for researchers and practitioners is to discover how to get more people to stay or become flourishing. Those in public health and governments who expect answers immediately as to how to best promote and protect are not being fair or realistic—it takes time and financial support. The National Institute of Mental Health (NIMH) in the United States was created by an Act of Congress in 1946, and it started its work in earnest in 1949. Today, billions of dollars annually (see http://www.nimh.nih.gov/about/budget/cj2010.shtmt) of taxpayer money are spent by well-intentioned leaders for the study and treatment of mental illness. If it wants good mental health in the population, the government must provide the same realistic time frame and financial support to MHPP—imagine where we might be today had we had started the "war" on mental illness 50 years ago by attempting to promote and protect the best in people—we just might have the flourishing society we all aspire to and need for the security and health of our nation.

References

Albee, G. W. (1959). *Mental health manpower trends*. New York: Basic Books.

Albee, G. W. (2006). Historical overview of primary prevention of psychopathology: Address to the 3rds world conference on the promotion of mental health and prevention of mental and behavioral disorders September 15–17, 2004, Auckland, New Zealand. *The Journal of Primary Prevention, 27*, 449–456.

Andrews, F. M., & Withey, S. B. (1976). *Social indicators of well-being: Americans' perceptions of life quality*. New York: Plenum.

Berger, M. L., Howell, R., Nicholson, S., & Sharda, C. (2003). Investing in healthy human capital. *Journal of Occupational and Environmental Medicine, 45*, 1213–1225.

Bloom, D. E., & Canning, D. (2000). The health and wealth of nations. *Science, 287*, 1207–1209.

Bradburn, N. M. (1969). *The structure of psychological well-being*. Chicago: Aldine.

Campbell, A., Converse, P. E., & Rodgers, W. L. (1976). *The quality of American life: Perceptions, evaluations, and satisfactions*. New York: Russell Sage.

Cantril, H. (1965). *The pattern of human concerns*. New Brunswick: Rutgers University Press.

Chisholm, D., Sanderson, K., Ayuso-Mateos, J. L., & Saxena, S. (2004). Reducing the global burden of depression: Population-level analysis of intervention cost-effectiveness in 14 world regions. *British Journal of Psychiatry, 184*, 393–403.

Davis, N. J. (2002). The promotion of mental health and the prevention of mental and behavioral disorders: Surely the time is right. *International Journal of Emergency Mental Health, 4*, 3–29.

Diener, E. (1984). Subjective well-being. *Psychological Bulletin, 95*, 542–575.

Diener, E., Suh, E. M., Lucas, R. E., & Smith, H. L. (1999). Subjective well-being: Three decades of progress. *Psychological Bulletin, 125*, 276–302.

Gallagher, M. W., Lopez, S. J., & Preacher, K. J. (2009). The hierarchical structure of well-being. *Journal of Personality, 77*, 1025–1049.

Greenspoon, P. J., & Saklofske, D. H. (2001). Toward an integration of subjective well-being and psychopathology. *Social Indicators Research, 54*, 81–108.

Gurin, G., Veroff, J., & Feld, S. (1960). *Americans view their mental health*. New York: Basic Books.

Headey, B., Kelley, J., & Wearing, A. (1993). Dimensions of mental health: Life satisfaction, positive affect, anxiety, and depression. *Social Indicators Research, 29*, 63–82.

Health and Welfare Canada. (1988). *Mental health for Canadians: Striking a balance*. Ottawa: Supply and Services Canada.

Huppert, F. A., & Whittington, J. E. (2003). Evidence for the independence of positive and negative well-being: Implications for quality of life assessment. *British Journal of Health Psychology, 8*, 107–122.

Insel, T. R., & Scolnick, E. M. (2006). Cure therapeutics and strategic prevention: Raising the bar for mental health research. *Molecular Psychiatry, 11*, 11–17.

Jahoda, M. (1958). *Current concepts of positive mental health*. New York: Basic Books.

Jané-Llopis, E., Barry, M., Hosman, C., & Patel, V. (2005). Mental health promotion works: A review. *Promotion and Education, 12*(Suppl 2), 9–25.

Kessler, R. C., Foster, C. L., Saunders, W. B., & Stang, P. E. (1995). Social consequences of psychiatric disorders, I: Educational attainment. *American Journal of Psychiatry, 152*, 1026–1032.

Kessler, R. C., Andrews, G., Mroczek, D., Ustun, B., & Wittchen, H.-U. (1998). The world health organization composite international diagnostic interview short form (CIDI–SF). *International Journal of Methods in Psychiatric Research, 7*, 171–185.

Kessler, R. C., DuPont, R. L., Berglund, P., & Wittchen, H.-U. (1999). Impairment in pure and comorbid generalized anxiety disorder and major depression at 12 months in two national surveys. *American Journal of Psychiatry, 156*, 1915–1923.

Keyes, C. L. M. (1998). Social well-being. *Social Psychology Quarterly, 61*, 121–140.

Keyes, C. L. M., & Ryff, C. D. (2000). Subjective change and mental health: A self concept theory. *Social Psychology Quarterly, 63*, 264–279.

Keyes, C. L. M. (2002). The mental health continuum: From languishing to flourishing in life. *Journal of Health and Social Behavior, 43*, 207–222.

Keyes, C. L. M. (2005a). The subjective well-being of America's youth: Toward a comprehensive assessment. *Adolescent and Family Health, 4*, 3–11.

Keyes, C. L. M. (2005b). Mental health *and/or* mental illness? Investigating axioms of the complete state model of health. *Journal of Consulting and Clinical Psychology, 73*, 539–548.

Keyes, C. L. M. (2006). Mental health in adolescence: Is America's youth flourishing? *American Journal of Orthopsychiatry, 76*, 395–402.

Keyes, C. L. M. (2007). Promoting and protecting mental health as flourishing: A complementary strategy for improving national mental health. *American Psychologist, 62*, 95–108.

Keyes, C. L. M. (2009a). The black-white paradox in health: Flourishing in the face of inequality. *Journal of Personality, 77*, 1677–1706.

Keyes, C. L. M. (2009b). The nature and importance of positive mental health in America's adolescents. In R. Gilman, E. S. Huebner, & M. J. Furlong (Eds.), *Handbook of positive psychology in schools* (pp. 9–23). New York: Routledge.

Keyes, C. L. M., Shmotkin, D., & Ryff, C. D. (2002). Optimizing well-being: The empirical encounter of two traditions. *Journal of Personality and Social Psychology, 82*, 1007–1022.

Keyes, C. L. M., Wissing, M., Potgieter, J. P., Temane, M., Kruger, A., & van Rooy, S. (2008). Evaluation of the Mental Health Continuum Short Form (MHC-SF) in Setswana speaking South Africans. *Clinical Psychology and Psychotherapy, 15*, 181–192.

Keyes, C. L. M., Dhingra, S. S., & Simoes, E. J. (2010). Change in level of positive mental health predicts risk of mental illness. *American Journal of Public Health, 100*, 2366–2371.

Kovacs, M. (1992). *Children's depression inventory manual.* North Tonawanda: Multi-Health Systems.

Lamers, S. M. A., Westerhof, G. J., Bohlmeijer, E. T., ten Klooster, P. M., & Keyes, C. L. M. (2010). Evaluating the psychometric properties of the Mental Health Continuum-Short Form (MHC-SF). *Journal of Clinical Psychology, 67*, 99–110.

Larsen, R. J., Diener, E., & Emmons, R. A. (1985). An evaluation of subjective well-being measures. *Social Indicators Research, 17*, 1–17.

Marsh, H. (1990). *Self-description questionnaire manual.* Macarthur: University of Western Australia.

Masse, R., Poulin, C., Dassa, C., Lambert, J., Belair, S., & Battaglini, A. (1998). The structure of mental health higher-order confirmatory factor analyses of psychological distress and wellbeing measures. *Social Indicators Research, 45*, 475–504.

McGregor, I., & Little, B. R. (1998). Personal projects, happiness, and meaning: On doing well and being yourself. *Journal of Personality and Social Psychology, 74*, 494–512.

Mroczek, D. K., & Kolarz, C. M. (1998). The effect of age on positive and negative affect: A developmental perspective on happiness. *Journal of Personality and Social Psychology, 75*, 1333–1349.

Robitschek, C., & Keyes, C. L. M. (2006). *Multidimensional well-being and social desirability.* Unpublished data.

Robitschek, C., & Keyes, C. L. M. (2009). The structure of Keyes' model of mental health and the role of personal growth initiative as a parsimonious predictor. *Journal of Counseling Psychology, 56*, 321–329.

Ryff, C. D. (1989). Happiness is everything, or is it? Explorations on the meaning of psychological well-being. *Journal of Personality and Social Psychology, 57*, 1069–1081.

Ryff, C. D., & Keyes, C. L. M. (1995). The structure of psychological well-being revisited. *Journal of Personality and Social Psychology, 69*, 719–727.

Secker, J. (1998). Current conceptualizations of mental health and mental health promotion. *Health Education Research, 13*, 57–66.
Severin, F. T. (1965). *Humanistic viewpoints in psychology*. New York: McGraw-Hill.
Sigerist, H. E. (1941). *Medicine and human welfare*. New Haven: Yale University Press.
Smith, M. B. (1959). Research strategies toward a conception of positive mental health. *American Psychologist, 14*, 673–681.
Suldo, S. M., & Shaffer, E. J. (2008). Looking beyond psychopathology: The dual-factor model of mental health in youth. *School Psychology Review, 37*, 52–68.
Sullivan, S. (2004). Making the business case for health and productivity management. *Journal of Occupational and Environmental Medicine, 46*, 56–61.
Ustun, T. B. (1999). The global burden of mental disorders. *American Journal of Public Health, 89*, 1315–1318.
Ustun, T. B., Ayuso-Mateos, J. L., Chatterji, S., Mathers, C. D., & Murray, C. J. L. (2004). Global burden of depressive disorders in the year 2000. *British Journal of Psychiatry, 184*, 386–392.
Watson, D., & Clark, L. A. (1997). The measurement and mismeasurement of mood: Recurrent and emergent issues. *Journal of Personality Assessment, 86*, 267–296.
Westerhof, G. J., & Keyes, C. L. M. (2008). Mental health is more than the absence of mental illness. *Monthly Mental Health* (In Dutch, Summary in English), *63*, 808–820.
Westerhof, G. J., & Keyes, C. L. M. (2010). Mental illness and mental health: The two continua model across the lifespan. *Journal of Adult Development, 17*, 110–119
World Health Organization. (2004). *Promoting mental health: Concepts, emerging evidence, practice* (Summary report). Geneva: Author.

Chapter 2
Complete Mental Health in South Australian Youth: Prevalence, Measurement, and Promotion

Anthony Venning, Jaklin Eliott, Lisa Kettler, and Anne Wilson

Seligman (2008) states that building psychological strengths to promote mental health may be the best approach to preventing or alleviating mental illness. According to the Australian Bureau of Statistics (ABS 1997), an individual with good mental health is considered to be able to handle day-to-day events and obstacles, function effectively among peers and society, and engage in health-promoting behavior. In contrast, the American Psychiatric Association (APA 2000) attests that an individual with mental illness is considered to exhibit a clinically significant behavioral or psychological set of symptoms (or is at significantly higher risk of these), and that such symptoms are associated with present distress, pain, disability, or a loss of freedom that impacts the individual's ability to function effectively.

At present, despite Seligman's call for a focus on building psychological strengths, most mental health information available to the public (e.g., brochures and general practitioner support) has focused on the elimination of mental illness, with little focus on psychological strengths and mental health. In order to address this broad issue, we set out to examine both mental health and mental illness within South Australian adolescents and to provide a baseline from which the mental health needs of young Australians may be better understood and met.

A. Venning (✉) • L. Kettler
School of Psychology, The University of Adelaide, Adelaide, Australia
e-mail: anthony.venning@adelaide.edu.au

J. Eliott
School of Population Health, The University of Adelaide, Adelaide, Australia

A. Wilson
School of Nursing, The University of Adelaide, Adelaide, Australia

C.L.M. Keyes (ed.), *Mental Well-Being: International Contributions to the Study of Positive Mental Health*, DOI 10.1007/978-94-007-5195-8_2,

Promotion of Mental Health in Australia

The promotion of mental and physical health has been, and remains, a priority of the Australian government. Promoting and maintaining good health is one of Australia's national research priorities, with AUD $5 billion dollars allocated to the National Action Plan on Mental Health 2006–2011 (Council of Australian Governments [COAG] 2006). There is evidence to suggest that attempts to improve the physical health of Australian adults have been successful: The Australian Institute of Health and Welfare (AIHW 2008) has reported that since the 1950s, rates of smoking in Australian males have fallen from 75 to <20%, and deaths from cardiovascular disease have fallen 76% from their peaks in the 1960s. However, attempts to promote mental health in Australia have not met with the same success, particularly among youth. At present, mental health problems remain the largest nonfatal burden of disease in Australia, with 14% of youth aged 4–17 years (Sawyer et al. 2000) and 26% of youth aged 16–24 years (ABS 2008) reporting a mental health problem. In relation to health-risk behavior in Australian youth, 11% of young Australians (ages 14–19 years) smoke, 25% (ages 5–17 years) are overweight or obese, 24% (ages 14–19 years) drink alcohol on a weekly basis, and 62% (ages 15–24 years) are engaged in very little or no exercise (ABS 2006, 2009; AIHW 2005, 2006). Given the well-established links between mental and physical health (Shaffer-Hawkins et al. 2010), these rates of health-risk behaviors among Australian youth are causes for significant concern in the quest to improve mental health in this population.

Numerous programs have been developed and employed with the avowed intent to promote mental health in young Australians, all of which acknowledge the need for engaging, appropriate, and comprehensive strategies to respond to the specific needs of young people (McGorry et al. 2006). Few programs, however, actually promote mental health. To qualify this, it appears that the vast majority of mental health strategies and initiatives in Australia focus on the prevention or alleviation of mental illness, despite theoretical and empirical evidence that indicates that mental health is not automatically increased when mental illness is prevented or as mental illness decreases (e.g., Keyes 2005a). For example, the four strategies in Australia's current Action Plan on Mental Health (Council of Australian Governments 2006), to which funding is allocated, are to (a) reduce the prevalence and severity of mental illness, (b) reduce risk factors that contribute to mental illness, (c) increase access to health care for people with mental illness, and (d) increase the opportunities for people with mental illness to participate in the community. Therefore, the primary focus in this strategy is on the prevention and alleviation of mental illness, with an implicit assumption that the prevention and treatment of mental illness will indirectly promote mental health.

Why the Need to Promote Mental Health in Adolescence?

Adolescence typically refers to the developmental period between the ages of 12 and 20 years, and is characterized by changes in biological appearance, self-esteem, social networks, autonomy, and sexual maturation (Graber et al. 1996; Petersen and Leffert 1995; Seifert et al. 2000). Thus, while adolescence—the age of onset for most mental disorders (Kessler et al. 2005)—may be an overwhelming and stressful time, it may also provide opportunities for growth and the development of protective factors (Maggs et al. 1997). Protective factors for mental health include those psychological strengths (e.g., self-esteem or hope), contexts (e.g., stable family environment), or health-promoting behaviors (e.g., exercise or healthy diet) that act to increase the likelihood of desirable outcomes and buffer or moderate the negative influence of exposure to risk factors (Luthar 1991; Rutter 1987). Risks to mental health arise from stressors or circumstances that act to increase the likeliness of negative outcomes and decrease the likeliness of positive outcomes (Braverman 1999). Health-risk behavior is defined as participating in those activities that have a negative effect on health or are associated with undesirable consequences, such as tobacco smoking or unprotected sex (Keeler and Kaiser 2010).

Adolescence is the developmental period most commonly associated with an increased exposure to risk factors and an increased vulnerability to mental illness and/or the adoption of health-risk behavior (AIHW 2006; Larson and Ham 1993; Rowling 2006; Rutter and Smith 1995). To some degree, however, risk-taking behavior is a normal part of development as young people attempt to discover and consolidate their identities (Carr-Gregg et al. 2003), but it becomes abnormal when the type or frequency of the behavior has the potential for serious, long-term, and negative health consequences (Irwin et al. 1997). Moffitt (1993) defines two patterns of risk-taking behavior: a continuous *life-persistent* course and a temporary *adolescent-limited* involvement. It is suggested that the majority of risk-taking that stems from the perceived rewards available is adolescent-limited (i.e., rebellious image), and abandoned when prosocial behavior becomes more rewarding (Moffitt 1993). However, the combined or individual effect of mental illness, risk factors, and/or health-risk behavior in adolescence can prevent the natural development of the protective factors that, if developed early, are more likely to persist and have enduring consequences for physical and mental health (Maggs et al. 1997).

Australian Programs Employed to Promote Mental Health in Young People

Numerous efforts have been made within the research community in Australia to identify the prevalence of mental health in young people; trial programs have been designed to improve the mental health of young people, and coordination of services have been aimed at supporting young people at risk for the development of mental illness. The effectiveness of these approaches at achieving these goals, however, is questionable due to their predominate focus on the identification and elevation of mental illness. Several noteworthy examples are introduced here, and their impacts are discussed below. The universal school-based Friends program was developed by Barrett and colleagues (Barrett et al. 2006), and has been trialed in Australia to determine whether it can help prevent the onset of anxiety and depression in young Australians. The Friends program aims to teach young people how to identify feelings, understand physiological responses, link thoughts to feelings, and develop the cognitive, physiological, and behavioral processes needed to prevent or cope with psychological distress. Roberts et al. (2003) conducted a trial of the Penn Prevention Program (PPP) to reduce the symptoms of depression in young Australians identified as being at risk of developing depression. The PPP was employed in a school setting and focused on teaching young people to identify feelings, subdue catastrophic thoughts, deal with family conflict, and develop coping skills.

Quayle et al. (2001) conducted a trial of a universal prevention program to reduce levels of depression and increase levels of self-esteem in young Australians. The program trialed by Quayle et al. focused on instructing young people about the link between thoughts and feelings, challenging pessimistic beliefs, and increasing coping skills, social skills, and problem solving. Headroom, launched in 2000, is an innovative website operated by the Child, Youth, and Women's Health Service (South Australia) that attempts to promote mental health in young Australians (ages 6–18 years), and increase health literacy and community awareness via games, information, and activities related to mental health (Headroom 2009). MindMatters, launched in 2000, is a government-funded approach targeted at young people while at school and is designed to enhance resilience; develop strategies to cope with change, loss, bullying, and harassment; and improve a child's overall understanding of mental illness (MindMatters 2009). Finally, Headspace, initially founded in 2006, is a federal government initiative that seeks to provide a national and coordinated approach to the mental health and social well-being of young Australians (ages 12–26 years), with a particular focus on the early identification of those at risk of developing mental illness (Headspace 2006).

The few studies that have attempted to describe the prevalence of mental health in Australian youth have predominately used indicators of negative functioning to do so (e.g., Sawyer et al. 2000; Zubrick et al. 1995). There is, moreover, some discrepancy evident in that some of the research has reported that up to a third of young people in Australia show significant psychological distress (Eckersley et al. 2005), while others have suggested that approximately 80% are satisfied with life and have good mental health (Smart and Sanson 2005). Thus, faced with this conflicting information, it is imperative that further information on a young person's complete mental health be obtained, and an alternative approach to assessing and promoting mental health be developed.

The main focus of the Friends program and PPP was to reduce the symptoms of anxiety and depression. While these programs were successful at achieving this in the short term, it is unclear whether or not levels of mental health were increased because no indictors of positive functioning were included in the studies that evaluated them (Barrett et al. 2006; Lowry-Webster et al. 2001; Roberts et al. 2003). Similarly, a holistic and treatment-based approach was adopted by the Headspace and MindMatters initiatives, with an aim to increase knowledge about mental illness. However, Headspace and MindMatters arguably stopped short of actively promoting mental health because they primarily focused on providing information about and treating the symptoms of mental illness. Therefore, we argue that strategies and programs that focus on the prevention or alleviation of mental illness may be successful at doing just that, but they do not actively propel a young person toward a sustainable state of mental health, and effectively support only those who have mental health problems. In contrast, the Headroom initiative and the universal program trialed by Quayle et al. (2001) are a step in the right direction and focus on developing psychological strengths to prevent the onset of mental health problems. However, the sustainability of the benefits provided by the universal program trialed by Quayle et al. (2001) is unclear, given that no follow-up period existed beyond 6 months and given that the online and informational platform of Headroom fails to provide any practical strategies for promoting mental health and may not reach those who do not have the time, resources, or inclination to access the website.

Despite the contribution of research and programs such as those cited above, a high proportion of young Australians still experience mental health difficulties, engage in health-risk behavior, and are at risk of developing comorbid mental illness. In some part, this less-than-ideal situation may be the result of the flawed assumption that appears to underpin the promotion of mental health in Australia (i.e., that mental health can be obtained by reducing levels of mental illness), and the limited mental health information *not* based on the absence of mental illness.

With a perceived lack of alternatives, it seems the current situation has led to a failure to develop alternative strategies of identifying or attaining mental health outside of eliminating mental illness, despite empirical evidence that mental health and mental illness are not polar opposites, and the prevention or alleviation of the latter does not necessarily indicate or increase levels of the former (Keyes 2005a, 2007; Keyes and Lopez 2002). The success of any strategy based on the assumption that mental illness and mental health are opposite ends of the same continuum is therefore questionable. That is not to say that we do not acknowledge the importance of addressing mental illness, particularly given that the annual cost of mental illness is approximately AUD $20 billion (COAG 2006). However, we suggest that a focus on mental illness is not a focus on mental health, nor does it promote mental health by default, and that the mental health needs of young Australians may be better served by an additional focus on a young person's psychological strengths.

An Alternative Approach to Mental Health

Since 1998, the field of positive psychology has contributed significantly to the conceptualization of mental health and has shown that increases in positive virtues or strengths are associated with better physical, psychosocial, and psychological

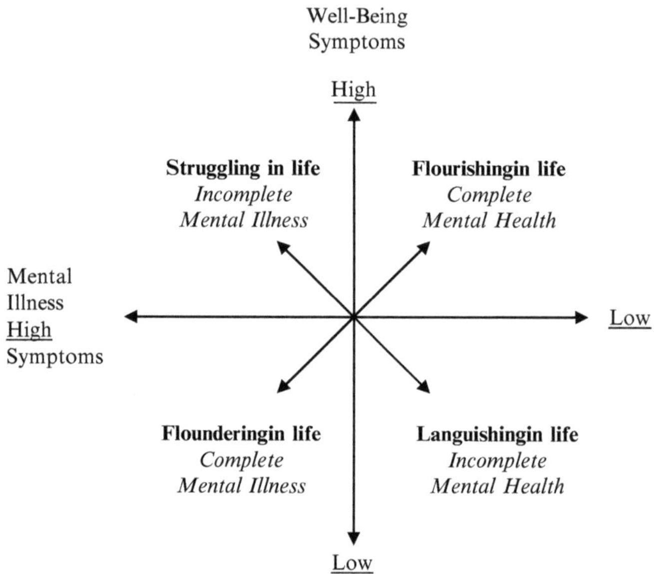

Fig. 2.1 Mental health and mental illness: the Complete State Model

functioning, and fewer symptoms of mental illness (Seligman and Csikszentmihalyi 2000; Seligman et al. 2005; Seligman 2005). It is suggested that if such a positive focus is adopted early in life, it can help develop a young person's psychological strengths and lay the foundations of a sustained healthy life in adulthood (Licence 2004). From this perspective, the Complete State Model (Keyes and Lopez 2002) provides a valuable therapeutic and diagnostic framework for clinicians, and Snyder's Hope Theory (Snyder et al. 1991) and Fredrickson's Broaden and Build Theory (1998) offer two processes that can be employed to propel an individual toward a sustainable state of mental health.

The Complete State Model of Mental Health

The Complete State Model (CSM) of mental health is a diagnostic framework that conceptualizes mental health and mental illness separately, and as complete or incomplete states, as seen in Fig. 2.1 (Keyes and Lopez 2002). In this framework, Complete Mental Health (CMH) (i.e., *flourishing* in life) is not just the absence of mental illness, nor is it just the presence of high levels of subjective well-being, but rather, CMH encompasses the absence of mental illness *and* the presence of high levels of subjective well-being. Alternatively, incomplete mental health (i.e., *languishing* in life) encompasses low levels of mental illness *and* low levels of subjective well-being; incomplete mental illness (i.e., *struggling* in life) encompasses high levels of mental illness *and* high levels of subjective well-being; and Complete Mental Illness (CMI) (i.e., *floundering* in life) encompasses high levels of mental illness *and* low levels of subjective well-being.

Practically speaking, an individual who is flourishing in life feels positive and is fulfilling their goals and aspirations, while an individual who is languishing in life lacks positive emotion and is not fulfilling their goals or aspirations in life (Grant and Cavanagh 2007). Research conducted by Keyes (2002, 2004, 2005b, 2006) has provided support for the CSM of mental health and has indicated that people classified as flourishing in life fare better than those who are not flourishing in terms of their physical, psychological, and psychosocial functioning.

In terms of a therapeutic framework, the CSM provides a way in which clinicians can organize and interpret an individual's cognitive, behavioral, and emotional functioning, and then translate aspects of these into objectives for therapy. Moreover, the CSM of mental health suggests that the objective of strategies to promote mental health must be to build those psychological strengths that can then shift people from poorer states of functioning (i.e., *languishing*, *struggling*, or *floundering*) toward a sustainable state of *flourishing* in life.

Hope Theory

The cognitive process of hope is an example of a positive psychological strength that can be employed as a mechanism to move young people toward a sustainable state of flourishing in life. According to Snyder's Hope Theory (Snyder et al. 1991), hopeful thinking consists of three elements: goal setting, *pathways* thinking, and *agency* thinking. Goals provide the anchor for the mental action sequences that are generated by successful hopeful thinking (Snyder 1994). Pathways and agency thinking are suggested to continually affect, and be affected by, each other during the goal pursuit process (Snyder 2000). Pathways thinking reflect an individual's capacity to conceptualize one or more avenues in order to arrive at a desired goal, while agency thinking reflects an individual's ability to initiate and sustain movement along a chosen pathway in order to reach that goal (Snyder et al. 1991). Successful hopeful thinking thus enables an individual to set goals, develop strategies to achieve those goals, and build and sustain the motivation to execute those strategies (Cheavens et al. 2006; Snyder et al. 1991). Hopeful thinking begins as children start to think about themselves and their goal pursuits (Snyder 2000). However, it is only upon reaching adolescence that an individual is suggested to have all the necessary cognitive resources required for successful hopeful thinking in all areas of life. According to Seifert et al. (2000), the development of formal operational thought enables a young person to emphasize the possible rather than the actual, reason systematically, and combine ideas skillfully. Relating this to hopeful thinking, it may be only during adolescence that young people can begin to envisage future goals, conceive possible and practical ways to obtain these, and envisage the practical benefits of goal pursuit in all aspects of their lives.

There is considerable evidence that high levels of hope promote physical and psychological health (Herth 1990; Nekolaichuk et al. 1999). When conceptualized cognitively, people high in hope—compared to those low in hope—not only believe that they can generate but actually generate more pathways to goals, sustain more energy to pursue goals, and view goal blockages merely as temporary setbacks (Snyder et al. 1991), even when faced with adversity (Cheavens 2000). In comparison, people low in hope set fewer goals, are more tenuous in their pursuit, are unlikely to produce alternative routes, and may view blockages as demoralizing (Snyder 2002). Thus, just as a generalized expectancy for failure can cause and sustain mental illness, it may be said that a generalized expectancy for goal success can promote mental health and protect against mental illness (Cheavens 2000). Furthermore, as hopeful thinking elicits emotion, people high in hope are suggested to experience enduring and positive emotions that are, in turn, accompanied by a zest for the pursuit of goals. This is in contrast to people low in hope, who are suggested to experience negative emotions accompanied by a lethargic attitude toward the pursuit of goals (Snyder 2002). Thus, the presence of high levels of hope appears to activate a positive upward spiral of functioning that better equips people with the skills and resources needed to overcome challenges and obtain a state of flourishing in life, while the presence of low levels of hope does not.

In terms of mental health promotion, this suggests that when faced with a challenging situation or a goal blockage, those low in hope may experience stress, which over time, elicits negative emotions. However, those high in hope will have the resources needed to redirect goal pursuit and alleviate any initial or subsequent stress that arises (Snyder 2002). There is evidence, moreover, that differences in hope levels have both short- and long-term effects. For example, compared to young people low in hope, young people high in hope report increased levels of physical and psychological functioning (Cheavens et al. 2006; Snyder et al. 2000, 1991), and the presence of high levels of psychological strengths when young is linked to positive mental health outcomes in adulthood (Arehart-Treichel 2006).

The Broaden and Build Theory of Positive Emotions

Fredrickson's Broaden and Build Theory of positive emotions (1998, 2002, 2008) states that the continued experience of positive emotions acts to broaden an individual's momentary thought–action responses (i.e., increase the range of responses available in a situation), build their enduring personal resources, and help people to cope more effectively with adversity (Fredrickson and Branigan 2005; Fredrickson and Joiner 2002; Fredrickson and Losada 2005; Fredrickson et al. 2003). Thus, while the experience of negative emotions may narrow the range of responses available in a situation and may also carry immediate adaptive benefits (i.e., fight or flight), the experience of positive emotions may widen the array of responses available and may carry indirect and long-term adaptive benefits. For example, *joy* creates the urge to play, push boundaries, be creative in one's activities, and expand involvement in life, while *interest* creates the urge to explore, learn, experience new things, and expand the self (Fredrickson 2002). Thus, in contrast to the experience of negative emotions that, if prolonged, may lead to depression, anxiety, aggression, and health-risk behavior, the experience of positive emotions has indirect and long-term adaptive benefits because these emotions help to develop the psychological strengths and positive resources an individual needs in order to reach and sustain a state of flourishing in life (Fredrickson 2002; Fredrickson and Joiner 2002).

The Hope Activation Cycle

Drawing together elements from the three concepts described above, it therefore follows that the ability to successfully hope provides the experiences that are capable of shifting young people from poorer states of mental health toward sustainable states of positive mental health (i.e., flourishing in life). High levels of hope, according to Fig. 2.2, result in the activation of a positive upward spiral in which increases in goal success lead to increases in the experience of positive emotion (e.g., happiness). This positive emotion, in turn, increases momentary thought–actions and builds enduring personal resources (e.g., resilience), buffers against the onset of mental illness (e.g., depression), activates health-promoting behavior (e.g., physical exercise), and ultimately leads to a state of flourishing in life. However, low levels of hope may lead to a state of languishing, struggling, or floundering in life. Low levels of hope, according to the model, may or may not result in the activation of a negative downward spiral. Nonetheless, the inability to successfully hope may leave an individual susceptible to mental illness.

The model depicted in Fig. 2.2 combines two related but increasingly disparate fields of investigation that have dominated research on well-being. The *hedonic* approach, traditionally aligned with positive psychology, conceptualizes well-being as a state with high levels of positive affect, low levels of negative affect, and a high degree of life satisfaction (i.e., subjective or short-term well-being; Boskovic and Jengic 2008). The *eudaimonic* approach, traditionally aligned with positive mental health, conceptualizes well-being as the processes that lead to the sustained fulfillment and/or realization of an individual's full potential (i.e., psychological or long-term well-being; Boskovic and Jengic 2008; Keyes et al. 2002). Ryan and Deci (2001), however, suggest that well-being is best conceptualized as incorporating elements of both the hedonic and eudaimonic approaches.

Consistent with this, Keyes et al. (2002) have empirically confirmed that subjective well-being and psychological well-being *are* related and *are not* mutually exclusive concepts. In line with this, the proposed model (Fig. 2.2) similarly assumes that feeling good in the short term (i.e., via increased levels of hope and the upward spiral of positive emotions that follow) may ultimately build the psychological resources needed to live well in the long term and provide clinicians with a mechanism to increase the mental health of young people.

The ability to successfully hope, an exemplar of a psychological strength, is an important element of mental health because it provides a young person with the

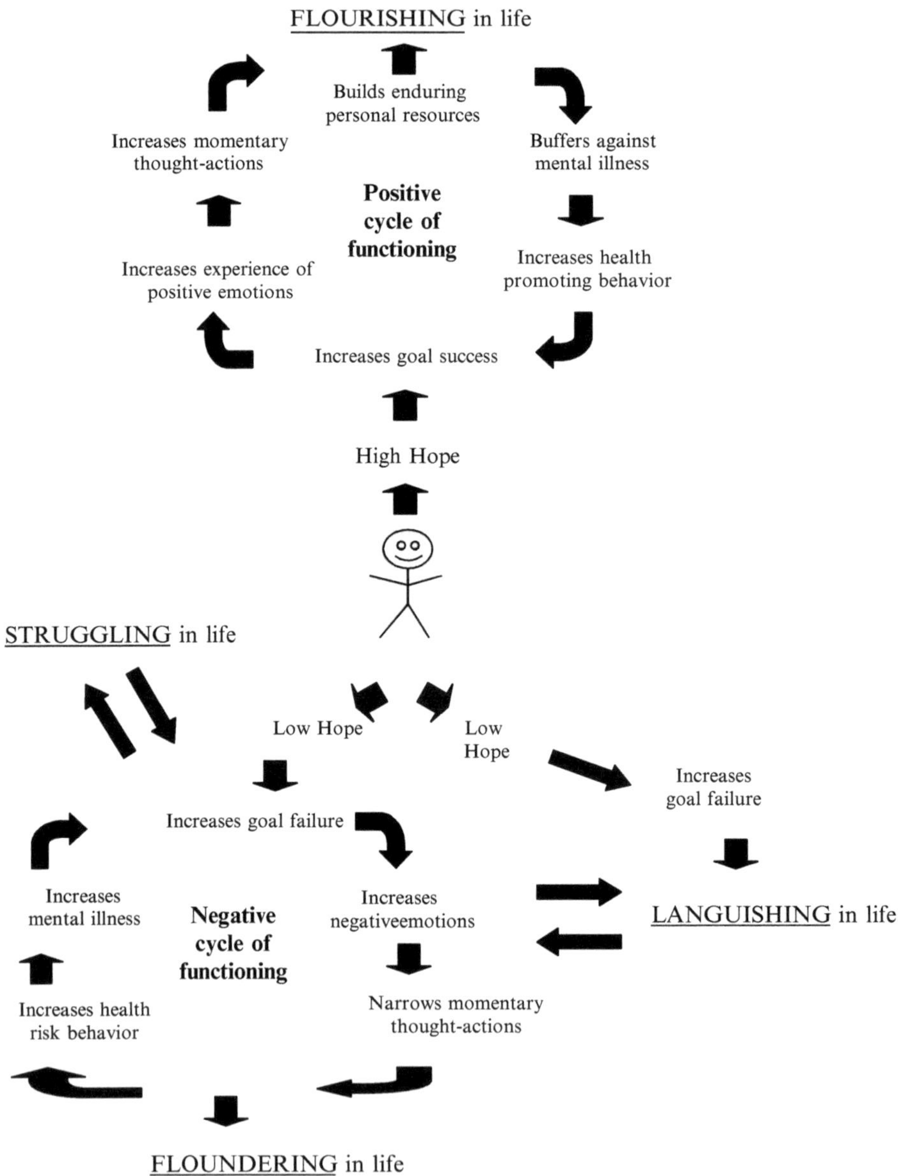

Fig. 2.2 The Hope activation cycle

skills and resources needed to reach and sustain an optimum state of mental health. This implies that psychological strengths, such as hope, can be developed to increase levels of mental health and prevent or reduce symptoms of mental illness. There is a counter argument, namely, that a baseline or genetically determined set point exists to which the symptoms of positive functioning always return following any short-term increases (Headey and Wearing 1992; Kahneman et al. 1999).

The *hedonic treadmill*, as this effect has been coined, suggests that any attempt to increase an individual's positive affect is futile, even though levels may fluctuate, as no sustained increase can ever be achieved (Brickman and Campbell 1971; Headey 2006; Headey and Wearing 1992). In contrast, research from a positive psychological perspective has indicated that (a) levels of life satisfaction can and do change over time (Fujita and Diener 2005); (b) strategies that focus on developing hopeful thinking increase subjective well-being and decrease the symptoms of mental illness (Cheavens et al. 2006); and (c) as goals change or are changed with time, a focus on goals may avoid the hedonic treadmill and ensure that increases in positive affect do not become routine, but remain a source of positive uplift (King 2008). This supports the assumptions that levels of hope—a future goal-orientated process—can be increased, and moreover, that developing hope may be an important new mental health strategies focus that is complementary to, and may be more effective than, the current focus on alleviating mental illness.

Research in Australia from a Complete Mental Health Perspective

Numerous studies in the United States have conceptualized mental health within a positive framework and reported its prevalence and relationship to various physical, social, and behavioral outcomes (Cheavens et al. 2006; Fredrickson and Branigan 2005; Fredrickson and Joiner 2002; Irving et al. 1998; Keyes 2004, 2005b, 2006; Lopez et al. 2000; Snyder 2002; Snyder et al. 1991). Excluding the research described below, very little research has adopted this focus in Australia, and none have operationalized the CSM of mental health (Keyes and Lopez 2002). Most Australian research has focused on the identification (Sawyer et al. 2000), prevalence (Boyd et al. 2000), and prevention of mental illness (Barrett et al. 2006; Lowry-Webster et al. 2001; Shochet et al. 2001), which was presumed to indirectly report mental health. Our own research aimed to expand this focus and thus to contribute to knowledge in the area of mental health from a positive psychological perspective, extending the platform from which positive mental health strategies can be developed and launched to meet the mental health needs of young Australians.

The next part of this chapter describes and summarizes the outcomes from our recent research program exploring the effective measurement of a CSM in Australian youth and the relationships between the cognitive asset of hope, complete mental health, and health-risk behaviors in young Australians.

Objectives of Research and Sample

Our research has three broad objectives. First, we have strived to describe the status of mental health in young Australians according to the four states outlined in the CSM of mental health (Keyes and Lopez 2002), to examine the relationship of these states to health-risk and health-promoting behavior, and to provide an example of

Table 2.1 Age and gender distribution of sample from SAYMHS (58% from metropolitan areas)

Age	Male n (%)	Female n (%)	Total N
13	502 (48)	537 (52)	1,039
14	475 (49)	496 (51)	971
15	418 (50)	414 (50)	832
16	296 (43)	392 (57)	688
17	172 (45)	211 (55)	383
Total	1,863 (48)	2,050 (52)	3,913

how multiple measures can be combined to diagnose young people as flourishing, languishing, struggling, or floundering in life. Second, we have explored the possibility that the cognitive process of hope—used as an exemplar of a psychological strength—may predict mental health in young Australians better than mental illness does and thereby support the argument for shifting the primary focus of health promotion toward building an individual's strengths.

Finally, we have attempted to establish normative scores for the Adult Hope Scale (AHS; Snyder et al. 1991) in a young Australian population. The AHS is an effective outcome measure that allows clinicians to assess an individual's hope levels and/or the effectiveness of therapeutic interventions. It was purported, however, that the AHS also has the potential to be used as an initial resource to identify young Australians who differ from the developmental norm in terms of their hope scores and, where appropriate, to guide interventions to help those in need of reaching and sustaining a state of flourishing in life.

The South Australian Youth Mental Health Survey (SAYMHS)

The SAYMHS was a predominantly online survey designed to collect indicators of positive and negative functioning from young people throughout rural and metropolitan South Australia (N=3,913; refer to Table 2.1). This age range was chosen to coincide with the ages during which a young person attends secondary school in Australia (years 8–12) and to make the results comparable to previous Australian research examining mental health in this population (Sawyer et al. 2000). The SAYMHS consists of five well-validated measures chosen to operationalize the CSM of mental health (Keyes and Lopez 2002), as well as demographic questions used to gather information on factors known to be associated with mental health, and questions on health-risk (smoking cigarettes and alcohol consumption) and health-promoting behavior (e.g., adequate sleep and exercise). The measures included were (a) the AHS (Snyder et al. 1991), (b) the Satisfaction with Life Scale (SWLS; Diener et al. 1985), (c) the Psychological Well-Being Scale (PWBS; Ryff 1989), (d) the Social Well-Being Scale (SWBS; Keyes 1998), and (e) the Depression Anxiety Stress Scale 21 (DASS-21; Lovibond and Lovibond 1995).

Details of the power analysis, sampling method, scale selection, and procedures followed during the SAYMHS have been published elsewhere (Venning et al. 2009,

2011a) but are briefly outlined below. Data collection took place in early 2007. In total, 129 schools were approached to participate (i.e., every secondary school in South Australia listed either with the Department of Education and Children's Services or listed in the 2005 Annual Report of the Advisory Committee on Non-Government Schools in South Australia that had a student population over 100 was approached). Data were recorded from 41 of the 129 schools canvassed, and while it was not possible under our funding constraints to obtain a stratified random sample, our data were drawn from schools that covered a wide geographical area and broad socioeconomic spectrum. Parental consent and student assent were gained before data collection began. Data were collected electronically from 38 schools ($n=3{,}315$; no missing values) and manually from three ($n=598$). Two approaches were taken to missing data collected via the manual version of the survey: if one or more of the measures were left completely blank, the entire data set for that individual was excluded; and if isolated missing values existed, mean imputation was used. No significant differences were found between the scores of participants who completed the online or the manual version of the survey, so data were merged for all analyses.

Outcomes of Research

Our first objective was to identify the prevalence and distribution of flourishing, languishing, struggling, and floundering in life in young South Australians, and to investigate the association of these states to health-risk behavior in order to better inform the development and targeting of mental health strategies. Data were drawn from the SAYMHS and combined to classify young people according to these diagnostic groups on the basis of their combined scores on the PWBS, SWBS, SWLS, and DASS-21. Results indicated that 42% of young people sampled were flourishing in life, 5% were languishing, 36% were struggling, and 17% were floundering in life. Therefore, contrary to what had been previously reported in Smart and Sanson's (2005) study (i.e., that 80% of young Australians have "good" mental health), these results suggest that <50% of young South Australians are flourishing in life.

In addition, flourishing in life was associated with more health-promoting and less health-risk behavior, while floundering in life was associated with more health-risk and less health-promoting behavior. There were, moreover, gender and regional differences in the uptake of health-risk or health-promoting behavior according to CMH states. Table 2.2 provides a description of the health behavior according to CMH states. Results have been reported in more detail elsewhere (Venning et al. 2012).

Our second objective was to examine the relationship between hope and mental health, and mental illness and mental health. It has been reported that, compared to young people low in hope, young people high in hope report increased levels of physical and psychological functioning (Snyder et al. 2000). However, whether hope predicts mental health in young people has remained empirically untested. Data were drawn from the SAYMHS, and scores from the PWBS, SWBS, and SLS were used to define the latent variable of mental health; scores from the DASS-21 comprised the latent variable of mental illness; and scores on the AHS comprised

Table 2.2 Health behavior of sample from SAYMHS (N=3,913) within Complete Mental Health States

	Smoke cigarettes		Consume alcohol		Exercise per week		Sleep per night	
	Yes	No	Yes	No	<5 h	>5 h	<8 h	>8 h
Flourishing (n=1,639) (%)	12	88	58	42	48	52	61	39
Languishing (n=202) (%)	18	82	62	38	61	39	72	28
Struggling (n=1,401) (%)	19	81	63	37	55	45	70	30
Floundering (n=671) (%)	27	73	69	31	61	39	76	24

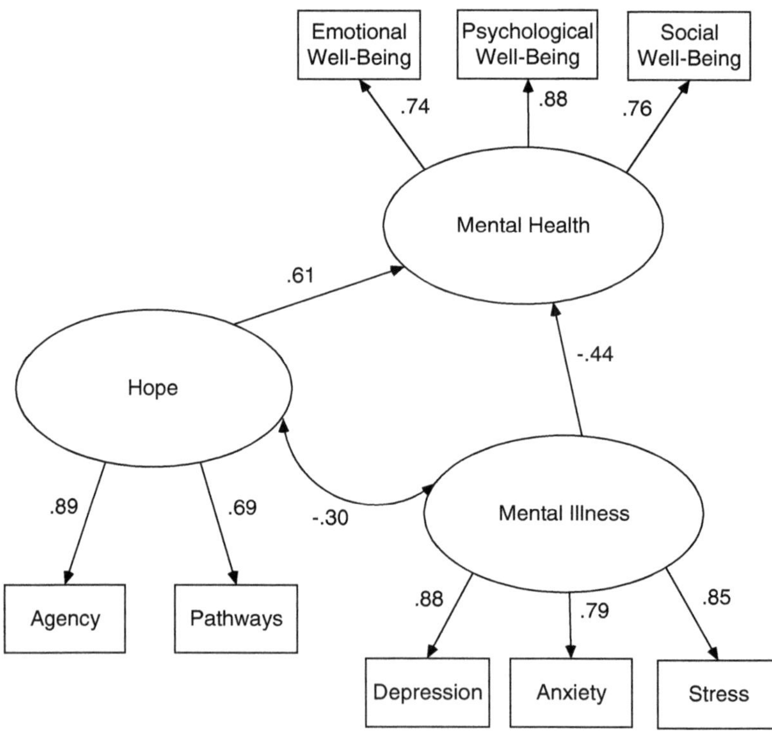

Fig. 2.3 Path-analytic model: the influence of hope and mental illness on mental health

the latent variable of hope. Confirmatory Factor Analysis (CFA) was then employed to confirm the independence of mental health and mental illness, and to examine the relationship between hope and mental health and mental illness and mental health, before the predictive nature of hope's components to mental health were examined separately. Results (reported in more detail elsewhere; Venning et al. 2011) indicated that hope was a better predictor of mental health than was mental illness (see Fig. 2.3), and, regardless of gender, agency explained significantly more of the variance in mental health than pathways.

Our final objective was to establish normative scores for the AHS (Snyder et al. 1991) in a young Australian population. Analysis of data indicated that there was a statistically significant difference in hope scores across age (i.e., scores rose from 13 to 16 years, but dropped at 17 years) and between regions (i.e., scores were consistently lower in rural compared to metropolitan areas), and a statistically significant difference in pathways scores existed between 17-year-old males and females (i.e., females reported lower scores than males). Results have been reported in detail elsewhere (Venning et al. 2009).

Promoting a Sustainable Mental Health in Australia

The research undertaken was based on the premise that a focus on developing one's strengths (e.g., hope), rather than on preventing or treating the symptoms of mental illness, is a better way to promote a sustainable mental health. As per the Hope Activation Cycle, it is purported that the successful and continued ability to hope (an exemplar of a psychological strength) may be a vital mechanism that activates a positive cycle of functioning, which ultimately leads to a sustainable state of mental health.

Prevalence and Measurement of Complete Mental Health in Young People

This study is the first to describe mental health in Australian youth according to the states outlined by the CSM of mental health (Keyes and Lopez 2002), and indicates that the prevalence of mental health in young people in Australia has been overestimated. Indirectly, the disparity between the current results and previous results based upon a more restricted definition of mental health may indicate that previous information has been, and is, insufficient to guide the development and targeting of strategies to promote mental health in Australia. In contrast, the current information may offer a more comprehensive picture of mental health that incorporates both positive and negative symptoms of functioning. The current results also suggest that a one-size-fits-all approach to mental health is not appropriate as age, gender, and regional variations were evident not only in the prevalence of all four mental health states but also in the engagement in health-promoting and health-risk behavior, and in the development or employment of hopeful thinking. Thus, while the findings of this study may inform the development of positive mental health strategies in Australia, it also suggests that such strategies need to be tailored to address variation across age, gender, and location. Further research is needed to explore the relationships between mental health and health-risk behavior, and hope and mental health.

It is argued that Australian programs that aim to promote mental health in young people, along with the Australian National Action Plan on Mental Health (2006), undervalue the importance of psychological strengths and, in isolation, may fail to identify those young Australians who require assistance in order to flourish in life, despite the absence of mental illness. The current research provided information about mental health in a young Australian population in an attempt to reduce the reliance on negative measures of functioning as indicators of mental health, and to provide a more comprehensive picture of mental health. Additionally, this study aimed to increase the awareness and use of positive measures of functioning in identifying young people who may need assistance in order to reach and sustain a state of flourishing in life. Specifically, the current research provides an example of how multiple, positive, and freely available psychological measures can be combined to diagnose people as flourishing, languishing, struggling, or floundering in life. Moreover, the provision of Australian normative scores for the AHS, broken down by age, gender, and region, may increase its usefulness in Australian clinical or health-care settings by making hope scores more meaningful in an Australian population and, in doing so, lessen the reliance on measures of mental illness as indicators of the presence or absence of mental health.

Promotion of Complete Mental Health in Young Australians

Our study found that hope predicted mental health better than did mental illness, and that the state of flourishing in life was associated with more health-promoting and less health-risk behavior than other states. Based on the Hope Activation Cycle, it is proposed that hope has the ability to activate a positive cycle of functioning that propels an individual toward a sustainable state of flourishing in life, and therefore, a focus on hope could be a useful element of any mental health strategy targeted at young Australians. Research has indicated that around 70% of patients relapse within the first 6 months following therapy to treat the symptoms of major depression (Ramana et al. 1995).

Keyes and Lopez (2002) have reported that the limited effectiveness of such therapies may be due to a narrow focus (i.e., mental illness, not mental health) that may effectively reduce the symptoms of mental illness in the short term but, in the absence of building positive strengths, only leaves individuals susceptible to their return. Accordingly, without an explicit focus on building psychological strengths (e.g., hope), Australian initiatives may overlook the strategies needed to effectively develop and promote mental health. The current research suggests, therefore, that a focus on hope may be a part of what is missing in these programs, and its addition may increase their effectiveness, promote a state of flourishing in life, and reduce the burden of mental illness in young Australians.

Future Directions

Clearly, further investigation into the role that hope plays in a young person's mental health (outlined in Fig. 2.3) is required. This may involve the development and trial of studies that not only examine the individual components of the proposed model and use Confirmatory Factor Analysis to examine the model (or the relationship) between variables if hope is substituted for other psychological strengths, but also promote mental health in young Australians through the development and trial of a hope-focused strategy. In regard to the latter, the AHS (Snyder et al. 1991), in conjunction with the newly developed Australian normative scores, may be used to identify young Australians who report low hope scores relative to the developmental norm and investigate the effectiveness of an individual or group strategy to increase hope and promote a state of flourishing in life.

Cheavens et al. (2006) reported that, following an 8-week hope-focused therapy, adults reported increases in agency, hope, and pathways scores, but more importantly, that these increases were associated with increases *and* decreases in other psychological constructs (e.g., increases in life meaning and self-esteem, and decreases in anxiety and depression). Such findings support the notion that a hope-focused approach to mental health may be a simple and useful way for clinicians to both identify young Australians in need of assistance and to activate a positive cycle of functioning in order to propel them toward a state of flourishing in life.

This research was not the first to have discussed and championed the role of hope in mental health. Nor is it the first to suggest that building mental health, rather than repairing mental illness, is a better focus of health promotion, simply because building mental health may directly or indirectly alleviate and undo the root causes of mental illness (Duckworth et al. 2005; Keyes and Lopez 2002). Nonetheless, this research was the first to lay the foundation from which a positive approach can be launched to meet the mental health needs of young Australians. There may be some reluctance to move toward a more comprehensive and positive view of mental health because doing so would increase the number of young people that could be diagnosed with poor mental health, such that the task of promoting mental health appears insurmountable, given existing resources. Such misgivings may be countered by the observation that a positive approach to mental health enables the identification of adolescents who may have previously gone unnoticed (i.e., by the absence of strengths rather than just the presence of mental illness) and indirectly reduces the future burden of mental illness by promoting a sustainable mental health (Venning et al. 2011b).

Conclusion

It has been claimed that promoting an individual's psychological strengths, such as hope or positive emotion, may be the best weapon against mental illness (Seligman 2008). The current research embraces this perspective and represents a first step to complement previous work based on a positive paradigm, thereby extending the platform in Australia from which positively focused strategies can be developed and launched in order to promote mental health in young people. Combined, the results suggest that a focus on positive strengths, such as hope, may play an important role in the mental health of young Australians and should be part of strategies designed to promote mental health. It is hoped that this research helps to redirect the focus of mental health policy and practice in Australia by highlighting the importance of positive symptoms of functioning—and by supporting claims that these *must* trump the negative—as a priority in developing strategies to promote a sustainable mental health and reduce the burden of mental illness, both in adolescence and beyond.

References

American Psychiatric Association. (2000). *Diagnostic and statistical manual of mental disorders* (5th ed., text rev.). Washington, DC: Author.

Arehart-Treichel, J. (2006). Teen personality traits can predict adult mental health. *Psychiatric News, 41*, 26.

Australian Bureau of Statistics. (1997). *Mentál health and well-being: Profile of adults, Australia. Cat. no. 4326*. Canberra: Author.

Australian Bureau of Statistics. (2006). *Physical activity in Australia: A snapshot 2004-05. Cat. no. 4835*. Canberra: Author.

Australian Bureau of Statistics. (2008). *National survey of mental health and wellbeing: Summary of results, 2997*. Canberra: Author.

Australian Bureau of Statistics. (2009). *Australian social trends, Australia. Cat. no. 4102*. Canberra: Author.

Australian Institute of Health and Welfare. (2005). *2004 national drug strategy household survey: Detailed findings, Cat. no. PHE 66*. Canberra: AIHW.

Australian Institute of Health and Welfare. (2006). *Australia's health 2006: Cat. no. AUS 73*. Canberra: AIHW.

Australian Institute of Health and Welfare. (2008). *Australia's health 2008 Cat. no. AUS 99*. Canberra: AIHW.

Barrett, P. M., Farrell, L. J., Ollendick, T. H., & Dadds, M. (2006). Long-term outcomes of an Australian universal prevention trial of anxiety and depression symptoms in children and youth: An evaluation of the friends program. *Journal of Clinical Child and Adolescent Psychology, 35*, 403–411.

Boskovic, G., & Jengic, Y. (2008). Mental health as eudaimonic well-being? *Psychiatria Danubina, 20*, 452–455.

Boyd, C. P., Kostanski, M., Gullone, E., Ollendick, T. H., & Shek, D. T. L. (2000). Prevalence of anxiety and depression in Australian adolescents: Comparisons with worldwide data. *The Journal of Genetic Psychology, 161*, 479–492.

Braverman, M. T. (1999). Research on resilience and its implications for tobacco prevention. *Nicotine & Tobacco Research, 1*, S67–S72.

Brickman, P., & Campbell, D. T. (1971). Hedonic relativism and planning the good society. In M. H. Appley (Ed.), *Adaptation-level theory*. New York: Academic.

Carr-Gregg, M. R., Enderby, K. C., & Grover, S. R. (2003). Risk-taking behaviours of young women in Australia: Screening for health-risk behaviours. *Medical Journal of Australia, 178*, 601–604.

Cheavens, J. S. (2000). Hope and depression: Light through the shadows. In C. R. Snyder (Ed.), *Handbook of hope: Theory, measures, and applications* (pp. 321–340). San Diego: Academic.

Cheavens, J. S., Feldman, D. B., Gum, A., Scott, T., & Snyder, C. R. (2006). Hope therapy in a community sample: A pilot investigation. *Social Indicators Research, 77*, 61–78.
Council of Australian Governments. (2006). *National action plan on mental health 2006-2011*. Canberra: Author.
Diener, E., Emmons, R. A., Larsen, R. J., & Griffen, S. (1985). The satisfaction with life scale. *Journal of Personality Assessment, 49*, 71–75.
Duckworth, A. L., Steen, T. A., & Seligman, M. P. (2005). Positive psychology in clinical practice. *Annual Review of Clinical Psychology, 1*, 629–651.
Eckersley, R. M., Wierenga, A., & Wyn, J. (2005). Life in a time of uncertainty: Optimising the health and wellbeing of young Australians. *Medical Journal of Australia, 183*, 402–404.
Fredrickson, B. L. (1998). What good are positive emotions? *Review of General Psychology, 2*, 300–319.
Fredrickson, B. L. (2002). Positive emotions. In C. R. Snyder & J. L. Lopez (Eds.), *Handbook of positive psychology* (pp. 120–134). New York: Oxford University Press.
Fredrickson, B. L. (2008). Promoting positive affect. In M. Eid & R. J. Larsen (Eds.), *The science of subjective well-being* (pp. 449–468). New York: Guilford Press.
Fredrickson, B. L., & Branigan, C. (2005). Positive emotions broaden the scope of attention and thought-action repertoires. *Cognition & Emotion, 19*, 313–332.
Fredrickson, B. L., & Joiner, T. (2002). Positive emotions trigger upward spirals toward emotional well-being. *Psychological Science, 13*, 172–175.
Fredrickson, B. L., & Losada, M. F. (2005). Positive affect and the complex dynamics of human flourishing. *American Psychologist, 7*, 678–686.
Fredrickson, B. L., Tugade, M. M., Waugh, C. E., & Larkin, G. R. (2003). What good are positive emotions in crisis? A prospective study of resilience and emotions following the terrorist attacks in the United States on September the 11th 2001. *Journal of Positive and Social Psychology, 84*, 365–376.
Fujita, F., & Diener, E. (2005). Life satisfaction set point: Stability and change. *Journal of Personality and Social Psychology, 88*, 158–164.
Graber, J., Brooks-Gunn, J., & Petersen, A. (1996). *Transitions through adolescence: Interpersonal domains and context*. Mahwah: Erlbaum.
Grant, A. M., & Cavanagh, M. J. (2007). Evidence-based coaching: Flourishing or languishing? *Australian Psychologist, 42*, 239–254.
Headey, B. (2006). Subjective well-being: Revisions to dynamic equilibrium theory using natural panel data and panel regression methods. *Social Indicators Research, 79*, 369–403.
Headey, B., & Wearing, A. (1992). *Understanding happiness: A theory of subjective well-being*. Melbourne: Longman Cheshire.
Headroom. (2009). *Headroom*. Retrieved June 22, 2009, from http://www.headroom.net.au/http://www.headroom.net.au/
Headspace. (2006). *Headspace: Where young minds come first*. Retrieved September 7, 2006, 2006, from http://www.headspace.org.au/www.headspace.org.au
Herth, K. (1990). Fostering hope in terminally-ill people. *Journal of Advanced Nursing, 15*, 1250–1259.
Irving, L. M., Snyder, C. R., & Crowson, J. J. (1998). Hope and coping with cancer by college women. *Journal of Personality, 66*, 195–214.
Irwin, C. E., Igra, V., Eyre, S., & Millstein, S. G. (1997). Risk taking: The paradigm. *Annals of the New York Academy of Sciences, 817*, 1–35.
Kahneman, D., Diener, E., & Schwarz, N. (1999). *Well-being: The foundations of hedonic psychology*. New York: Russell Sage.
Keeler, H. J., & Kaiser, M. M. (2010). An integrative model of adolescent health risk behaviour. *Journal of Pediatric Nursing, 25*, 126–137.
Kessler, R. C., Berglund, P. A., Demler, O., Jin, R., Merikangas, K. R., & Walters, E. E. (2005). Lifetime prevalence and age-of-onset distributions of DSM-IV disorders in the National Comorbidity Survey replication (NCS-R). *Archives of General Psychiatry, 62*, 593–602.
Keyes, C. L. M. (1998). Social well-being. *Social Psychology Quarterly, 61*, 121–140.

Keyes, C. L. M. (2002). The mental health continuum: From languishing to flourishing in life. *Journal of Health and Social Research, 43*, 207–222.
Keyes, C. L. M. (2004). The nexus of cardiovascular disease and depression revisited: The complete mental health perspective and the moderating role of age and gender. *Aging and Mental Health, 8*, 266–274.
Keyes, C. L. M. (2005a). Mental illness and/or mental health? Investigating axioms of the complete state model of mental health. *Journal of Consulting and Clinical Psychology, 73*, 539–548.
Keyes, C. L. M. (2005b). Chronic physical conditions and aging: Is mental health a potential protective factor? *Ageing International, 30*, 88–104.
Keyes, C. L. M. (2006). Mental health in adolescence: Is America's youth flourishing? *American Journal of Orthopsychiatry, 76*, 395–402.
Keyes, C. L. M. (2007). Promoting and protecting mental health as flourishing. *American Psychologist, 62*, 95–108.
Keyes, C. L. M., & Lopez, S. J. (2002). Towards a science of mental health. In C. R. Snyder & J. L. Lopez (Eds.), *Handbook of positive psychology* (pp. 45–59). New York: Oxford University Press.
Keyes, C. L. M., Ryff, C. D., & Shmotkin, D. (2002). Optimizing well-being: The empirical encounter of two traditions. *Journal of Personality and Social Psychology, 82*, 1007–1022.
King, L. A. (2008). Interventions for enhancing subjective well-being: Can we make people happier, and should we? In M. Eid & R. J. Larsen (Eds.), *The science of subjective well-being* (pp. 431–448). New York: The Guilford Press.
Larson, R. W., & Ham, M. (1993). Stress and "storm and stress" in early adolescence: The relationship of negative events with dysphoric affect. *Developmental Psychology, 29*, 130–140.
Licence, K. (2004). Promoting and protecting the health of children and young people. *Child: Care Health and Development, 30*, 623–635.
Lopez, S. J., Floyd, R. K., Ulven, J. C., & Snyder, C. R. (2000). Hope therapy: Helping clients build a house of hope. In C. R. Snyder & J. L. Lopez (Eds.), *Handbook of hope: Theory, measures, and applications* (pp. 123–150). San Diego: Academic.
Lovibond, S. H., & Lovibond, P. F. (1995). *Manual for the depression, anxiety and stress scales* (2nd ed.). Sydney: Psychology Foundation.
Lowry-Webster, H. M., Barrett, P. M., & Dadds, M. R. (2001). A universal prevention trial of anxiety and depressive symptomatology in childhood: Preliminary data from an Australian study. *Behaviour Change, 18*, 36–50.
Luthar, S. S. (1991). Vulnerability and resilience: A study of high-risk adolescents. *Child Development, 62*, 600–616.
Maggs, J. L., Schulenberg, J., & Hurrelmann, K. (1997). Developmental transitions during adolescence: Health promotion implications. In J. Schulenberg, J. L. Maggs, & K. Hurrelmann (Eds.), *Health risks and development transitions during adolescence* (pp. 522–546). New York: Cambridge University Press.
McGorry, P., Parker, A., & Purcell, R. (2006). Australian Psychological Society, *Youth Mental Health Services*. Retrieved October 2011, from http://www.psychology.org.au/
MindMatters. (2009). *MindMatters*. Retrieved June 22, 2009, from http://www.mindmatters.edu.au/default.asphttp://www.mindmatters.edu.au/default.asp
Moffitt, T. E. (1993). "Adolescence-limited" and "life-course-persistent" antisocial behaviour: A developmental taxonomy. *Psychological Review, 100*, 674–701.
Nekolaichuk, C. L., Jevne, R. F., & Maguire, T. O. (1999). Structuring the meaning of hope in health and illness. *Social Science & Medicine, 48*, 591–605.
Petersen, A. C., & Leffert, N. (1995). What is special about adolescence? In M. Rutter (Ed.), *Psychosocial disturbances in young people: Challenges for prevention* (pp. 3–36). New York: Cambridge University Press.
Quayle, D., Dziuraweic, S., Roberts, C., Kane, R., & Ebsworthy, G. (2001). The effect of an optimism and lifeskills program on depressive symptoms in preadolescence. *Behaviour Change, 18*, 194–203.

Ramana, R., Paykel, E. S., Cooper, Z., Hayhurst, H., Saxty, M., & Surtees, P. G. (1995). Remission and relapse in major depression: A two-year prospective follow-up study. *Psychological Medicine, 25*, 1161–1170.

Roberts, C., Kane, R., Thomson, H., Bishop, B., & Hart, B. (2003). The prevention of depressive symptoms in rural school children: A randomized controlled trial. *Journal of Consulting and Clinical Psychology, 71*, 622–628.

Rowling, L. (2006). Adolescence and emerging adulthood (12-17 years and 18-24 years). In M. Cattan & S. Tilford (Eds.), *Mental health promotion: A lifespan approach* (pp. 100–136). New York: Open University Press.

Rutter, M. (1987). Psychosocial resilience and protective mechanisms. *American Journal of Orthopsychiatry, 57*, 316–331.

Rutter, M., & Smith, D. J. (1995). *Psychosocial disorders in young people: Time trends and their causes*. Chichester: Wiley.

Ryan, R. M., & Deci, E. L. (2001). On happiness and human potential: A review of research on hedonic and eudaimonic well-being. *Annual Review of Psychology, 52*, 141–146.

Ryff, C. D. (1989). Happiness is everything, or is it? Explorations on the meaning of psychological well-being. *Journal of Personality and Social Psychology, 57*, 1069–1081.

Sawyer, M. G., Kosky, R. S., Graetz, B. W., Arney, F., Zubrick, S. R., & Baghurst, P. (2000). The national survey of mental health and well-being: The child and adolescent component. *Australian and New Zealand Journal of psychiatry, 34*, 214–220.

Seifert, K. L., Hoffnung, R. J., & Hoffnung, M. (2000). *Lifespan development*. New York: Houghton Mifflin Company.

Seligman, M. P. (2005). Positive psychology, positive prevention, and positive therapy. In C. R. Snyder & J. L. Lopez (Eds.), *Handbook of positive psychology* (pp. 3–9). New York: Oxford University Press.

Seligman, M. P. (2008). Positive health. *Applied Psychology: An International Review, 57*, 3–18.

Seligman, M. P., & Csikszentmihalyi, M. (2000). Positive psychology. *American Psychologist, 55*, 5–14.

Seligman, M. P., Steen, T. A., Park, N., & Petersen, C. (2005). Positive psychology progress: Empirical validation of interventions. *American Psychologist, 60*, 410–421.

Shaffer-Hudkins, E., Suldo, S. March, A., & Loker, T. (2010). How adolescents' mental health predicts their physical health: Unique contributions of subjective wellbeing and psychopathology. *Applied Research in Quality of Life, 5*(3), 203–217.

Shochet, I. M., Dadds, M., Holland, D., Whitefield, K., Harnett, P. H., & Osgarby, S. M. (2001). The efficacy of a universal school-based program to prevent adolescent depression. *Journal of Clinical Child Psychology, 30*, 303–315.

Smart, D., & Sanson, A. (2005). What is life like for young Australians today, and how well are they faring? *Family Matters, 70*, 46–53.

Snyder, C. R. (1994). *The psychology of hope: You can get there from here*. New York: The Free Press.

Snyder, C. R. (2000). Genesis: The birth and growth of hope. In C. R. Snyder (Ed.), *Handbook of hope: Theory, measures, and applications* (pp. 25–38). San Diego: Academic.

Snyder, C. R. (2002). Hope theory: Rainbows in the mind. *Psychological Inquiry, 13*, 249–275.

Snyder, C. R., Harris, C., Anderson, J. R., Holleran, S. A., Irving, L. M., Sigmon, S. T., et al. (1991). The will and the ways: Development and validation of an individual-differences measure of hope. *Journal of Personality and Social Psychology, 60*, 570–585.

Snyder, C. R., Feldman, D. B., Taylor, J. D., Schroeder, L. L., & Adams, V. H. (2000). The roles of hopeful thinking in preventing problems and enhancing strengths. *Applied and Preventative Psychology, 15*, 262–295.

Venning, A., Eliott, J., Kettler, L., & Wilson, A. (2009). Normative data for the Hope Scale using Australian adolescents. *Australian Journal of Psychology, 61*, 100–106.

Venning, A., Kettler, L., Zajac, I., Wilson, A., & Eliott, J. (2011). Is hope or mental illness a stronger predictor of mental health? *International Journal of Mental Health Promotion, 13*, 31–38.

Venning, A., Wilson, A., Kettler, L., & Eliott, J. (2012). Mental Health among Youth in South Australia :A survey of Flourishing, Languishing, Struggling, and Floundering. Australian Psychologist. Published online 28 March. doi:10.1111/j.1742-9544.2012.00068.x.

Zubrick, S., Silburn, S., Garton, A., Burton, P., Dalby, R., Carlton, J., et al. (1995). *Western Australian child health survey 1993: Developing health and well-being in the nineties* (No. ABS Cat. no. 4303.5). Perth: Australian Bureau of Statistics and the institute for Child Health research.

Chapter 3
The Complete Mental Health Model: The Social Distribution of Mental Health and Mental Illness in the Dutch Population

Gerben J. Westerhof

Mental health care has undergone a vigorous process of professionalization during the past few decades. Epidemiological studies have provided a wealth of information on the distribution of mental health problems in the general population and have identified important risk factors for developing mental disorders. Nowadays, the diagnostic process is supported by well-defined classifications of disorders, such as the Diagnostic and Statistical Manual, as well as valid instruments to assess them. Mental health treatments have become rationalized thanks to careful trials of their effectiveness. Lately, the ideal of the psychologist as a scientist-practitioner appears to be more alive than ever, at least within educational training. Taken together, this process has resulted in more evidence-based approaches, as well as in transparency and control in mental health care. This has also brought more widespread and, indeed, legal recognition of mental health professions.

One might wonder, however, what might be the cost associated with this professionalization process. To being, one of the most prevalent and noticeable costs is that mental health care focuses almost exclusively on malfunctioning and disorders (Maddux 2009; Vaillant 2003). Even though mental health is a positive term, it is basically defined as the absence of disease. Over the past 50 years, all efforts in public mental health care have been directed toward the prevention and treatment of mental illness (Keyes 2007). Yet, evidence is accumulating that the absence of mental illness does not imply that individuals are functioning optimally. In other words, mental health is more than the absence of disorders. The promotion and protection of mental health as a positive state is therefore a promising new goal in mental health care (Fledderus et al. 2010).

Epidemiological studies on positive mental health provide an important foundation for this new goal as they make clear just what, exactly, the state of mental health in a given population is and how mental health is socially distributed in that

G.J. Westerhof (✉)
Psychology, Health, and Technology, University of Twente, Enschede, The Netherlands
e-mail: g.j.westerhof@utwente.nl

C.L.M. Keyes (ed.), *Mental Well-Being: International Contributions to the Study of Positive Mental Health*, DOI 10.1007/978-94-007-5195-8_3,

population. In this chapter, we propose a theory for studying positive mental health, its relation to the absence of mental illness, and the social distribution of mental health and illness using a longitudinal, nationally representative survey of Dutch adults.

Mental Health Combines Two Traditions of Happiness

The World Health Organization (WHO) has recently drawn attention to mental health as a positive state. Mental health is described as "a state of well–being in which the individual realizes his or her own abilities, can cope with the normal stresses of life, can work productively and fruitfully, and is able to make a contribution to his or her community" (WHO 2004, p. 12). The three core elements in this definition are (1) well-being, (2) effective functioning of an individual, and (3) effective functioning within a community. A further conceptual and empirical translation of subjective evaluations of these core elements can be found in the research literature on different aspects of well-being (Westerhof and Keyes 2008, 2010).

Two traditions of well-being research are distinguished in present-day social psychology: the one focusing on hedonic well-being and the other on eudaimonic well-being (Keyes et al. 2002; Ryan and Deci 2001; Waterman 1993). Traditional studies of hedonic well-being focus on feelings of satisfaction, happiness, pleasure, and interest in life. Waterman (1993) has argued that this tradition shares similarities with the old Greek philosophy of hedonism, incorporated, among others, by Aristippus. In hedonism, the pursuit of pleasure is the central aim in life. In social sciences, the study of hedonic aspects of well-being dates back to survey research in the 1960s and 1970s. Scholars like Andrews and Withey (1976), Bradburn (1969), Campbell et al. (1976), Cantril (1965) and Gurin et al. (1960) were interested in the quality of American life from the perspective of American citizens themselves. To stress this perspective, the concept of subjective well-being was used (Diener 1984). At present, there is a widespread consensus that subjective well-being is a multidimensional concept, including cognitive evaluations of life in general (i.e., life satisfaction); positive affects such as pleasure, interest, and happiness; and the absence of negative affects such as depression, anxiety, nervousness, and hostility (Diener 1984; Diener et al. 1999).

Building on this tradition, we focus on positive states of subjective well-being because the negative states share similarities with mental illness. As other aspects of well-being also refer to individuals' subjective interpretations, we prefer to use the concept *emotional well-being* rather than subjective well-being. Emotional well-being thus refers to positive emotions as well as positive emotion-laden cognitions.

In the 1980s and early 1990s, there was some discomfort with the largely empirical way in which well-being was defined in the hedonic tradition (Ryff 1989; Waterman 1993). Psychologists started to reflect on the notion of well-being in terms of individual strivings and optimal functioning. This gave rise to the second strand of research, called *eudaimonic well-being*. The concept of eudaimonia dates back to Aristotle, for whom not happiness, but the realization of one's own potential, was the essential element of a good life (Waterman 1990, 1993, 2008). Although the eudaimonic tradition is too short to have developed a crystallized set of indicators such as those for hedonic well-being, the conceptual and empirical work of Ryff has become most influential (Ryff 1989; Ryff and Essex 1991; Ryff and Keyes 1995; Ryff and Singer 2008). Ryff studied earlier psychological theories on optimal lifespan development (Erikson, Jung, Neugarten), on optimal functioning and self-actualization (Allport, Maslow, Rogers), and on positive mental health (Jahoda). She found six elements of positive functioning from this literature. Together, these make up what she calls *psychological well-being*: self-acceptance, personal growth, purpose in life, environmental mastery, autonomy, and positive relations with others (Ryff 1989; Ryff and Keyes 1995). Each of these six dimensions is important in the striving to become a better person and to realize one's potential:

1. Self-acceptance—a positive and acceptant attitude toward aspects of self in past and present
2. Purpose in life—goals and beliefs that affirm a sense of direction and meaning in life
3. Autonomy—self-direction as guided by one's own socially accepted internal standards
4. Positive relations with others—having satisfying personal relationships in which empathy and intimacy are expressed
5. Environmental mastery—the capability to manage the complex environment according to one's own needs
6. Personal growth—the insight into one's own potential for self-development

The work of Ryff, like other psychological work on eudaimonic well-being, focuses mainly on optimal functioning in terms of individual fulfillment (Deci and Ryan 2008; Ryan and Deci 2001; Waterman 1990, 1993, 2008). It thereby neglects the societal embedding of a person. Just like Ryff studied the classical psychologists, Keyes (1998) studied the work of major sociologists and social psychologists, such as Marx, Durkheim, Seeman, and Merton, to find indicators of what it means to prosper in a social way. His conceptual analysis indicates that *social well-being* consists of at least five dimensions:

1. Social coherence—being able to make meaning of what is happening in society
2. Social acceptance—a positive attitude toward others while acknowledging their difficulties
3. Social actualization—the belief that the community has potential and can evolve positively
4. Social contribution—the feeling that one's activities contribute to and are valued by society
5. Social integration—a sense of belonging to a community

Emotional, psychological, and social well-being together make up positive mental health (Keyes 2005). This conceptualization nicely fits the WHO definition of positive mental health (Westerhof and Keyes 2008, 2010): Emotional well-being corresponds to the notion of well-being as used in the WHO definition, psychological well-being is a subjective appraisal of one's effective individual functioning toward self-realization, and social well-being is a subjective evaluation of one's effective functioning in the community.

The Tripartite Structure of Mental Health

Now that the concept of mental health has been elucidated, an important question becomes how different aspects of mental health relate to each other. Some have claimed that hedonic well-being is qualitatively different from eudaimonic well-being (Ryff 1989; Waterman 1993), whereas others argue that they are related (Ryan and Deci 2001) or even indistinguishable (Kashdan et al. 2008). The present study helps to accumulate more evidence about the relations between the different forms of well-being that make up the subjective evaluation of positive mental health.

There are theoretical reasons why hedonic and eudaimonic well-being are related to each other. On the one hand, fulfilling the need for self-realization and being part of a society that values your person and your contributions leads to higher levels of satisfaction and happiness in life. Positive affects are a kind of by-product of eudaimonic involvement in life. However, the process might also function the other way around: Positive affect may make it easier for individuals to achieve fulfillment.

There are also theoretical reasons why different forms of well-being are distinct. It is possible that leading a life toward fulfillment and social value does not always bring emotional well-being. On the one hand, working toward self-realization or being engaged in social life might call for personal sacrifices in terms of hedonic feelings. On the other hand, being happy and satisfied with one's present life might divert one's attention from striving toward individual and social fulfillment or even lead to some sort of inertia. Similarly, psychological and social well-being might contribute to each other's fulfillment, but they might also be somewhat antagonistic: Focusing only on self-realization might come with a cost in terms of societal commitments, and vice versa.

Factor-analytic approaches have typically provided evidence for the distinction between hedonic and eudaimonic well-being. Studies focusing on emotional and psychological well-being have consistently shown that a two-factor model describes well-being data better than a one-factor model (Compton et al. 1996; Kafka and Kozma 2002; Keyes et al. 2002; King and Napa 1998: McGregor and Little 1998; Ryff and Keyes 1995; Waterman 1993; Waterman et al. 2008). Similarly, studies on emotional, psychological, and social well-being have typically found three distinct factors (Gallagher et al. 2009; Keyes 2005, 2006; Keyes et al. 2008; Lamers et al. 2011). Furthermore, research has shown that hedonic and eudaimonic well-being have different correlates (Vittersø et al. 2009) and accumulate differently over time (Huta 2005).

Given their integration in one model of mental health, we believe that there is reason for different forms of well-being to be related to each other. However, these relationships are only moderate, and it is, therefore, also important to distinguish the different forms. High levels of mental health demand high levels of all three forms of well-being: emotional, psychological, *and* social. Keyes and Annas (2009) have provided evidence that it is indeed important to have high levels of different forms of well-being in order to function optimally in other psychological, social, and biological domains.

The Two-Continua Model of Mental Health and Mental Illness

An important next question is how positive mental health relates to mental illness. Traditionally, mental illness and mental health were seen as the opposite poles of one dimension. Lower levels of mental illness would therefore be the same as higher levels of mental health, and vice versa. There is, however, increasing evidence that this model is not true. Rather, mental illness and mental health are distinct dimensions, even though they tend to be related. The two-continua model of mental illness and health holds that one continuum indicates the presence or absence of mental health and the other, the presence or absence of mental illness (Keyes 2005). Complete mental health is therefore best viewed as a complete state: not merely the absence of mental illness but also the presence of mental health.

Keyes (2005) studied the relation between mental health and mental illness using data from the study on Midlife Development in the United States (MIDUS), a representative survey of 3,032 American adults between the ages 25 and 74. The data provide strong support for the two-continua model: A confirmatory factor model with two related factors proved to be superior to the single-factor model and provided a nearly perfect fitting model to the MIDUS data (Keyes 2005). Recently, this model has also been replicated in US adolescents (ages 12–18; Keyes 2006), US college students (Keyes et al. 2012), Dutch adults (Lamers et al. 2011), and South African adults (Keyes et al. 2008). Using other measures of mental health and mental illness, other studies have come to similar conclusions (Compton et al. 1996; Greenspoon and Saklofske 2001; Headey et al. 1993; Masse et al. 1998; Suldo and Shaffer 2008).

Further evidence for the validity of the two-continua model is given by studies on the relations of mental health and mental illness with other criteria. Findings consistently show that adults and adolescents who are diagnosed as anything less than a state of complete mental health are functioning worse in terms of health-care utilization, work productivity, and psychosocial functioning (Keyes 2002, 2005, 2006, 2007).

The Social Distribution of Mental Health and Illness

To further validate the distinction between mental health and mental illness and between the different forms of well-being, we have analyzed the social distribution in the Dutch population. If mental illness and different components of mental health have the same social distribution, one might argue that it is not much use to distinguish among them. Those with a higher risk for mental illness would be the same as those with a higher chance for positive mental health. Efforts toward the prevention and treatment of mental illness would thus be directed toward the same groups as efforts toward the promotion and protection of mental health. Similarly, it would not be necessary in public mental health care to distinguish between different components of mental health when the same adults who have a higher chance of experiencing emotional well-being also have a higher chance of experiencing psychological and social well-being. In contrast, when the pattern of social distribution differs between mental illness and mental health, as well as between the three components of mental health, this would lend further evidence to the importance of treating them as distinct. This would also have implications for public mental health care, as this would demand approaches which are more specifically targeted toward different aspects of mental illness and mental health in specific groups.

Previous studies have shown differentiated patterns of relations between mental illness and well-being with sociodemographic factors. With regard to mental illness, a recent large-scale Dutch study showed that disorders on Axis I of the DSM-IV (mood, anxiety, and substance disorders) have an uneven social distribution (De Graaf et al. 2010). Younger adults, those with lower educational levels, those without a partner, and those who are considered unemployed, have higher chances of experiencing any disorder during a 12-month period. No differences between men and women were found. Furthermore, studies have shown the mutual relations between physical and mental health (e.g., Moussavi et al. 2007; Prince et al. 2007).

Diener et al. (1999) reviewed the findings from many studies on emotional well-being. A higher education, being married, being employed, and being in good physical health related positively to emotional well-being, whereas gender tends to be unrelated to emotional well-being. The relation of age with emotional well-being depends on the measure used: Positive affects tend to be lower in older age groups, but life satisfaction tends to be equally high, or even higher, in older age groups.

Ryff and Singer (2008) describe the following pattern for psychological well-being. A higher education tends to go with higher levels of psychological well-being, in particular, personal growth and purpose in life. Women tend to score higher on positive relations than men, but there are few other gender differences in psychological well-being. Lastly, studies have shown that older adults score higher on autonomy and environmental mastery, lower on purpose in life and personal growth, and similar on self-acceptance and positive relations as younger adults. Similar results have been found in Canada (Clarke et al. 2001) and Sweden (Lindfors et al. 2006). There are few studies that relate psychological well-being to resources, such as employment or marriage, but one study has shown a complex relation of marital status and changes therein to psychological well-being (Marks and Lambert 1998). Last, chronic illness tends to be related to lower levels of psychological well-being (Mangelli et al. 2002), and there are studies showing that psychological well-being has various neurobiological correlates (Ryff and Singer 2006).

The social distribution of social well-being is least often studied, so we have to depend mainly on findings from the MIDUS study (Keyes 1998; Keyes and Shapiro 2004). A higher education is consistently related to higher social well-being, whereas poor physical health is consistently related to lower social well-being. Men tend to be higher on social coherence and women on social acceptance. Marriage is particularly related to a higher level of social integration. Age shows a complex pattern, with older adults having higher levels of social integration and acceptance and younger adults experiencing higher social coherence and contribution.

Usually, these sociodemographic factors explain, at best, 10% of the variance in well-being measures (Veenhoven 1996; Keyes and Shapiro 2004; Ryff and Singer 2008). Nevertheless, the existing findings show that sociodemographic factors hold different relations to different dimensions of mental illness and mental health. These findings support the idea that it is important to distinguish between mental illness and mental health as well as between the three components of positive mental health.

The Present Study

The present study contributes to the existing knowledge in three ways. First, few studies have addressed the three components of positive mental health simultaneously. Hence, it is difficult to know whether one's social position is related in a similar or different way to emotional, psychological, and social well-being. For example, gender tends to be related to some aspects of psychological and social well-being, but not to emotional well-being. However, we do not know whether gender is related in a *significantly* different way to these three forms of well-being. On the other hand, education is related to lower levels of emotional, psychological, and social well-being, but still, these relations may differ in strength. Our study can therefore contribute to the existing knowledge by including a measure for all three aspects of well-being and by investigating the relation of the three types of well-being with indicators of one's societal position (age, gender, and education) as well as with indicators of living conditions (marital status, employment, and physical health).

Second, this chapter provides further validation of the two-continua model, by analyzing the relationship of mental health and mental illness with sociodemographic variables. Although there have been many epidemiological studies addressing mental illness, there is still a lack of knowledge about the social distribution of mental health. Most importantly, it is still unknown whether the relation of mental health to sociodemographical variables differs from the relation of mental illness to these variables.

Lastly, few studies addressed the social distribution of mental health and mental illness over time. In our study, we followed the participant over 9 months, measuring their mental health and mental illness four times, with intervals of 3 months. This makes it possible to address whether the relation of sociodemographics to the three components of mental health and mental illness is stable over time.

Method

Procedures and Sample

In this chapter, data from the LISS panel of CentERdata are used. The LISS panel (Longitudinal Internet Study in the Social sciences) comprises Dutch-speaking noninstitutionalized individuals from 5,000 households in the Netherlands. Members answer Internet-based questionnaires on a monthly basis. Participants who did not have a computer or Internet were provided with the necessary means to cooperate in the study.

A *module on mental health and mental illness* (MMHMI; Westerhof and Keyes 2008) was presented to one person per household in one-third of the households at four points in time (December 2007 and March, June, and September 2008). This subsample was stratified according to age (18–29, 30–49, 50–64, 65+ years), gender, and migratory status (being Dutch versus being born abroad, or having at least one parent born abroad). This procedure resulted in a sample of 1,662 respondents who filled out the questionnaire in December 2007 (a response of 76% of those who were asked to participate in the panel). To gather additional information on the physical health of the respondents, we used a core module on health issues administered in November 2007 ($N=1{,}340$; 80.6%). These 1,340 respondents served as our baseline for the analyses in this chapter. Of those 1,340 participants, 1,220 filled out the MMHMI in March 2008 (91.0%), 946 in June 2008 (70.6%), and 1,086 in September 2008 (81.0%). Almost two-thirds of the respondents ($N=850$; 63.4%) filled out the questionnaires at all four measurement points. A logistic regression analysis showed that all variables used in this chapter (age, gender, migratory status, educational status, marital status, employment status, physical health, psychopathology, and emotional, psychological, and social well-being) explained only 2% of the variance between respondents who did or did not complete all measurements. Those who completed all four measures were somewhat less likely to be married ($\text{Exp}(B)=.751$; $p=.020$) or employed ($\text{Exp}(B)=.671$; $p=.002$) than those who did not.

To replace the missing data of those who did not complete the MMHMI at a given point in time, we carried out a regression analysis of that measurement at the previous point in time for those who did have complete data. We used the resulting regression equation to replace the missing values for those who did not complete the MMHMI at the corresponding point in time. In this way, we could analyze data for all 1,340 participants of our baseline sample.

Some basic characteristics of the sample are presented in Table 3.1. The age of the respondents varied between 18 and 85 (Mean = 48.32 years; SD = 17.66). Half of the sample was female. Fourteen percent were born abroad or had at least one parent born abroad. About one-third of them came from Western countries and two-thirds from non-Western countries. One-third had 10 years of education or less. Somewhat more than half of them were married, and half of them had paid work.

Instruments

The *Brief Symptom Inventory* (BSI; Derogatis 1975), one of the most often used instruments in mental health care, was used for assessment of psychopathology. The BSI consists of 53 items on symptoms of psychopathology, to be rated on a 5-point Likert scale (*not at all–a lot*) to the degree to which the respondent experienced these symptoms in the past week. The BSI measures somatization, obsessive-compulsive complaints, interpersonal sensitivity (social phobia), depression, anxiety, hostility, phobic anxiety, paranoid ideation, and psychoticism. Examples are "During the past 7 days, how much were you distressed by nervousness and shakiness inside?" and "During the past 7 days, how much were you distressed by feeling afraid to travel on buses, subways, or trains?" The Dutch translation has recently been validated (de Beurs and Zitman 2006). The reliability of the total scale in the present sample at baseline is .95 (Cronbach alpha). We computed the mean total score on the BSI, with higher scores indicating more psychopathology.

The *Mental Health Continuum – Short Form* (MHC-SF; Keyes et al. 2008; Lamers et al. 2011; Westerhof and Keyes 2008) consists of 14 items which correspond to our theoretical formulation of emotional, psychological, and social well-being. This innovative instrument was derived from the Mental Health Continuum – Long Form, which consists of longer scales measuring the three types of well-being. Sample items for the three types of well-being are "[i]n the past month, how often did you feel: happy; that your life has a sense of direction or meaning to it; that people are basically good?" There were six answering categories ranging from *almost never* to *every day*. The MHC-SF was translated into Dutch and back into English and subsequently used in four pilot studies. These pilot studies gave reason to reformulate some Dutch items. The final version was used in the LISS sample. Confirmatory factor analysis showed that the scale was empirically made up of three theoretical scales on emotional, psychological, and social well-being (Lamers et al. 2011). The internal consistency (Cronbach alpha) for the three scales at the baseline measurement in December 2007 was .83 for emotional well-being, .83 for psychological well-being, and .74 for social well-being. The scales also proved to have good concurrent and discriminatory validity (Lamers et al. 2011). Lastly, an analysis of the four measurement points based on item response theory showed that there is no substantial differential item functioning across sociodemographic variables, physical and mental illness, or time. Hence, the items are interpreted in a similar way by people from various backgrounds in Dutch society at different points in time (Lamers et al. 2012). We computed mean scores for emotional, psychological, and social well-being with higher scores indicating higher levels of well-being.

Background variables included age, gender, migration status, educational level, marital status, and employment status. Furthermore, we computed a composite index for physical health. We used three measures from the core module on health, developed for the LISS panel: number of physical conditions, number of limitations in activities of daily living, and subjective health. The number of physical conditions was measured with a checklist, asking whether a physician had told the

Table 3.1 Major characteristics of the respondents (N=1,340)

		Percent
Gender	Female	50.0
	Male	50.0
Migrant	No	86.0
	Yes, Western country	5.0
	Yes, non-Western country	9.0
Education	Max. 10 years	32.1
	11–14 years	35.7
	15 or more years	32.3
Marital status	Married	54.3
	Divorced	9.3
	Widowed	6.3
	Never married	30.1
Employment status	Paid work	50.7
	Unemployed	1.9
	Disabled	2.8
	School or study	7.2
	Retired	23.5
	Household	10.5
	Other	3.5

respondent during the last year that the respondent had suffered from any of 18 possible physical conditions (Mean=0.79; SD=1.31). Limitations in basic and instrumental activities of daily living were measured as the mean on 23 activities (from 1=*without problems* to 4=*only with help from others*; Mean=1.16; SD=0.26). Subjective health was measured with a single question asking how respondents rate their present health (1=*bad* to 5=*excellent*; Mean=3.13; SD=0.76). We carried out a factor analysis on subjective health, number of physical conditions, and number of limitations and saved the factor score as an overall measure of physical health (Mean=0.0; SD=1.0).

Analyses

We first carried out a MANOVA for repeated measures. The seven independent variables were age, gender, migratory status (*Dutch origin*=0, *other*=1), educational attainment (six categories as in Table 3.1), marital status (*married*=1, *not married*=0), employment status (*paid work*=1, *other*=0), and physical health (the composite index described above). The scores on the BSI and the three subscales of the MHC-SF at the four measurement points made up the 16 repeated measures. The scores on the BSI were reversed in this analysis so that they indicated more absence of mental illness and carried a similar meaning to that of the mental health scales. The 16 repeated measures were divided over two factors with four levels each: The first factor was called *scales* and concerned the four different dimensions of mental illness and mental health (absence of psychopathology and presence of emotional well-being, psychological well-being, and social well-being), and the second factor was called *time* and concerned the four measurement points (December 2007 and March, June, and September 2008). We used Helmert contrasts to make comparisons between the scales: Psychopathology was compared to all other scales, emotional well-being to both eudaimonic well-being measures, and psychological to social well-being. We used repeated contrasts for the second factor (time), comparing each time point to the previous time point. After examining the results of this MANOVA, we further analyzed the data with four ordinary least-squares regression analyses to assess the relation between sociodemographics and the four indicators of mental illness and mental health. Last, for those results which differed over time, we carried out post hoc paired t-tests to assess which time differences were significant.

Results

Table 3.2 presents the basic findings for mental illness and mental health across the four points in time. We carried out the MANOVA with repeated measures to analyze this pattern of findings and to find out whether the background variables had any effect on it. When looking at the multivariate tests, we found that the factor scales was significant ($F_{3,1330}=47.60$; $p < .001$). That is to say, the mean scores on the different scales differ from each other, independent of the time of measurement. The Helmert contrasts were all significant ($p < .001$). The absence of psychopathology differs significantly from the presence of mental health, but this is a result of the different answering scales used (a four-point format for psychopathology and a six-point format for mental health). It can be seen in Table 3.2 that the sample scored rather low on psychopathology: approximately 0.35 on a scale from 0 to 3. More interesting is the finding that the means of emotional, psychological, and social well-being differed from each other. On the mental health measure, participants scored highest on emotional well-being, followed by psychological well-being, and lowest on social well-being (Table 3.2). The factor time is not significant ($F_{3,1330}=0.78$; $p=.506$), nor is the interaction between scales and time ($F_{9,1324}=1.59$; $p=.113$). As can be seen in Table 3.2, the means are remarkably stable across time and so are the differences between the scales.

How is this pattern qualified by the background variables? First, all background variables (age, gender, migratory status, educational attainment, being married, having paid work, and being in good physical health; all $p < .05$) showed a significant interaction with the factor scales. Hence, the predictive value of each of these variables was different for the four scales used. We will analyze these differences in more detail below. Furthermore, none of the interactions between the factor time and the background variables were significant (all $p > .05$). The stability in time observed in Table 3.2 is therefore similar for all characteristics of the participants considered here. However, age showed a significant three-way interaction with scales and time ($F_{9,1324}=2.54$; $p=.007$). A similar finding pertains to education

Table 3.2 Frequency distribution of measures of mental illness and health across time ($N=1,340$)

		T0	*T1*	*T2*	*T3*	All
Mental illness	Mean	.37	.35	.34	.34	.35
	SD	.34	.33	.32	.32	.30
Mental health						
Emotional well-being	Mean	4.68	4.66	4.56	4.61	4.63
	SD	.93	.94	.92	.87	.77
Psychological well-being	Mean	4.17	4.20	4.12	4.16	4.16
	SD	.98	.97	.92	.95	.81
Social well-being	Mean	3.32	3.31	3.33	3.41	3.50
	SD	1.00	1.01	.94	.93	.78

Table 3.3 Ordinary least-squares regression of mental illness and mental health on background variables ($N=1,340$)

	Mental illness	Emotional well-being	Psychological well-being	Social well-being
	Beta	Beta	Beta	Beta
Age	–.28***	.08*	–.12***	–.01
Gender: female	.01	.07*	.07*	.00
Migration: yes	.06*	–.05	.02	.04
Education	–.03	–.01	.07*	.06*
Married: yes	–.07*	.12***	.01	–.02
Employed: yes	–.07*	–.03	.05	.02
Physical health	–.41***	.27***	.12***	.15***
Adjusted R^2	.19	.08	.06	.03

*p<.05;
***p<.001

($F_{9,1324}=2.53$; $p=.007$). These findings indicate that participants with a different age and those with a different educational background show a somewhat different pattern across time on some scales than other scales. We will also analyze these differences in more detail below.

To further analyze the relations of the different background variables with mental illness and mental health, we carried out a regression analysis for each of the four dimensions of mental illness and mental health. We used the mean score of each dimension across the four time points as the dependent variable and age, gender, migration, education, marital status, employment status, and physical health as the independent variables. The results are presented in Table 3.3.

It can be seen that age, migration, marital status, employment status, and physical health were related to mental illness: Being young, being a migrant, not being married or employed, and having poor physical health were all related to more mental illness complaints. Together, these variables account for 19% of the explained variance in mental illness. Emotional well-being was related to age, gender, marital status, and physical health: Being older, being female, being married, and having a better physical health were related to better emotional well-being. These variables account for 8% of the variance in emotional well-being. Six percent of the variance of psychological well-being can be explained by age, gender, education, and physical health: A younger age, being female, higher educational achievement, and good physical health were related to better psychological well-being. Finally, the variables explain 3% of the variance in social well-being: Higher educational achievement and good physical health were related to higher social well-being. To conclude, the mean score across time for each dimension of mental illness and mental health was differently related to different background variables.

The within-subjects contrasts in the MANOVA with repeated measures give some more information with regard to the different relations of the background variables with mental illness and mental health. It can be seen in Table 3.3 that an older age was related to less mental illness problems and higher emotional and lower psychological well-being, but it was unrelated to social well-being. All three Helmert contrasts were significant for age. That is to say that the relation of age to mental illness differed from that of mental health, the relation of age to emotional well-being differed from the relation to eudaimonic well-being, and the relation of age to psychological well-being differed from that of social well-being. Being female was related to more emotional and psychological well-being, but not to social well-being and mental illness. The Helmert contrasts were only significant for the comparison between psychological and social well-being. For the other variables, only the Helmert contrast between emotional and eudaimonic well-being was significant. It can be seen that being a migrant and being employed were negatively related to emotional well-being, but positively to psychological and social well-being. Furthermore, higher education was related to more psychological and social well-being, but not to emotional well-being. Being married was related to more emotional well-being, but not to both measures of eudaimonic well-being. Lastly, good physical health was more strongly related to emotional than to psychological and social well-being.

Two three-way interactions were significant: age by scales and time as well as education by scales and time. We carried out post hoc t-tests in order to compare the changes between any two adjacent points in time per scale and age/education group. Figure 3.1 presents the findings for three age groups: a younger group between 18 and 39 years, a middle-aged group between 40 and 59 years, and an older group aged 60 years and over. The scores for mental health range from 1 to 6, those for mental illness from 0 to 3. Straight lines refer to scores on mental illness, dotted lines to mental health. The thicker lines refer to two adjacent means, which were significantly different in the post-hoc paired *t*-test. It can be seen that the two younger groups (18–39 and 40–50 years) had somewhat less mental illness complaints at the second than the first time of measurement (*T*0 and *T*1). Between *T*1 and *T*2, we found a significant drop in mental illness complaints and an increase in emotional well-being. Furthermore, the youngest group decreased in emotional but increased in social well-being, whereas the middle age group showed a decrease in psychological well-being. Finally, the oldest age group showed an increase in social well-being and the two youngest groups in emotional well-being. It can be concluded that mental illness and mental health have a somewhat different longitudinal pattern for different age groups. Most important, however, is the finding that a change in one dimension does not always go together with changes in other dimensions.

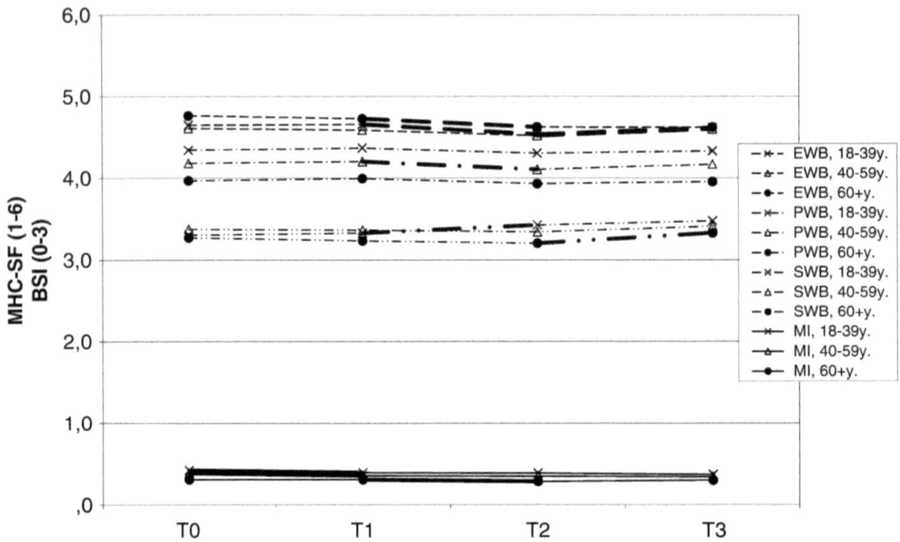

Fig. 3.1 Mean of mental illness and mental health across time for three different age groups. *EWB* emotional well-being, *PWB* psychological well-being, *SWB* social well-being, *MI* mental illness, *MHC-SF* Mental Health Continuum – Short Form, *BSI* Brief Symptom Inventory

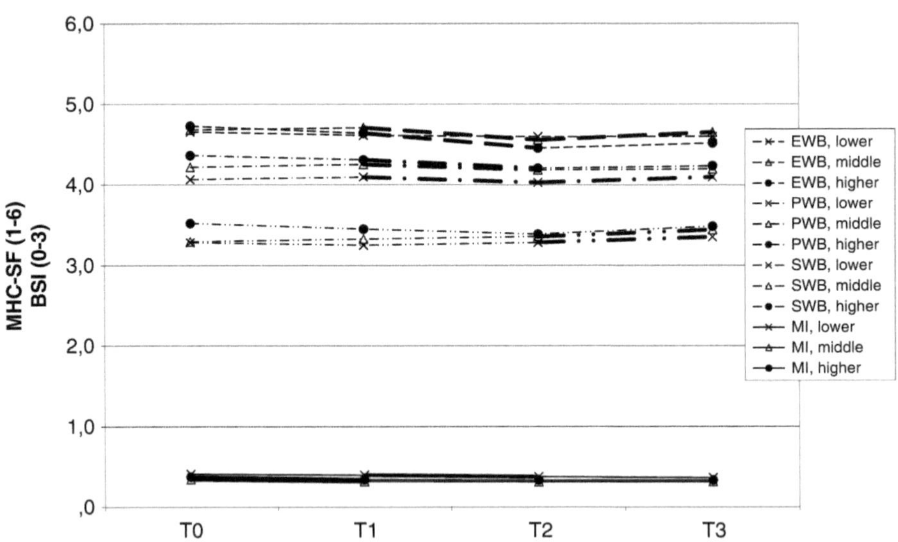

Fig. 3.2 Mean of mental illness and mental health across time for three different educational groups. *EWB* emotional well-being, *PWB* psychological well-being, *SWB* social well-being, *MI* mental illness, *MHC-SF* Mental Health Continuum – Short Form, *BSI* Brief Symptom Inventory

Figure 3.2 presents the findings for three educational groups: lower educated (10 years or less), middle (11–14 years), and higher (15 years and more). There was a decrease in mental illness between the first and second measurement for the middle- and higher educated groups. The lowest educated group showed a significant decrease in mental illness problems 3 months later. Furthermore, all groups declined in psychological well-being, but only the two highest educated groups also declined in emotional well-being. Between *T2* and *T3*, there was a significant increase in well-being: The lowest educated group rose in social and psychological well-being, and the middle group in social and emotional well-being. It can be concluded that mental illness and mental health have a somewhat different longitudinal pattern for different educational groups. Most important, again, is the finding that a change in one dimension does not always go together with changes in other dimensions. These findings therefore provide further evidence for the distinction between the different measures of mental illness and mental health.

Conclusion

The promotion and protection of mental health are new goals in public mental health care, which has traditionally been focused on the treatment and prevention of mental illness. In line with the basic definition of positive mental health given by the WHO (2004), we argued that mental health consists of the experience of emotional well-being in combination with the experience of personal and social fulfillment. In this chapter, we provided important information about the social distribution of mental illness and different components of mental health in the Dutch population. The three most important findings are (1) that sociodemographic variables hold different relations with different indicators of mental illness and mental health, (2) that these relations are remarkably stable across time, and (3) that the exceptions to this stability for age and educational level showed distinct time trajectories for the different indicators of mental health and illness. Taken together, these findings show that it is important to distinguish among the three different components of mental health, i.e., emotional, psychological, and social well-being. Furthermore, the findings provide further support for the two-continua model of mental health and illness.

In the following two paragraphs, we will interpret the findings in relation to previous studies on mental illness and different aspects of well-being. We found that younger adults, migrants, unmarried or unemployed persons, and those with poor physical health experienced more mental illness complaints. These findings generally match the findings from the studies discussed in the introduction, with the exception that we found no relation between education and mental illness. However, post hoc analyses showed that there is a bivariate relation of lower education with mental illness, but this relation is mediated by the poorer physical health condition of those with lower educational levels.

We also found that emotional well-being is better among older adults, women, married persons, and those with good physical health. In contrast to the studies mentioned in the introduction, we found no relations of educational attainment or unemployment to emotional well-being. These lacking correlations might be specific for Dutch society, which is more egalitarian and has a stronger social security net than the United States, where most studies have been carried out. Furthermore, we found a difference between men and women which was not always found in previous studies; however, this finding appears to be the result of a suppression effect of the poorer health condition of women. Psychological well-being is explained by a lower age, being female, and having higher education and good physical health. Previous studies have shown somewhat differentiated patterns for age and gender, but these did not examine psychological well-being in total. Apparently, the differentiated patterns account for small differences in the advantage of younger adults and women. Education and physical health were related to psychological well-being in previous studies as well. Social well-being is explained only by higher education and better physical health. These were the two strongest predictors of social well-being in previous studies as well.

Our study added to the existing knowledge as we were also able to compare the ways in which sociodemographic variables are related to the different indicators of mental illness and health. Physical health was the only predictor that was significantly related to mental illness as well as to all three well-being measures. Even physical health showed a differentiated pattern across the four indicators: It was more strongly related to mental illness than to emotional well-being and more strongly to emotional well-being than to psychological and social well-being. The stronger relation with mental illness might be explained by the fact that the mental illness measure also contains a somatization subscale including items with psychophysiological symptoms, such as pain and breathing difficulties. By contrast, age has the most contradictory pattern: Older adults experience less mental illness problems, more emotional well-being, less psychological well-being, but equal levels of social well-being as younger adults. This pattern might be related to better emotion regulation capacities of older adults, yet a lack of societal possibilities for self-realization or societal participation (cf. Westerhof and Keyes 2010). Marriage is related to less mental illness problems and higher well-being but not to both forms of eudaimonic well-being, whereas the opposite is true for education. Apparently, marriage does not help in individual and social fulfillment, whereas a better education is an important resource for fulfillment. Education might not be related to emotional regulation, whereas marriage is an important resource there.

It is interesting to see that the relations of sociodemographic background with mental illness and health are remarkably stable across time. We only found some differential time trajectories for age and education, contributing to our knowledge about the relative independence of the indicators for mental illness and health used here. Further studies should clarify which aspects of mental illness and mental health change and under what conditions. One might think of critical life events here, but also of far-reaching societal changes, such as the recent economic recession which came just after our survey concluded. The present study also suggests that for certain age and educational groups, changes in mental illness precede later changes in well-being. Further studies should clarify whether and how mental illness and mental health influence each other across time. For example, Keyes et al. (2010a) found that mental health is an important predictor of mental illness 10 years later in time.

Even though measures were taken to provide underprivileged groups with a computer and Internet access in order to participate in the LISS panel, certain groups remained underrepresented in the panel. Compared with national statistics, the LISS panel shows some underrepresentation of older adults, single, never married persons, widowers, and immigrants (Knoef and de Vos 2009). Furthermore, not all participants were equally conscientious in filling out all questionnaires every month. However, this did not lead to a substantial distortion in the variables used in this chapter. Finally, sociodemographic status explained only some of the variance in mental illness and mental health. As noted in the introduction, this is known from other studies as well. It is therefore important to search for other explanations of individual differences, such as genetics (Keyes et al. 2010b), personality (Joshanloo and Nosratabadi 2009), and psychological processes, such as coping or psychological flexibility (Fledderus et al. 2010).

Despite these limitations, we can conclude that mental health is more than the absence of mental illness. Given the differential relations of background characteristics to mental health and illness, public mental health care is best served by a differentiated approach in the treatment and prevention of mental illness, as well as by the promotion and protection of mental health. Such a differentiated approach should be tailored to groups with different backgrounds.

References

Andrews, F. M., & Withey, S. B. (1976). *Social indicators of well-being: Americans' perceptions of life quality*. New York: Plenum.

Bradburn, N. M. (1969). *The structure of psychological well-being*. Chicago: Aldine.

Campbell, A., Converse, P. E., & Rodgers, W. L. (1976). *The quality of American life: Perceptions, evaluations and satisfactions*. New York: Russell Sage.

Cantril, H. (1965). *The pattern of human concerns*. New Brunswick: Rutgers University Press.

Clarke, P., Marshall, V., Ryff, C., & Wheaton, B. (2001). Measuring psychological well-being in the Canadian study of health and aging. *International Psychogeriatrics, 13*, 79–90.

Compton, W. C., Smith, M. L., Cornish, K. A., & Qualls, D. L. (1996). Factor structure of mental health measures. *Journal of Personality and Social Psychology, 76*, 406–413.

De Beurs, E., & Zitman, F. (2006). De Brief Symptom Inventory (BSI): De betrouwbaarheid en validiteit van een handzaam alternatief. [Reliability and validity of a practical alternative to the SCL 90]. *Maandblad Geestelijke Volksgezondheid, 61*, 120–141.

De Graaf, R., ten Have, M., & van Dorsselaer, S. (2010). *De psychische gezondheid van de Nederlandse bevolking: NEMESIS-2, Opzet en eerste resultaten*. Utrecht: Trimbos.

Deci, E., & Ryan, R. (2008). Hedonia, eudaimonia, and well-being: An introduction. *Journal of Happiness Studies, 9*, 1–11.

Derogatis, L. R. (1975). The brief symptom inventory. Baltimore, MD:Clinical Psychometric Research.

Diener, E. (1984). Subjective well-being. *Psychological Bulletin, 95*, 542–575.

Diener, E., Suh, E. M., Lucas, R., & Smith, H. L. (1999). Subjective well-being: Three decades of progress. *Psychological Bulletin, 125*, 276–302.

Fledderus, M., Bohlmeijer, E. T., Smit, F., & Westerhof, G. J. (2010). Mental health promotion as a new goal in public mental health care: A randomized controlled trial of an intervention enhancing psychological flexibility. *American Journal of Public Health, 100*, 2372–2378.

Gallagher, M., Lopez, S., & Preacher, K. (2009). The hierarchical structure of well-being. *Journal of Personality, 77*, 1025–1050.
Greenspoon, P. J., & Saklofske, D. H. (2001). Toward an integration of subjective well-being and psychopathology. *Social Indicators Research, 54*, 81–108.
Gurin, G., Veroff, J., & Feld, S. (1960). *Americans view their mental health*. New York: Basic Books.
Headey, B., Kelley, J., & Wearing, A. (1993). Dimensions of mental health: Life satisfaction, positive affect, anxiety, and depression. *Social Indicators Research, 29*, 63–82.
Huta, V. (2005). *Pursuing pleasure versus growth and excellence: Links with different aspects of well-being*. Dissertation, McGill University, Montreal.
Joshanloo, M., & Nosratabadi, M. (2009). Levels of mental health continuum and personality traits. *Social Indicators Research, 90*, 211–224.
Kafka, G., & Kozma, A. (2002). The construct validity of Ryff's Scales of Psychological Well-Being (SPWB) and their relationship to measures of subjective well-being. *Social Indicators Research, 57*, 171–190.
Kashdan, T. B., Biswas-Diener, R., & King, L. A. (2008). Reconsidering happiness: The costs of distinguishing between hedonics and eudaimonia. *Journal of Positive Psychology, 3*, 219–233.
Keyes, C. L. M. (1998). Social well–being. *Social Psychology Quarterly, 61*, 121–140.
Keyes, C. L. M. (2002). The mental health continuum: From languishing to flourishing in life. *Journal of Health and Social Behavior, 43*, 207–222.
Keyes, C. L. M. (2005). Mental illness and/or mental health? Investigating axioms of the complete state model of health. *Journal of Consulting and Clinical Psychology, 73*, 539–548.
Keyes, C. L. M. (2006). Mental health in adolescence: Is America's youth flourishing? *American Journal of Orthopsychiatry, 76*, 395–402.
Keyes, C. L. M. (2007). Promoting and protecting mental health as flourishing: A complementary strategy for improving national mental health. *American Psychologist, 62*, 95–108.
Keyes, C. L. M., & Annas, J. (2009). Feeling good and functioning well: Distinctive concepts in ancient philosophy and contemporary science. *Journal of Positive Psychology, 4*, 197–201.
Keyes, C. L. M., & Shapiro, A. D. (2004). Social well-being in the United States: A descriptive epidemiology. In O. G. Brim, C. D. Ryff, & R. C. Kessler (Eds.), *How healthy are we: A national study of well-being at midlife* (pp. 350–373). Chicago: University of Chicago Press.
Keyes, C. L. M., Shmotkin, D., & Ryff, C. D. (2002). Optimizing well-being: The empirical encounter of two traditions. *Journal of Personality and Social Psychology, 82*, 1007–1022.
Keyes, C. L. M., Wissing, M., Potgieter, J., Temane, M., Kruger, A., & van Rooy, S. (2008). Evaluation of the Mental Health Continuum – Short Form (MHC-SF) in Setswana-speaking South Africans. *Clinical Psychology and Psychotherapy, 15*, 181–192.
Keyes, C. L. M., Dhingra, S. S., & Simoes, E. J. (2010a). Change in level of positive mental health as a predictor of future risk of mental illness. *American Journal of Public Health, 100*, 2366–2371.
Keyes, C. L. M., Myers, J. M., & Kendler, K. S. (2010b). The structure of the genetic and environmental influences on mental well-being. *American Journal of Public Health, 100*, 2379–2384.
Keyes, C. L. M., Eisenberg, D., Perry, G. S., Dube, S. R., Kroenke, K., & Dhingra, S. S. (2012). The relationship of level of positive mental health with current mental disorders in predicting suicidal behavior and academic impairment in college students. *Journal of American College Health, 60*(2), 126–133.
King, L. A., & Napa, C. (1998). What makes a life good? *Journal of Personality and Social Psychology, 75*, 156–165.
Knoef, M., & Vos, K. de. (2009). *The representativeness of LISS, an online probability panel*. RetrievedAugust31,2012,fromhttps://www.lisspanel.nl/assets/uploaded/representativeness_LISS_panel.pdf
Lamers, S. M. A., Westerhof, G. J., Bohlmeijer, E. T., ten Klooster, P. M., & Keyes, C. L. M. (2011). The psychometric properties of the Mental Health Continuum-Short Form (MHC- SF) in the Dutch population. *Journal of Clinical Psychology, 67*, 99–110.

Lamers, S. M. A., Glas, C. A. W., Westerhof, G. J., & Bohlmeijer, E. T. (2012, online first). Longitudinal evaluation of the Mental Health Continuum-Short Form (MHC-SF): Item functioning across demographics, physical illness and mental illness. *European Journal of Psychological Assessment*. doi:10.1027/1015-5759/a000109

Lindfors, P., Berntsson, L., & Lundberg, U. (2006). Factor structure of Ryff's psychological well-being scales in Swedish female and male white-collar workers. *Personality and Individual Differences, 40*, 1213–1222.

Maddux, J. (2009). Stopping the 'madness': Positive psychology and deconstructing the illness ideology and the DSM. In S. J. Lopez & C. R. Snyder (Eds.), *Oxford handbook of positive psychology* (2nd ed., pp. 61–69). New York: Oxford University Press.

Mangelli, L., Gribbin, N., Büchi, S., Allard, S., & Sensky, T. (2002). Psychological well-being in rheumatoid arthritis: Relationship to 'disease' variables and affective disturbance. *Psychotherapy and Psychosomatics, 71*(2), 112–116.

Marks, N. F., & Lambert, J. D. (1998). Marital status continuity and change among young and midlife adults: Longitudinal effects on psychological wellbeing. *Journal of Family Issues, 19*, 652–686.

Masse, R., Poulin, C., Dassa, C., Lambert, J., Belair, S., & Battaglini, A. (1998). The structure of mental health higher-order confirmatory factor analyses of psychological distress and wellbeing measures. *Social Indicators Research, 45*, 475–504.

McGregor, I., & Little, B. R. (1998). Personal projects, happiness, and meaning: On doing well and being yourself. *Journal of Personality and Social Psychology, 74*, 494–512.

Moussavi, S., Chatterji, S., Verdes, E., Tandon, A., Patel, V., & Ustun, B. (2007). Depression, chronic diseases, and decrements in health: Results from the World Health Surveys. *Lancet, 370*, 851–858.

Prince, M., Patel, V., Saxena, S., Maj, M., Maselko, J., Phillips, M. R., et al. (2007). No health without mental health. *Lancet, 370*, 859–877.

Ryan, R. M., & Deci, E. L. (2001). On happiness and human potentials: A review of research on hedonic and eudaimonic well-being. *Annual Review of Psychology, 52*, 141–166.

Ryff, C. D. (1989). Happiness is everything, or is it? Explorations on the meaning of psychological well-being. *Journal of Personality and Social Psychology, 57*, 1069–1081.

Ryff, C. D., & Essex, M. J. (1991). Psychological well-being in adulthood and old age: Descriptive markers and explanatory processes. *Annual Review of Gerontology and Geriatrics, 10*, 144–171.

Ryff, C. D., & Keyes, C. L. M. (1995). The structure of psychological well-being revisited. *Journal of Personality and Social Psychology, 69*, 719–727.

Ryff, C. D., & Singer, B. (2006). Best news yet on the six-factor model of well-being. *Social Science Research, 35*, 1103–1119.

Ryff, C. D., & Singer, B. (2008). Know thyself and become what you are: A eudaimonic approach to psychological well-being. *Journal of Happiness Studies, 9*, 13–39.

Suldo, S. M., & Shaffer, E. J. (2008). Looking beyond psychopathology: The dual-factor model of mental health in youth. *School Psychology Review, 37*, 52–68.

Vaillant, G. E. (2003). Mental health. *American Journal of Psychiatry, 169*, 1373–1384.

Veenhoven, R. (1996). Developments in satisfaction research. *Social Indicators Research, 37*, 1–46.

Vittersø, J., Oelmann, H., & Wang, A. (2009). Life satisfaction is not a balanced estimator of the good life: Evidence from reaction time measures and self-reported emotions. *Journal of Happiness Studies, 10*, 1–17.

Waterman, A. (1990). The relevance of Aristotle's conception of eudaimonia for the psychological study of happiness. *Theoretical & Philosophical Psychology, 10*(1), 39–44.

Waterman, A. (1993). Two conceptions of happiness: Contrasts of personal expressiveness (eudaimonia) and hedonic enjoyment. *Journal of Personality and Social Psychology, 64*, 678–691.

Waterman, A. (2008). Reconsidering happiness: A eudaimonist's perspective. *The Journal of Positive Psychology, 3*(4), 234–252.

Waterman, A. S., Schwartz, S. J., & Conti, R. (2008). The implications of two conceptions of happiness (hedonic enjoyment and eudaimonia) for the understanding of intrinsic motivation. *Journal of Happiness Studies, 9*, 41–79.
Westerhof, G. J., & Keyes, C. L. M. (2008). Geestelijke gezondheid is meer dan de afwezigheid van geestelijke ziekte. *Maandblad Geestelijke Volksgezondheid, 63*, 808–820.
Westerhof, G. J., & Keyes, C. L. M. (2010). Mental illness and mental health: The two continua model across the lifespan. *Journal of Adult Development, 17*, 110–119.
World Health Organization. (2004). *Promoting mental health: Concepts, emerging evidence, practice* (Summary report). Geneva: WHO.

Chapter 4
The Prevalence of Levels of Well-Being Revisited in an African Context

Marié P. Wissing and Q. Michael Temane

The last decade has seen the evolution of many conceptualizations and operationalizations of psychosocial well-being, or mental health, since the shift in focus to mental well-being instead of merely on mental ill-being. However, very little is known about the prevalence of various levels of psychosocial well-being in communities and in various contexts. Such baseline knowledge is important for health and wellness promotion, not only for individuals but also for communities and societies. This chapter will report on some findings with regard to the prevalence of levels of psychosocial well-being within an African context against the theoretical backdrop of Keyes' mental health continuum model.

According to the World Health Organization (1998), *health* is a state of complete physical, mental, and social well-being. However, very little is known about the prevalence of such high levels of functioning in communities. In the past, the focus in epidemiological studies was mainly on *risk factors* and *pathology* and on *physical ill-health*, with an aim to decide where, and for which risk factors or diseases, interventions should be planned for the sake of health promotion in communities. Major studies on the epidemiology of diseases do exist. However, as far as levels of psychosocial well-being on the upper end of a mental health continuum are concerned, very little information is available. Only Keyes' research (2002, 2005, 2006a, 2007) in the United States on the distribution or prevalence of strengths and characteristics of psychosocial well-being in communities, and the findings of So and Huppert (2009), could be found. In order to approach the ideal of complete mental health that is more than the absence of symptoms, we also need information on the nature of complete psychosocial health and on the prevalence of levels of *psychosocial well-being* in communities, in order to decide where, when, and for whom interventions may be indicated (and should be planned) as part

M.P. Wissing (✉) • Q.M. Temane
School for Psychosocial Sciences: Psychology, North-West University,
Potchefstroom Campus, Private Bag X6001, 2520 Potchefstroom, South Africa
e-mail: Marie.Wissing@nwu.ac.za

C.L.M. Keyes (ed.), *Mental Well-Being: International Contributions to the Study of Positive Mental Health*, DOI 10.1007/978-94-007-5195-8_4,

of public health promotion. Therefore, it is also necessary to understand and measure the prevalence of levels of well-being in groups and communities.

Recently, the possible value of national indicators of psychological well-being has been highlighted (e.g., Diener 2000; Diener and Seligman 2004; Keyes 2007; Lyobomirsky et al. 2005). Diener et al. (2008) argued that accounts of well-being may be highly useful for policymakers and may add value beyond existing social and economic indicators. Previous research has indicated that psychological well-being and life satisfaction are associated with many positive outcomes on both individual and societal levels (e.g., Pressman and Cohen 2005; Keyes 2005, 2007).

Accounts of well-being may help a government to identify groups in the greatest need of interventions in a given society (Diener et al. 2008; Higgs 2007). These previous findings, however, do not indicate what theoretical model and measure would be the most appropriate for use in epidemiological studies and why or how various models and measures compare in predictions of outcomes. Neither are levels of well-being distinguished nor are critical cutoff points for positive outcomes indicated, except for indications in the work of Keyes (2002, 2007) with his mental health continuum measure in the United States and to a limited extent, categories for the Satisfaction with Life Scale (Pavot and Diener 1993). Currently, no national or regional systematically collected data on levels of psychological health over time exist, and in South Africa in particular, very little is known about the prevalence of various levels of well-being in different contexts. Some epidemiological data does exist for symptoms and syndromes of psychopathology in South Africa (e.g., Williams et al. 2007) but very little on levels of psychological well-being, although some data are available on quality of life (e.g., Higgs 2007).

Conceptual Challenges

Measuring the prevalence of levels of well-being in epidemiological studies poses several conceptual (and practical) challenges that need to be considered: Firstly, there is no word to indicate the distribution of strengths in a community. The construct *epidemiology* refers to the *distribution of diseases*. It is suggested that we use a new word such as "epidemiofortology" to indicate the distribution of (levels or patterns of) wellness and strengths in communities (*forte* = strength). This option is preferable to that of just broadening the meaning of the word epidemiology to also include the distribution of strengths, as that may strengthen the dominance of the medical model, which may not be the best suitable option in all instances.

Secondly, there is no consensus as to what model, strengths, characteristics, patterns, or levels of psychosocial well-being and measure should be considered in the development of an epidemiofortology of psychological well-being. There are many constructs that refer to facets of psychological well-being, for example, sense of coherence (Antonovsky 1987), self-efficacy (Chen et al. 2001; Schwarzer and Jerusalem 1993), positive affect (Fredrickson 2001), fortitude (Pretorius 1998), satisfaction with life (Diener et al. 1985, 2008), but very few refer to levels or cutoff points for various levels of wellness. A further problem is that the same construct is sometimes defined in different ways; for example, Keyes (2002) developed the idea of *flourishing* as the positive end of the mental health dimension which is part of a holistic model of a mental health continuum, and specified criteria on his Mental Health Continuum Scale. However, the same construct is used by So and Huppert (2009), explicating it in terms of other core and peripheral features of well-being, as developed in the European Social Survey's (ESS) well-being module. To be flourishing, a participant must have scores above a specific level on all three identified core features (positive emotions, engagement/interest, and meaning/purpose) and at least three additional features (self-esteem, optimism, resilience, vitality, self-determination, and positive relationships; So and Huppert 2009). Huppert et al. (2009) refer to similar (but not the same) features in the well-being module of the European Social Survey, and this is also the case in Tennant et al.'s (2007) validation of the Warwick–Edinburg Mental Well-Being Scale (WEMWBS). However, the latter two publications do not refer to the construct of flourishing as an overarching concept.

In the selection of a model and measure to explore the prevalence of various levels of well-being in epidemiological/epidemiofortological studies, it makes intuitive sense to use a holistic model that includes various facets of wellness but is also operationalized with a relatively short, but comprehensive, measure of criteria for various levels/patterns of wellness. Such a possible suitable model and measure is Keyes' mental health continuum model (Keyes 2002, 2005, 2007), which includes emotional, social, and psychological/personal well-being facets, represents both hedonic and eudaimonic components of wellness, and for which scoring criteria for three levels of wellness are indicated on the measure (the distinguished categories are languishing, moderate mental health, and flourishing). However, a question on how findings on this scale correlate with those on other measures of psychosocial well-being (criterion-related validity) representing other theoretical perspectives of wellness still persists.

Theoretical Model and Measure as Point of Departure

For purposes of the current study, Keyes' (2002, 2005, 2007) mental health continuum model is taken as the theoretical backdrop. According to this model, mental health can be viewed as existing on a continuum from pathology to optimal functioning. Keyes proposed that psychopathology and psychological well-being are two different, but negatively correlated, dimensions of human functioning. At the upper end of the positive health dimension (upper part of the continuum), he distinguishes three levels of well-being (or mental health), namely, *languishing* (i.e., low levels of emotional, social, and psychological well-being), *moderate mental health*, and *flourishing* (i.e., high levels of emotional, social, and psychological well-being). Individuals who are moderately psychologically healthy have scores between flourishing and languishing. The positive dimension of the mental health continuum model is operationalized with the Mental Health Continuum Scale for which a short form of 14 items exists (MHC-SF), with which the various levels of well-being can be established. Criteria for levels are as follows: To be flourishing, participants must report that they experience "every day" or "almost every day" at least seven of the characteristics, where one of them is from the hedonic (i.e., emotional well-being) cluster (i.e., happy, interested in life, or satisfied) and the others from the social and personal/psychological well-being clusters. To be identified as languishing, participants must report that they "never" or "once or twice" experienced at least seven of the characteristics, where one of them is from the hedonic (i.e., emotional well-being) cluster and the others from the eudaimonic clusters. Participants who do not fit these criteria for flourishing or languishing are moderately mentally healthy. Keyes (2005, 2007, 2010) has shown that languishing and moderately mentally healthy people in the United States have more chronic diseases, more days lost at work, and a generally higher morbidity and mortality rate than those who are flourishing, with an associated loss of quality of life for the individual and higher financial expenditure to the state. This supports the value of this model and measure for further use in studies on the prevalence of levels of well-being.

Previous Findings on the Prevalence of Levels of Well-Being

Keyes (2006a, 2007) found in a large representative sample of US adults ($N=3{,}032$) that 18% were flourishing as measured with the MHC scale–long form, 65% were moderately mentally healthy, and 17% were languishing. For US youth ($N=1{,}234$) between 12 and 18 years of age, he determined with the MHC-SF that 38% were flourishing, 56% were moderately mentally healthy, and 6% were languishing. He warned that it seems as if flourishing diminishes from adolescence to adulthood and that the number of languishing people increases—which has implications for public policy on the promotion of mental health.

In a South African context, Keyes et al. (2008) established with a Setswana version of the 14-item MHC-SF that 20% of a random sample ($N=1{,}050$) of Setswana-speaking people in the North West province were flourishing, 67.8% were moderately mentally healthy, and 12.2% were languishing. These percentages are roughly in line with those reported by Keyes (2007) for US adults but also different from those for adolescents reported in the United States. Van Schalkwyk and Wissing (2010) found prevalence levels for well-being in the case of a multicultural (but predominantly white) group of secondary school children ($N=665$) between 15 and 17 years of age in the Cape Province of South Africa that corresponded to that of US youth, as reported by Keyes (2006a), namely, 42% flourishing, 53% moderately mentally healthy, and 5% languishing. The question is, however, whether adolescents and adults in other South African contexts and specific cultural groups show the same prevalence and whether this prevalence is more or less stable over time.

Possible Contributions of This Study

Very little is known about the prevalence of levels of well-being in various contexts. This chapter will contribute to further filling this gap. The exploration of the prevalence of levels of psychosocial well-being in communities is also important because health promotion is part of public health responsibilities. Baseline information is necessary to enhance well-being not only for individuals but also for communities and for the majority of people in a broader population, as argued by Huppert (2009) and Keyes (2007). This study is one step in the direction of providing such baseline data.

Aims

The aims of this study were (a) to explore the congruence of Keyes' measure with other operationalizations of psychosocial well-being and (b) to explore the prevalence of various degrees (or levels) of psychosocial health (languishing, moderate mental health, and flourishing) in various South African samples against the backdrop of Keyes' model.

Method

For purposes of this study, analyses were done on data obtained in various projects with other objectives. All studies had a cross-sectional survey design as far as the psychological data are concerned. All protocols were approved by the relevant ethics committees.

Participants

Group 1: FET 1 (FET = further education and training) college students (N = 568). This availability multicultural group consisted of 75% black African participants. Students were between 16 and 35 years of age (mean age = 21 years) and were from four different campuses of an FET (further education training) institution (overlapping between secondary and tertiary education). Two were situated in middle-income-level areas and two in lower socioeconomic areas. On all campuses, students varied in mean income levels within their families. Data were collected at the end of the 2007 academic year, close to the examination period and were part of the FORT2 (FORT2 = Understanding and promoting psychosocial health, resilience, and strengths in an African context; Wissing 2005) and FORT3 projects (FORT3 = The prevalence of levels of psychosocial health: Dynamics and relationships with biomarkers of (ill)health in South African social contexts; *forte* = strength; Wissing 2008).

Group 2: FET 2 college students (N = 1,480). This availability multicultural sample consisted of 75% African students. Students were from four campuses and had a mean age of 20 years. Data were collected at the beginning of the 2008 academic year as part of the FORT3 project.

Group 3: FET 3 Setswana-speaking college students (N = 185). This was an availability sample consisting of only black students from a deep rural area (Taung). The mean age of participants was 22 years. Data were collected in the middle of academic year, 2009, as part of the FORT3 project.

Group 4: FET 4 college students (N = 263). This was a multicultural sample of mainly black participants in an urban area, with a mean age of 20 years. Data were collected at the beginning of the academic year, 2010, as part of the FORT3 project.

Group 5: University students (N = 293). This was an availability multicultural sample consisting of predominantly white students. The mean age of students was 19 years. Data were collected in 2010 as part of the FORT3 project.

Group 6: Adults, Afrikaans speaking (N = 122). This was an availability sample of Afrikaans-speaking adults between 30 and 51 years of age, with equal numbers of males and females in each of the age groups 30–40 and 41–51 years. Data were collected in 2008 as part of the South African leg of the Eudaimonic-Hedonic Happiness Investigation (EHHI; Delle Fave et al. 2011) and the FORT3 project (cf. Coetzee et al. 2010).

Group 7: Adults, English, and Afrikaans speaking (N = 204). This was an availability multicultural sample of mainly white participants with a mean age of 35.9 years. Data were collected in 2007 and 2008 as part of the FORT2 and FORT3 projects.

Group 8: Teachers (N = 409). This randomized sample of South African teachers consisted of 200 black and 209 white adult teachers at a secondary school and were part of the multidisciplinary SABPA project (SABPA = Sympathetic Activity and Ambulatory Blood Pressure in Africans; Malan 2007; Potgieter et al. 2010) and FORT3 projects. Fifty percent in each of the black and white groups were males. Data were collected in 2008 and 2009.

Group 9: Adults, Setswana speaking (N = 296). This random sample of black Setswana-speaking adults from an urban area were between 18 and 80 years of age and consisted of 104 males and 192 females. Data were collected in 2008 as part of the FORT3 project (cf. Khumalo et al. 2010).

Group 10: Adults, Setswana speaking (N = 459). This was a randomly selected sample of Setswana-speaking adults from urban (*N* = 249) and rural (*N* = 210) areas in the North West province between 31 and 60 years of age, with 21% being between 30 and 40 years of age. It consisted of 141 males and 318 females. Data were collected in 2009 as part of the FORT3 project (cf. Khumalo et al. 2010).

Group 11: Adults, Setswana speaking (N = 1,050). This was a stratified community sample of black Setswana-speaking adults from rural (*N* = 599) and urban (*N* = 451) areas in the North West province. It consisted of 392 males and 649 females. Data were collected in 2005 as part of the multidisciplinary PURE-SA project (PURE = Prospective Urban and Rural Epidemiology; Kruger 2005) and the FORT2 project (cf. Keyes et al. 2008).

Group 12: Adults, Setswana speaking (N = 1,275). Data were collected from this stratified randomly selected community sample of urban (*N* = 581) and rural (*N* = 694) Setswana-speaking adults as part of the multidisciplinary PURE-SA project and the FORT3 project in 2010. This was a follow-up study in the community in which the 2005 data collection took place, described in group 11 (mostly the same participants). Data collection for the urban group took place in March and April 2010 and in April and May 2010 for the rural group.

Measures

Mental Health Continuum–Short Form (MHC-SF). The 14-item MHC-SF measures the degree of (a) emotional well-being (EWB; items 1–3) as defined in terms of positive affect/satisfaction with life, (b) social well-being (SWB; items 4–8) as described in Keyes' (1998, 2006b) model of social well-being (one item on each of the facets of social acceptance, social actualization, social contribution, social coherence, and social integration), and (c) psychological well-being (PWB; items 9–14) as described in Ryff's (1989) model (including one item on each of the dimensions of autonomy, environmental mastery, personal growth, positive relations with others, purpose in life, and self-acceptance).

Sense of Coherence Scale (SOC). The SOC 29-item scale was implemented, which measures an individual's way of experiencing the world and life within it. Core components are comprehensibility, manageability, and meaningfulness (Antonovsky 1987, 1993).

Affectometer 2 (short version; AFM). The AFM was developed to measure a general sense of well-being (or general happiness) and measures positive affect (PA), negative affect (NA), and affect balance (PA–NA). The 20-item scale was used in the present research. The more that positive affect predominates over negative affect, the higher the overall level of well-being (Kammann and Flett 1983).

Satisfaction with Life Scale (SWLS). The 5-item SWLS measures a person's general satisfaction with life on a cognitive–judgmental level and as evaluated according to self-reported criteria (Diener et al. 1985).

General Health Questionnaire (GHQ). The 28-item GHQ was implemented. It aims to detect common symptoms indicative of various syndromes of mental disorder and differentiates between individuals with psychopathology as a general class and those who are considered to be normal. Subscales are somatic symptoms (SS), anxiety and insomnia (AI), social dysfunction (SD), and severe depression (DS; Goldberg and Hillier 1979).

New General Self-Efficacy Scale (NGSE). This 8-item scale measures individuals' tendency to view themselves as capable of meeting task demands in various contexts (Chen et al. 2001).

Self-Regulation Scale (SRS). The 7-item SRS measures participants' post-intentional self-regulation when they are in the process of goal pursuit and facing difficulties in maintaining their action. Attention as well as emotion regulation are reflected in the scale items (Schwarzer et al. 1999).

Coping Self-Efficacy Scale (CSE). This 26-item scale measures a person's confidence (or perceived self-efficacy) in performing coping behaviors when facing life challenges or threats and can also be implemented to assess changes in coping self-efficacy (CSE) over time (Chesney et al. 2006).

The Fortitude Questionnaire (FORQ). The 20-item FORQ measures the extent to which a person feels able to handle stress and experiences support from family and friends (Pretorius 1998).

Patient Health Questionnaire: Depression Symptoms (PHQ-9). The 9-item PHQ measures the extent of symptoms of major depression as conceptualized in the DSM-IV criteria (Kroenke et al. 2001).

General Psychological Well-Being Scale (GPWS). This 20-item scale measures general psychological well-being as conceptualized by Wissing and Van Eeden (2002) and measures hedonic and eudaimonic facets of well-being (Khumalo et al. 2010).

Warwick–Edinburg Mental Well-Being Scale (WEMWBS). The WEMWBS is a 14-item questionnaire on a 5-point scale (1 = *none of the time* to 5 = *all the time*; Stewart-Brown et al. 2009). It measures hedonic as well as eudaimonic components of well-being and includes facets of positive affect and emotional well-being (optimism, cheerfulness, relaxation), satisfying interpersonal relations, and positive functioning (energy, self-acceptance, personal development, competence, autonomy; Tennant et al. 2007).

Procedure

Participants completed the MHC-SF as well as the various other questionnaires measuring facets of psychological well-being after informed consent was obtained in each of the specific subgroups. In the community sample, trained field-workers administered the questionnaires in a structured interview format. All groups completed the MHC-SF, but other measures of psychosocial well-being varied in the different studies. Groups 3, 9, 10, 11, and 12 completed the validated Setswana version (cf. Keyes et al. 2008) of the MHC-SF, as well as other validated Setswana measures. All other groups completed the English versions of the measures.

Analyses

Descriptive statistics for the MHC-SF in the various groups were determined, as well as correlations between the MHC-SF and other measures of psychosocial well-being, the percentage of languishing, and the amount of moderately mentally healthy and flourishing participants in each group.

Results

Descriptive Statistics for the MHC-SF in All Groups

The descriptive statistics (mean, standard deviation, range, skew, and kurtosis) and Cronbach's alpha reliability indices for the MHC-SF in all samples are shown in Table 4.1.

The MHC-SF measured consistently in all groups, as indicated by Cronbach's alpha coefficients from 0.71 for the Setswana version as completed by adult Setswana speakers in group 11 (2005) to 0.91 for the English version as completed by Afrikaans- and English-speaking adults. Most of the other reliability indices were between 0.80 and 0.90. Mean scores vary between 36.5 for the Setswana

Table 4.1 Descriptive statistics and reliability of the MHC-SF in the various subgroups

Subgroup	Mean	SD	Min-max	Skewness	Kurtosis	Cronbach's alpha
Group 1 (N=568)	46.4	11.3	4–70	–.61	.28	.83
FET1 college students 2007						
Group 2 (N=1,480)	48.0	10.4	10–70	–.53	.32	.82
FET2 college students 2008						
Group 3 (N=185)	43.0	10.4	15–63	–.31	–.51	.74
FET3 Setswana-speaking college students 2009						
Group 4 (N=263)	48.3	10.6	5–68	–.78	.84	.83
FET4 college students 2010						
Group 5 (N=293)	46.6	10.5	14–67	–.63	.03	.90
University students 2010						
Group 6 (N=122)	43.9	10.8	6–66	–.57	.75	.90
Adults, Afrikaans speaking 2008						
Group 7 (N=204)	45.1	11.6	8–69	–.49	.23	.91
Adults, English and Afrikaans speaking 2007/8						
Group 8 (N=409)	48.2	10.9	11–70	–.42	–.18	.89
Teachers multicultural 2008/9						
Group 9 (N=296)	46.2	13.1	6–70	–.49	–.35	.82
Adults, Setswana speaking 2008						
Group 10 (N=459)	43.4	12.8	2–69	–.29	–.52	.84
Adults, Setswana speaking 2009						
Group 11 (N=1,050)						
Adults, Setswana speaking						
A. Urban 2005	41.0	9.2	8–63	–.36	–.11	.71
B. Rural 2005	36.5	9.3	6–67	.52	.86	.76
Group 12 (N=1,275)						
Adults, Setswana speaking						
A. Urban (N=581) 2010	45.9	12.1	7–70	–.59	.30	.80
B. Rural (N=694) 2010	46.4	11.9	4–70	–.86	.53	.78

Table 4.2 Correlations between the MHC-SF and other measures[a] of psychosocial health in student/youth subgroups

Measures	Group 1 FET1 $N=568$	Group 2 FET2 $N=1,480$	[b]Group 3 FET3 $N=185$	Group 4 FET4 $N=263$	Group 5 University $N=293$
SWLS					.50
GHQ	−.23	−.30	−.29	−.31	
PHQ-9	−.24	−.31	−.28	−.32	
NGSE	.31	.38	.26	.40	
SRS	.46	.49		.40	
CSE	.49	.50		.56	
FORQ	.42	.51	.30	.55	
GPWS				.58	

MHC-SF Mental Health Continuum-Short Form, *SWLS* Satisfaction with Life Scale, *GHQ* General Health Questionnaire, *PHQ-9* Patient Health Questionnaire: Depression Symptoms, *NGSE* New General Self-Efficacy Scale, *SRS* Self-Regulation Scale, *CSE* Coping Self-Efficacy Scale, *FORQ* Fortitude Questionnaire, *GPWS* General Psychological Well-Being Scale

[a]Measures varied in the different groups

[b]Setswana version

version as determined in a rural sample (2005) and 48.3 for the English version in a college student group as completed in 2010. Standard deviations vary between 9.2 and 13.1. In all instances (except that of the adult rural Setswana-speaking group of 2005), scores were negatively skewed, indicating more scores to the positive/higher side though all the values were within the suggested range of −1 to 0,which indicates a moderate deviation from the normal distribution curve (Field 2005). The kurtoses for the various groups range from steep (groups 1, 2, 4, 5, 6, 7, 11, and 12) to shallow (groups 3, 8, 9, 10), with group 5 almost nearing a normal curve (Howitt and Cramer 2008).

Correlations Between the MHC-SF and Other Measures of Psychosocial Well-Being

The correlations between the MHC-SF, on the one hand, and other measures of psychosocial well-being on the other are shown in Table 4.2 for the student/youth groups and in Table 4.3 for the adult groups.

As can be noted in Tables 4.2 and 4.3, the MHC-SF correlates significantly with other indices of psychosocial well-being and negatively with indices of symptoms as measured by the GHQ and PHQ-9. The magnitude of correlations of the MHC-SF with a particular scale varied slightly in the different groups. The strongest positive correlations are found with positive affect, sense of coherence, coping self-efficacy, fortitude, and general psychological well-being. The correlations can be classified as ranging from large to medium effect (Field 2005) in terms of the practical significance of the correlations. Satisfaction with life in group 5 has a significant correlation of 0.50 with MHC-SF, which explains 25% of the variance.

Table 4.3 Correlations between the MHC-SF and other measures[a] of psychosocial health in adult samples

Measures	Group 6 Afrikaans N=122	Group 7 English N=204	Group 8 Teachers N=409	Group 9 Setswana N=296	Group 10 Setswana N=459	Group 11 Setswana N=1,050 U–R	Group 12 Setswana N=1,275 U–R
SOC	.57				.46	.30–.31	
AFM:PA	.70				.56	.51–.51	
AFM:NA	−.54				−.18	−.25 to −.29	
SWLS				.49	.34	.39–.39	.40–42
GHQ		−.56	−.30		−.37	−.22 to −.21	−.37 to −.37
PHQ-9		−.53	−.25	−.25	.38		−.19 to −.20
NGSE						.31–.35	
SRS		.31					
CSE		.70		.47	.45		.50–.39
FORQ	.65	.59	.46		.48		
GPWS				.53	.52		.50–.50
WEMWBS							.42–.42

U urban, *R* rural, *MHC-SF* Mental Health Continuum-Short Form, *SOC* Sense of Coherence Scale, *AFM* affectometer 2, *PA* positive affect, *NA* negative affect, *SWLS* Satisfaction with Life Scale, *GHQ* General Health Questionnaire, *PHQ-9* Patient Health Questionnaire: Depression Symptoms, *NGSE* New General Self-Efficacy Scale, *SRS* Self-Regulation Scale, *CSE* Coping Self-Efficacy Scale, *FORQ* Fortitude Questionnaire, *GPWS* General Psychological Well-Being Scale, *WEMWBS* Warwick–Edinburg Mental Well-Being Scale
[a]Measures varied in the different groups

Prevalence of Levels of Psychosocial Well-Being

The percentages of participants who were flourishing, languishing, or moderately mentally healthy in each of the subgroups are shown in Table 4.4.

As can be seen from Table 4.4, the prevalence of flourishing in groups varied from 28% in teachers to 61.7% in a rural Setswana-speaking group of adults and between 1.5% (teachers) and 9% (urban Setswana-speaking adults) for languishing. The variation in percentage of groups that were flourishing was relatively large.

Discussion

The main finding of this study is that there are considerable differences in the prevalence of levels of well-being, as measured with the Mental Health Continuum–Short Form (MHC-SF) among the various groups explored in this study. This variation is, in some instances, greater than previously reported and needs to be explained and explored further.

Table 4.4 The prevalence of the various levels of mental health in all groups

Subgroup	Number of participants	Flourishing	Moderate mental health	Languishing
Group 1	568	60	34	6
FET1 college students 2007				
Group 2	1,480	60.2	34.3	3.5
FET2 college students 2008				
Group 3	185	43.9	47.6	7.5
FET3 Setswana-speaking college students 2009				
Group 4	263	60.8	35.4	3.8
FET4 college students 2010				
Group 5	293	51.5	45.1	2.7
University students 2010				
Group 6	122	38.5	57.4	4.1
Adults, Afrikaans speaking 2008				
Group 7	204	51.5	45.1	3.4
Adults, English and Afrikaans. speaking 2007/8				
Group 8	409	28.0	70.5	1.5
Teachers multicultural 2008/9				
Group 9	296	52.0	42.6	5.4
Adults, Setswana speaking Urban 2008				
Group 10	459	47.4	43.6	9.0
Adults, Setswana speaking Urban and Rural 2009				
Group 11				
Adults, Setswana speaking				
A. Urban 2005	443	29.6	66.1	3.6
B. Rural 2005	583	13.9	78.9	7.2
Group 12				
Adults, Setswana				
A. Urban 2010	581	52.8	40.6	6.5
B. Rural 2010	694	61.7	32.4	5.9

The Measure and Model of Levels of Well-Being

Both the English and Setswana versions of the MHC-SF measured reliably in all the groups of participants and showed comparable descriptive statistics. In both the student and adult groups, findings showed moderate to strong positive correlations between the MHC-SF, on the one hand, and all other measures of (facets of) psychosocial well-being as implemented in the specific project on the other hand, especially with positive affect, coping self-efficacy, perceived social support, and general psychological well-being. The MHC-SF also showed negative correlations with indices of symptoms and pathology. These findings support the criterion-related validity of the MHC-SF as a measure of well-being in these various groups, which differ—in some instances—in cultural contexts, and are in line with the conclusions of Keyes et al. (2008). The positive correlations, with a variety of other measures of different facets of well-being, also support the assumption that this model is appropriate for establishing (levels of) psychosocial well-being from a relatively holistic perspective.

The Prevalence of Levels of Well-Being in Youth

The findings of this study are in line with that of Keyes (2006a, 2007) in so far as youth, in general, show a higher percentage of flourishing than adults. However, the findings differ from the findings in the United States, as participants in some of the five convenience samples of young people in the South African context showed much higher percentages of flourishing. Whereas Keyes (2006a, 2007) reported a prevalence of approximately 38% flourishing in US youth, the current student samples showed prevalence between 43 and 61% of flourishing. Of course, it may be because the South African groups were convenience samples, whereas Keyes used larger and more representative samples, but it is probably also because they are student samples. Students at colleges and universities are highly selected, and in some instances, quite privileged, and may therefore report relatively higher levels of flourishing and the same or smaller levels of languishing. Another possible explanation for the difference between the current findings and that of Keyes for youth may perhaps be because the student groups are slightly older (mean age of 20 years) than youth in the Keyes sample (12–18 years of age). Percentages of flourishing youth in Keyes' (2006a) sample are more in line with those found in secondary school children (between 15 and 17 years of age) in the South African context; for example, Van Schalkwyk and Wissing (2010) found 42% flourishing in a multicultural group, and Brink (2010) found 32% flourishing in a primarily white group.

Of the student samples included in the current study, group 3 (a Setswana-speaking group from a deep rural area with very little resources and poor infrastructure) showed the smallest percentage of flourishing (43%), which is still slightly higher than that reported by Keyes. The relatively lower prevalence of flourishing in this group may indicate the possible role of context and sociodemographic variables. Groups 1, 2, and 4, for which data were gathered from 2007 to 2010, showed a very high percentage of flourishing (60%). These groups are multicultural samples with approximately 75% black participants from urban areas. This high level of flourishing was unexpected, as most of the participants in these samples had many socioeconomic and other challenges to cope with. However, it is in line with findings of Rugiera et al. (submitted) in a Tanzanian group of students who also showed an unexpected 72% of flourishing. University students (group 5), of which approximately 70% were white, also manifested high percentages of flourishing (51%); however, this is lower than that of the primarily black groups of students. It may thus be that black African participants show a higher prevalence of flourishing, as suggested by Keyes (2007), but this needs to be explored further, as well as the role of contextual factors and sociodemographic variables determined in the South African context.

In order to obtain a further perspective on the discrepancy between percentages of flourishing youth in the United States and South African samples, post hoc analyses were conducted on the percentage participants in each level of well-being who also manifested symptoms of major depression, as diagnosed with the PHQ-9, in the various student groups where data were available. Keyes (2005) reported that 5%, 13%, and 28% of adults in the flourishing, moderate mentally healthy, and languishing groups, respectively, experienced major depression. The flourishing participants in the South African college student groups 1, 2, and 3 showed symptoms of major depressive disorder of 21%, 14%, and 13%, respectively; the moderately mentally healthy level participants showed major depression of 32%, 19%, and 27%, respectively, in the various samples; and the languishing participants showed 56%, 34%, and 29% of depressive disorder in groups 1, 2, and 3, respectively. The high levels of depressive symptoms in group 1 in comparison to the other two groups may be due to data being collected directly before the end-of-the-year exams, whereas the other groups completed the questionnaires in the beginning (group 2) and middle (group 3) of the year. The tendency reported by Keyes (2005) for adults with higher percentages of depression in languishing groups was also found in the South African data with college students, but the students showed a higher incidence of depression. It should, however, be taken into account that depression was not evaluated in the same way in the US and South African studies. What is important to note for the purposes of the current study is that the South African groups showed both higher percentages of flourishing and more depression. This raises the question of whether these findings are the result of a response artifact or whether other, perhaps cultural, explanations are possible. Further research is necessary, for example, on the role of response style and specific contexts of the identification of levels of well-being and pathology. Possibly, measurement equivalence to exclude bias could be tested in various contexts.

The Prevalence of Levels of Well-Being in Adults

Adults in the South African context, as evaluated in groups 6–12, showed notably higher percentages of flourishing and lower levels of languishing than the 18% and 17%, respectively, found by Keyes (2007) in a US sample. The subgroup with the lowest percentage of flourishing participants in this study was found in group 11 for Setswana-speaking people in a deep rural area where only approximately 14% were flourishing (but at the same time also only 7% languishing) during data gathering in 2005. This is the same area where the college students in group 3 were evaluated in 2009 and which showed lower levels of well-being than other student groups in the same educational system. Context and sociodemographic variables may thus play a role and should be further explored. The other adult group that showed a notably lower percentage of flourishing in comparison to other groups in this study (but still slightly higher than adults as found by Keyes in the United States) is the multicultural group of secondary school teachers (group 8) with 28% flourishing. The explanation for this relatively lower percentage of flourishing in comparison to other South African groups of adults in the current study may be due to teachers experiencing relatively high levels of stress, especially in the South African context, because of various factors such as high pressure, high workloads, little resources, low salaries, many curricula changes, overcrowded classes, etc. (Naring et al. 2006). It is, however, also noteworthy that this group manifested the lowest percentage of languishing. It may be because people who could not cope in the educational system had left. In the instance of this group of comparable (age, gender, socioeconomic status; cf. Malan 2007; Potgieter et al. 2010) black and white teachers, the mean scores on the MHC- SF did not differ significantly between black (M=48.3, SD=10.9) and white (M=47.8, SD=9.8) teachers.

The other adult groups (excluding groups 8 and 11) showed prevalence rates for flourishing between approximately 40% and 60% and languishing between 4% and 9%, which differ from Keyes' (2007) adult sample and with generally little differences between primarily black and white samples. Results from group 11 showed that urban versus rural contexts are important, as was also suggested by the findings for students in urban versus rural contexts. Other South African studies have also indicated that people in rural areas are far worse off as far as psychosocial well-being is concerned, in comparison to people from urban areas, and different from the trend in developing countries (cf. Vorster et al. 2000; Wissing et al. 2010).

An unexpected finding that is difficult to explain is that the rural subgroup in group 12 showed 61% flourishing, whereas the rural group in group 11 showed only 13% flourishing (findings were double checked, from data collection to coding and statistical analyses). Data for group 12 were collected in 2010 as part of a multidisciplinary follow-up study on the same participants who participated in the 2005 data collection wave (group 11), with only a few new participants in the sample. The urban subgroup also showed a notable increase in percentage of flourishing participants, but not to the same extent as the rural group. Although circumstances in South Africa might have improved in some regards from 2005 to 2010, very little has changed in the rural areas, which still have fewer resources, poor infrastructures, poor health facilities, high unemployment, high poverty rates, etc., and where recent protests took place because of the lack of facilities. However, the ministry of rural development and land reform, with its planning, may have given more hope to people in rural areas in terms of agrarian transformation, land reform, and consequent development (Parliamentary Monitoring Group 2009). A further possible explanation for the much higher percentages of flourishing in the rural participants of group 12 is that the soccer World Cup, which took place in South Africa during June–July 2010 generated a very positive mood in the country as reported by various social commentators such as *esprit de temps* and by Harris as part of her follow-up study of optimism in South Africa (Harris 2007). This explanation links to Haybron's (2007) argument that people's evaluations of their lives are influenced by the perspectives they are taking at that moment and that these are influenced by contextual factors. But why was there more incidence of flourishing in rural areas than in urban areas? It may be because there is so little going on in the rural areas that the World Cup festivities in the rural areas made such a huge difference to people's lives—more than in the case of urban participants, who also have other distractions and recreational opportunities. However, further research is necessary, especially qualitative research, to understand the 2010 findings in the rural group.

Limitations

The current study has several limitations; for example, only some of the samples were probabilistic whereas others were not. The role of age, gender, time of data collection, and sociodemographic variables has not been systematically controlled for. Possible concomitant psychopathology was also not taken into account, and therefore, findings cannot be generalized. But still, the findings suggest that the prevalence of levels of well-being may vary in different contexts and that the prevalence of levels of flourishing, as measured with the MHC-SF, is higher in an African context than in the United States, despite the fact that South Africa is only a developing country with many challenges ahead of it.

Further Research

Future research could explore the prevalence of psychosocial well-being in typically probabilistic national surveys, such as the US General Social Survey and the European Social Survey. These types of studies could explore the role of sociodemographic variables and the urban–rural divide in psychosocial well-being, as prevalence differentials are indicated in various studies. In this way, national probabilistic samples may clarify the distribution of psychosocial well-being in various contexts in order to enable a body of knowledge in epidemiofortology.

Programs to enhance strengths, coping self-efficacy, and flourishing for various specifically targeted groups may be developed and evaluated. Van Schalkwyk and Wissing (in press) show that such a program can significantly enhance the number of flourishing participants in a multicultural secondary school sample of children, but further research is still necessary. This is true for adult groups, as well.

Further Conceptual Issues for Consideration

Keyes' mental health continuum model conceptualizes mental health from pathology to flourishing and can be viewed as an idealistic, hermeneutic model, or a critical approach model, with a pragmatic focus on health promotion. However, the distinction of levels (or categories) of mental health on the positive end/dimension (languishing to flourishing) and their measurement with the MHC-SF also suggest a statistical, nomothetic model. This raises the question of whether psychological health is normally distributed in a community and/or whether it is realistic to optimize psychological functioning for all people to levels of flourishing or close to that. Conceptual clarification of such issues is important for standardizing cutoff points and norms for levels of well-being and percentages of flourishing.

Another issue to be considered is that it may be worthwhile to distinguish between levels (degrees) of well-being and *patterns* of well-being (analogous to patterns or syndromes of psychopathology) and to further explore both in epidemiological and epidemiofortological studies. Keyes refers in his description of the categories flourishing, moderate mental health, and languishing sometimes as levels (or degrees) of well-being, and then again as *syndromes*, to make it comprehensible in a medical context. The problem with this is, firstly, that a degree and a syndrome are not the same thing, and secondly, a syndrome is a combination of symptoms and thus part of a medical model. We suggest that patterns of well-being may exist that may also vary in different cultural contexts (cf. Wissing and Temane 2008), and that these should be further explored, described, and researched in epidemiofortological studies.

Conclusion

The prevalence of levels of well-being is not the same in all the groups included in this study, and various contextual, sociodemographic, or group-specific characteristics may play a role and should be explored in future studies. The percentages of flourishing in most of these South African groups are higher than those in the United States, particularly in students and black African participants, whereas the percentages of languishing are similar. Further empirical research is required to determine the role of contextual, historical, and sociodemographic variables. Qualitative research may help to provide a deeper understanding of the shift in well-being in rural areas, as found from 2005 to 2010, in order to capitalize thereupon for consolidation and further facilitation of psychosocial health. Further conceptualization and exploration with regard to possible patterns of well-being (different from *levels* of well-being but analogous to syndromes of pathology) may be a next step in building a base of knowledge for mental health from a positive perspective.

Acknowledgements The following colleagues and students are thanked for their inputs, organization, data collection, and/or supervision of fieldwork: Johan Potgieter, Tumi Khumalo, Alida Nienaber, Tertia Oosthuizen, Heleen Coetzee, Mabet van Wyk, Annamarie Kruger, Leoné Malan, and all the field-workers.

Funding: The following organizations are recognized for financial assistance for conducting the PURE and/or FORT2 and 3 projects: the National Research Foundation (NRF) of South Africa, the Medical Research Council (MRC) of South Africa, the North-West University, SANPAD, and the Population Health Research Institute (PHRI) of Canada.

References

Antonovsky, A. (1987). *Unravelling the mystery of health: How people manage stress and stay well.* San Francisco: Jossey-Bass.

Antonovsky, A. (1993). The measure and properties of the Sense of Coherence Scale. *Social Science and Medicine, 36*, 725–733.

Brink, A. (2010). *Evaluering van 'n program ter fasilitering van positiewe jeugontwikkeling* [Evaluation of a program for facilitating positive youth development]. Unpublished doctoral dissertation, North-West University, South Africa.

Chen, G., Gully, S. M., & Eden, D. (2001). Validation of a new general self-efficacy scale. *Organizational Research Methods, 4*(1), 62–83.

Chesney, M. A., Neilands, T. B., Chambers, D. B., Taylor, J. M., & Folkman, S. (2006). A validity and reliability study of the Coping Self-efficacy Scale. *British Journal of Health Psychology, 11*(3), 421–437.

Coetzee, H. K., Wissing, M. P., & Temane, Q. M. (2010). Die belewing van betekenisvolheid deur 'n groep Suid-Afrikaners (Meaningfulness as experienced by a group of South Africans). *Tydskrif vir Geesteswetenskappe/Journal of Humanities, 50*(3), 293–312.

Delle Fave, A., Brdar, I., Freire, T., Vella-Brodrick, D., & Wissing, M. P. (2011). The eudaimonic and hedonic components of happiness. *Social Indicators Research, 100*(2), 158–207.

Diener, E. (2000). Subjective well-being: The science of happiness and a proposal for a national index. *American Psychologist, 55*(1), 34–43.

Diener, E., & Seligman, E. P. (2004). Beyond money: Toward an economy of well-being. *Psychological Science in the Public Interest, 5*(1), 1–31.

Diener, E., Emmons, R., Larsen, R. J., & Griffin, S. (1985). The satisfaction with life scale. *Journal of Personality Assessment, 49*(1), 71–75.

Diener, E., Kesebir, P., & Lucas, R. (2008). Benefits of accounts of well-being: For societies and for psychological science. *Applied Psychology, 57*(1), 37–53.

Field, A. (2005). *Discovering statistics using SPSS.* London: Sage.

Fredrickson, B. L. (2001). The role of positive emotions in positive psychology: The broaden-and-build theory of positive emotions. *American Psychologist, 56*(3), 218–226.

Goldberg, D. P., & Hillier, V. F. (1979). A scaled version of the General Health Questionnaire. *Psychological Medicine, 9*, 139–145.

Harris, M. (2007). Monitoring optimism in South Africa. *Social Indicators Research, 81*(2), 435–454.

Haybron, D. (2007). Life satisfaction, ethical reflection, and the science of happiness. *Journal of Happiness Studies, 8*, 99–138.

Higgs, N. T. (2007). Measuring and understanding the well-being of South Africans: Everyday quality of life in South Africa. *Social Indicators Research, 81*, 331–356.

Howitt, D., & Cramer, D. (2008). *Introduction to statistics in psychology* (4th ed.). London: Pearson Education.

Huppert, F. A. (2009). A new approach to reducing disorder and improving well-being. *Perspectives on Psychological Science, 4*(1), 108–111.

Huppert, F. A., Marks, N., Clark, A., Siegrist, J., Stutzer, A., Vitters, J., & Wahrendorf, M. (2009). Measuring well-being across Europe: Description of the ESS well-being module and preliminary findings. *Social Indicators Research, 91*, 301–315.

Kammann, R., & Flett, R. (1983). Affectometer 2: A scale to measure current levels of general happiness. *Australian Journal of Psychology, 35*, 259–265.

Keyes, C. L. M. (1998). Social well-being. *Social Psychology Quarterly, 61*, 121–140.

Keyes, C. L. M. (2002). The mental health continuum: From languishing to flourishing in life. *Journal of Health and Social Research, 43*, 207–222.

Keyes, C. L. M. (2005). Mental illness and/or mental health? Investigating the axioms of the complete state model of health. *Journal of Consulting and Clinical Psychology, 73*(3), 539–548.

Keyes, C. L. M. (2006a). Mental health in adolescence: Is America's youth flourishing? *American Journal of Orthopsychiatry, 76*, 395–402.

Keyes, C. L. M. (2006b). *If health matters: When will we stop saying one thing and doing another?* Keynote address presented at the South African Conference on Positive Psychology: Individual, social and work wellness. Potchefstroom, South Africa.

Keyes, C. L. M. (2007). Promoting and protecting mental health as flourishing: A complementary strategy for improving national mental health. *American Psychologist, 62*(2), 95–108.

Keyes, C. L. M. (2010). *Stopping the insanity: Promoting positive mental health is sanity in a world needing better mental health.* Keynote address at the 5th European Conference on Positive Psychology, Copenhagen, Denmark.

Keyes, C. L. M., Wissing, M. P., Potgieter, J., Temane, Q. M., Kruger, A., & Van Rooy, S. (2008). Evaluation of the Mental Health Continuum Short Form (MHC-SF) in Setswana speaking South Africans. *Clinical Psychology and Psychotherapy, 15*, 181–192.

Khumalo, I. P., Temane, Q. M., & Wissing, M. P. (2010). Development and initial validation of a General Psychological Well-being Scale (GPWS) in an African context. *Journal of Psychology in Africa, 20*(1), 13–22.

Kroenke, K., Spitzer, R. L., & Williams, J. B. (2001). The PHQ-9: Validity of a brief depression severity measure. *Journal of General Internal Medicine, 16*, 606–613.

Kruger, A. (2005). *Prospective urban and rural epidemiological study (PURE): Instruction manual for South Africa* (2nd draft). Unpublished document, North-West University, Potchefstroom.

Lyobomirsky, S., King, L., & Diener, E. (2005). The benefits of frequent positive affect: Does happiness lead to success? *Psychological Bulletin, 131*(6), 803–855.

Malan, L. (2007). *The SABPA study. (SABPA = Sympathetic activity and Ambulatory Blood Pressure in Africans).* Unpublished research protocol, North West University, South Africa.

Naring, G., Briet, M., & Brouwers, A. (2006). Beyond demand and control: Emotional labor and symptoms of burnout in teachers. *Work and Stress, 20*(4), 303–315.

Parliamentary Monitoring Group. (2009). Rural development & land reform minister on strategic plan & budget 2009/10. Retrieved from http://www.pmg.org.za/report/20090623-minister%E-2%80%99s-briefing-department-rural-development-land-reform-strategi

Pavot, W., & Diener, E. (1993). Review of the Satisfaction with Life Scale. *Psychological Assessment, 5*(2), 164–172.

Potgieter, J. C., Malan, L., Hamer, M., & Harvey, B. H. (2010). Overview of biomedical pathophysiology relevant to stress and disease: Active coping, stroke risk factors and target organ damage (TOD): The Sympathetic Activity and Ambulatory Blood Pressure in Africans Study (SABPA). 68th Annual Meeting of the American Psychosomatic Society, Portland, Oregon, USA (invited symposium).

Pressman, S. D., & Cohen, S. (2005). Does positive affect influence health? *Psychological Bulletin, 131*, 925–971.

Pretorius, T. B. (1998). *Fortitude as stress-resistance: Development and validation of the Fortitude Questionnaire (FORQ).* Bellville: University of the Western Cape.

Rugiera, J., Nienaber, A. W., & Wissing, M. P. (submitted). *The prevalence of various degrees of psychological well-being among Tanzanian university students.*

Ryff, C. D. (1989). Happiness is everything, or is it? Explorations on the meaning of psychological well-being. *Journal of Personality and Social Psychology, 57*(6), 1069–1081.

Schwarzer, R., & Jerusalem, M. (1993). *Measurement of perceived self-efficacy: Psychometric scales for cross-cultural research.* Berlin: Freie Universität.

Schwarzer, R., Diehl, M., & Schmitz, G. S. (1999). *Self-regulation.* Retrieved from http://userpage.fu-berlin.de/~health/selfreg_e.htm

So, T. T. C., & Huppert, F. A. (2009). *What percentage of people in Europe are flourishing and what characterises them?* Philadelphia: First World Congress on Positive Psychology.

Stewart-Brown, S., Tennant, A., Tennant, R., Platt, S., Parkinson, J., & Weich, S. (2009). Internal construct validity of the Warwick-Edinburgh Mental Well-being Scale (WEMWBS): A rash analysis using data from the Scottish Health Education Population Survey. *Health and Quality of Life Outcomes, 7*(15). doi:doi:10.1186/1477-7525-7-15.

Tennant, R., Hiller, L., Fishwick, R., Platt, S., Joseph, S., Weich, S., Parkinson, J., Secker, J., & Stewart-Brown, S. (2007). The Warwick-Edinburgh Mental Well-being Scale (WEMWBS): Development and UK validation. *Health and Quality of Life Outcomes, 5*, 63. doi:10.1186/1477-7525-5-63.

Van Schalkwyk, I., & Wissing, M. P. (2010). Psychosocial well-being in a group of South African adolescents. *Journal of Psychology in Africa, 20*(1), 53–60.

Van Schalkwyk, I., & Wissing, M. P. (in press). *Evaluation of a programme to enhance flourishing in adolescents*. In M. P. Wissing (Ed.). Well-Being Research in South Africa.

Vorster, H. H., Wissing, M. P., Venter, C. S., Kruger, H. S., Kruger, A., Malan, N. T., et al. (2000). The impact of urbanization on physical and mental health of Africans in the Northwest Province of South Africa: The THUSA study. *South African Journal of Science, 96*, 505–514.

Williams, D. R., Herman, A., Stein, D. J., Heeringa, S. G., Jackson, P. B., Moomal, H., & Kessler, R. C. (2007). Twelve-month mental disorders in South Africa: Prevalence, service use and demographic correlates in the population-based South African stress and health study. *Psychological Medicine, 38*(2), 211–220.

Wissing, M. P. (2005). *Understanding and promoting psychosocial health, resilience and strengths in an African context (FORT2)*. Unpublished research protocol. Funded by the National Research Foundation of South Africa.

Wissing, M. P. (2008). *The prevalence of levels of psychosocial health: Dynamics and relationships with biomarkers of (ill)health in the South African contexts (FORT3)*. Unpublished research protocol. Funded by the National Research Foundation of South Africa.

Wissing, M. P., & Temane, Q. M. (2008). The structure of psychological well-being in cultural context: Towards a hierarchical model of psychological health. *Journal of Psychology in Africa, 18*(1), 45–56.

Wissing, M. P., & Van Eeden, C. (2002). Empirical clarification of the nature of psychological well-being. *South African Journal of Psychology, 32*, 32–44.

Wissing, M. P., Temane, M., Khumalo, T., Kruger, A., & Vorster, E. (2010). *Urbanization and psychosocial wellbeing: the case of rural versus urban health*. Paper at the 5th European Conference on Positive Psychology, Copenhagen, Denmark.

World Health Organization. (1998). *Health promotion glossary*. Geneva: Author. Retrieved from http://www.who.int/hpr/NPH/docs/hp_glossary_en.pdf

Chapter 5
Prevalence and Correlates of Complete Mental Health in the South Korean Adult Population

Young-Jin Lim, Young-Gun Ko, Hee-Cheon Shin, and Yongrae Cho

This chapter investigates the prevalence and correlates of complete mental health in South Korea using the 2010 Mental Health Index Survey data. According to recent research on traditional mental health (or mental illness) in South Korea (Cho et al. 2010), the lifetime and 12-month prevalence rates for DSM-IV major mental disorders were 29.0 and 16.9%, respectively. Those for specific disorders were as follows: (a) alcohol use, 16.2 and 5.6%; (b) nicotine use, 9.0 and 6.0%; (c) specific phobia, 3.8 and 3.4%; (d) major depressive disorder, 5.6 and 2.5%; and (e) generalized anxiety disorder, 1.6 and 0.8%. Data related to nicotine and alcohol use revealed a very high male to female ratio, whereas mood and anxiety disorders were more prevalent in females than in males. Cho and his colleagues (2010) indicated that about 1 in 10 South Korean adults have a disorder related to alcohol or nicotine use each year and that 3 in 10 experience one serious mental illness in their lifetime.

Though mental illness is common in South Korea, about 70% of the adult population will remain free from mental illness. This raises a difficult question. Can those adults who are left untroubled by mental illness be regarded as mentally healthy? This is a core issue for positive psychologists, who present a model of

---

The present research has been conducted by the Research Grant of the Korean Psychological Association in 2010.

Y.-J. Lim, Ph.D.
Department of Psychology, Daegu University, Daegu, South Korea

Y.-G. Ko, Ph.D.
Department of Psychology, Korea University, Seoul, South Korea

H.-C. Shin, Ph.D.
Department of Psychology, Ajou University, Suwon, South Korea

Y. Cho, Ph.D. (✉)
Department of Psychology, Hallym University, 1 Hallymdaehak-gil,
Chuncheon, Gangwon-do 200-702, South Korea
e-mail: yrcho@hallym.ac.kr

C.L.M. Keyes (ed.), *Mental Well-Being: International Contributions to the Study of Positive Mental Health*, DOI 10.1007/978-94-007-5195-8_5,

mental health in which mental health is not simply the absence of mental disorder (Keyes 2002).

Recently, some researchers have regarded high levels of subjective well-being as a symptom of mental health (Keyes and Lopez 2002). Whereas in the past, mental health was viewed as the lack of mental illness or psychopathology, there is now a great deal of evidence to suggest that mental health can, and indeed should, be defined as not only the absence of mental illness but also the presence of something positive (Ryff and Singer 1998) and that mental health and mental illness are not the opposite poles of a single continuum of measurement (Keyes 2002, 2003).

However, to achieve a comprehensive understanding of what it means to be fully mentally healthy, further information is needed about the assessment of healthy functioning as opposed to simply the assessment of happiness or emotional well-being. In the traditional hedonic approach to subjective well-being, emotional well-being or happiness has been emphasized, whereas the functional aspects of subjective well-being were less focused upon, or regarded as less important. Hedonic, or emotional, well-being is a specific dimension of subjective well-being which consists of perceptions of avowed interest in life, happiness, satisfaction with life, and the balance of positive to negative affect (Diener and Emmons 1985; Diener et al. 1985). In contrast, eudaimonic well-being, sometimes referred to as positive functioning, consists of an individual's evaluation of their psychological well-being (Ryff 1989; Ryff and Keyes 1995).

In short, mental health is conceived of as a complete state in which individuals are free of mental illness and *flourishing* with high levels of emotional well-being (EWB, e.g., happiness or satisfaction), psychological well-being (PWB, e.g., personal growth), and social well-being (SWB, e.g., social integration) (Keyes and Lopez 2002). While we now have some knowledge about mental illness in South Korea, we do not have adequate information about subjective well-being, especially eudaimonic well-being which consists of PWB and SWB.

How much subjective well-being exists in South Korea? While we lack information about subjective well-being, we do have good information about objective well-being. As South Korea's economic, political, and technical development has been realized, the objective quality of life in South Korea has improved significantly (Park 2009). From an economic standpoint, South Korea is now the 13th largest economy in the world. According to the latest Human Development Report (United Nations Development Programme 2010) in 2007, the combined primary, secondary, and tertiary gross enrollment ratio (each equally weighted) was 98.5%; GDP per capita (as measured by purchasing power parity) was US$24,801; and life expectancy at birth was 79.2 years. As a consequence, South Korea is ranked 26th among 182 countries on the Human Development Index, implying that South Koreans generally attain higher education levels, have a higher standard of living, and have healthier and longer lives than most of the other people in the world.

From a political standpoint, South Korea meets the criteria for a democratic country in terms of free and fair elections, multiparty competition, civil and political rights, universal suffrage, and a free press. On the indices from Freedom House in 2010, South Korea received a score of 1 on the political rights scale and 2 on the civil liberties scale (seven-point scales with 7 defined as least free), indicating that South Korea's democracy has sound institutions and processes. The 2008 World Bank Worldwide Governance Indicators awarded South Korea sound evaluations in all six categories: voice and accountability (+0.59), rule of law (+0.79), political stability (+0.41), government effectiveness (+1.26), control of corruption (+0.45), and regulatory quality (+0.73) (Kaufman et al. 2009). These indicators, which are measured on a scale ranging from −2.5 to 2.5, with higher values indicating higher quality of governance in a particular category, show that South Korea has improved the overall quality of public administrations and bureaucracy.

From a technical standpoint, South Korea is one of the most advanced countries in the world in terms of the percentage of Internet users and broadband Internet penetration rate. The National Internet Development Agency of Korea reported that the number of Internet users in Korea had reached 77.1% of Korea's total population aged 6 years or older as of December 31, 2008. The number of Internet users per 100 persons almost doubled in just 6 years (from 40.5 in 2000 to 77.1 in 2008). In addition, the number of subscribers to broadband in South Korea was approaching 30 per 100 people as of December 31, 2008, and Korea had one of the highest broadband Internet penetration rates among the OECD countries (OECD Factbook 2008). Due to the high broadband Internet penetration rate and the growing popularity of the Internet, South Korea ranks 1st out of 181 countries in terms of the International Telecommunication Union's Digital Opportunity Index, suggesting that South Koreans live in a richer variety of digital information environments than do any other people in the world.

Objective quality of life, however, cannot be regarded as comparable to *subjective* quality of life. Previous studies have demonstrated that those who have a very high objective quality of life did not report a comparable level of subjective quality of life or subjective well-being. We therefore primarily deal with the subjective quality of life, or subjective well-being, directly and subjectively experienced by the South Korean people and then report the findings of a cross-cultural application of the mental health continuum (MHC) (Keyes 2002, 2005) to the South Korean adults. The MHC represents a clinical approach to the continuous assessment and categorical diagnosis of states of mental health as *something positive* rather than solely the absence of psychopathology.

The MHC model has been bolstered by research on diverse populations, including samples from South Africa and the Netherlands (Keyes et al. 2008; Strümpfer et al. 2009; Westerhof and Keyes 2010). However, Asian people were not included in their cross-cultural studies. Furthermore, there have been no studies, to date, which have examined the validity of the MHC model in Asian samples. Previous studies have indicated two major differences between East Asian and European and American population samples in the reporting of subjective well-being. Firstly, subjective well-being in North America is achieved by means of a sense of personal achievement and self-esteem, whereas subjective well-being in East Asia is attained through satisfying social relationships (Diener et al. 2003). Secondly, North Americans reported that subjective well-being is relevant to a strong positive feeling, whereas East Asians emphasized the idea of balance in the conceptualization of subjective well-being (Lu and Gilmour 2004). These differences between two cultures could affect the pattern of responses on the MHC. For example, differences between East Asian and European and American samples could emerge in terms of the prevalence and correlates of complete mental health, the relationship between the categories of mental health, the levels of psychosocial assets, and the relationship between mental health and mental illness.

We therefore administered the Mental Health Continuum–Short Form (MHC–SF) to a sample of South Koreans in order to investigate the cross-cultural application of the MHC model. The aims of this study were (a) to verify whether measures of mental health and mental illness belong to separate latent factors, (b) to examine if the diagnostic categories of mental health distinguish between different levels of psychosocial functioning, and (c) to find out which socioeconomic factors determine the levels of mental health.

Findings reviewed below are the results of the analysis of data from the Korean Mental Health Index survey. This survey was conducted in 2010 using online or off-line methods with a nationwide sample of South Korean adults. The respondents who participated in the online survey included 467 adults between the ages of 18 and 54, and 48.8% of them were female (mean age = 35.83 years, SD = 10.39). The off-line participants included 1,000 adults between the ages of 19 and 80, and 50.5% of them were female (mean age = 43.73 years, SD = 14.11). The samples were stratified by age, gender, and region.

Two measures of mental health were used in the survey. The first was the Mental Health Continuum–Short Form (MHC–SF), which assesses subjective well-being. The MHC–SF consists of 14 items and measures the degree of (a) EWB (items 1–3) as defined in terms of positive affect (PA) and satisfaction with life; (b) SWB (items 4–8) as described in Keyes's (1998) model of SWB (one item on each of the facets of social acceptance, social actualization, social contribution, social coherence, and social integration); and (c) PWB (items 9–14) as described in Ryff's (1989) model (including one item on each of the dimensions of autonomy, environmental mastery, personal growth, positive relations with others, purpose in life, and self-acceptance). This measure was used in both the online and off-line surveys.

The second measure was the Patient Health Questionnaire (PHQ), which diagnoses mental illness. The PHQ is a 4-page questionnaire that can be entirely self-administered by the respondent. The questionnaire assesses eight diagnoses, separated into threshold disorders (disorders that correspond to specific diagnoses in the Diagnostic and Statistical Manual of Mental Disorders, Fourth Edition; specifically major depressive disorder, panic disorder, other anxiety disorder, and bulimia nervosa) and subthreshold disorders (disorders for which criteria include fewer symptoms than are required for any specific diagnoses in Diagnostic and Statistical Manual of Mental Disorders, Fourth Edition; specifically other depressive disorder, probable alcohol abuse or dependence, and somatoform and binge eating disorders). For this study, we used a shortened version of the PHQ, which included only the questions related to the four diagnoses (major depressive disorder, panic disorder, other anxiety disorder, and probable alcohol abuse or dependence) from the original PHQ. This measure was used only in the online survey.

Table 5.1 Fit indices of alternative factor models of theories about the latent structure of the measures of mental health and mental disorders

Model	χ^2	df	TLI	CFI	RMSEA
Adults sample ($N=467$)					
One factor	281.389	14	0.602	0.734	0.202
Orthogonal two factor	78.263	14	0.904	0.936	0.099
Correlated two factor	41.933	13	0.971	0.954	0.069

TLI Tucker-Lewis index, *CFI* comparative fit index, *RMSEA* root mean square error of approximation

Mental Health: Prevalence and Comorbidity

Table 5.1 reports the indices of fit for the various confirmatory factor models, which represent different theories about the latent structure of the measures of mental health and mental illness. Three subscales served as indicators of the latent construct of mental health: the summed scales that reflected EWB (i.e., three items of the MHC–SF), PWB (i.e., seven items of MHC–SF), and SWB (i.e., five items of MHC–SF). Four summary measures served as indicators of the latent construct of mental illness: the number of symptoms of major depressive disorder, panic disorder, other anxiety disorder, and probable alcohol abuse or dependence. Based on previous studies, we specified three models for comparison by a confirmatory factor analysis (CFA), i.e., a single-factor model (Model I), a two orthogonal factor model (Model II), and a two correlated factor model (Model III). Model I was found to be a poor fit. The two correlated factor solution (Model III) provided the best fit (Table 5.1).

The results of our CFA showed that a correlated two-factor solution provided a suitable fit for the present data. This is consistent with the factor structure found by Keyes (2005). In sum, our data strongly support the structural axiom hypothesis that measures of mental health and mental illness clearly form separate, correlated factors (Keyes 2005) and that this model applies to a South Korean population.

Figure 5.1 reports the prevalence of mental health using the MHC–SF as diagnosed categorically and assessed continuously according to the suggestions by Keyes (2005). Only 7.9% fit the categorical diagnosis of flourishing (a state in which an individual feels positive emotion toward life and is functioning well psychologically and socially). Moreover, only 6.2% fit into the highest range of the continuous assessment of mental health (i.e., 50–70), which was the fifth most prevalent range of mental health scores. Most South Koreans, roughly 7 in 10 according to the categorical diagnosis, were moderately mentally healthy. The most prevalent range of mental health scores was the approximate midpoint of the continuous assessment (i.e., 20–30 scores, 30.0%; 30–40 scores, 27.6%). Although only one in five South Koreans were *languishing*, a state in which an individual is devoid of positive emotion toward life and is not functioning well psychologically or socially (about 21% according to the categorical diagnosis), it is important to note that more South Koreans were mentally unhealthy (i.e., languishing) than were mentally healthy (i.e., flourishing).

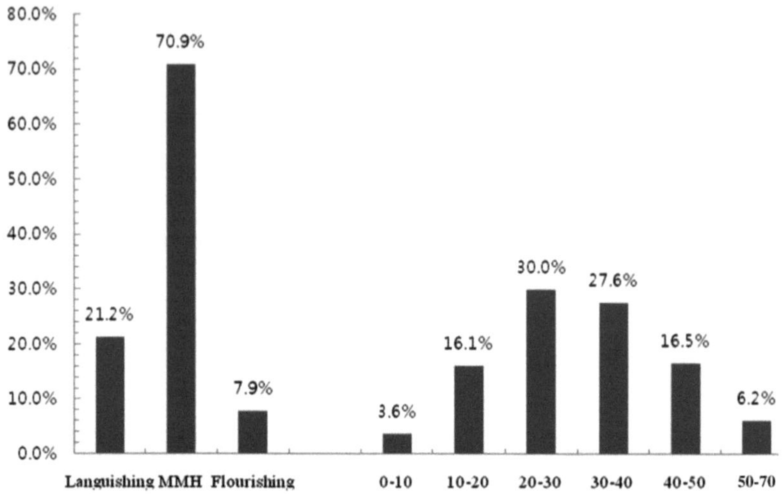

Fig. 5.1 Prevalence of mental health diagnosis (Note: *MMH* Moderately Mentally Healthy)

To obtain the estimates of the states of complete mental health, whether individuals had any of the mental disorders was cross-tabulated against the categorical mental health diagnosis (Fig. 5.2). The prevalence of complete mental health was nearly 6.2%, whereas 51.4% were moderately mentally healthy, and 13.1% had a form of pure languishing, which is languishing without any of the four mental disorders. Of the 29.3% of adults who had any of the four mental illnesses, 8.1% were also languishing, whereas 21.2% had a pure form of mental illness, indicating that this latter group had either moderate mental health or was flourishing.

Mental Health: Psychosocial Functioning

Cross-tabulation of the four DSM-IV mental disorders and the mental health diagnoses revealed that flourishing individuals were at the lowest risk of three of the four mental disorders and that the prevalence of each mental disorder decreased as the level of mental health increased. For example, 23% of languishing and 22% of moderately mentally healthy individuals, compared with 10% of flourishing adults, had probable alcohol abuse or dependence, which is the most common diagnosis in South Korea. Moderately mentally healthy adults were about three times less likely than languishers to have a major depressive disorder. Moderately mentally healthy individuals also were about four times less likely than languishers to have comorbid mental disorders.

Respondents were asked to evaluate their *physical health* on a scale from *poor*, *fair*, *very good*, to *excellent*. Figure 5.3 shows that the diagnosis of complete mental

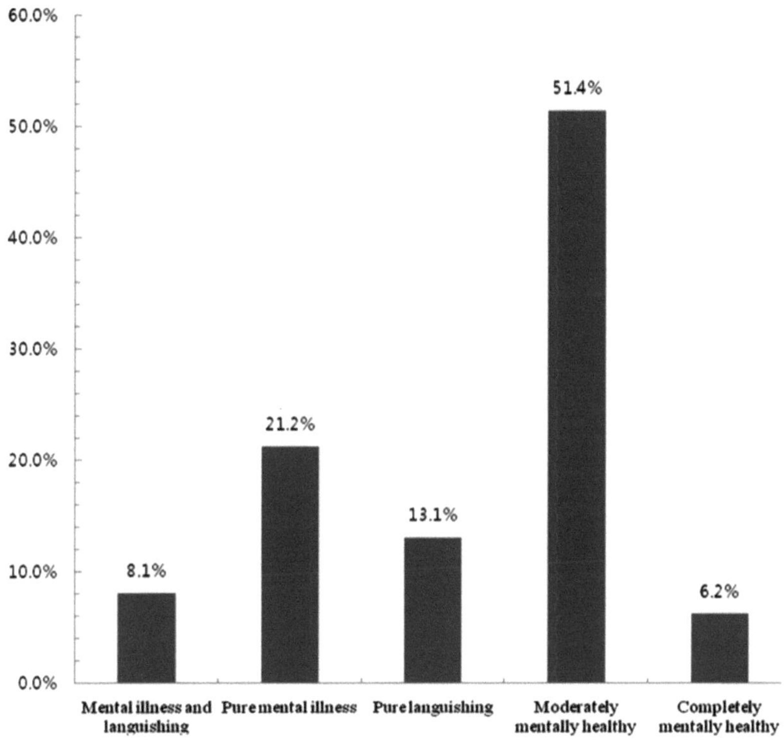

Fig. 5.2 Point prevalence of complete mental health in South Korea in 2010

health is consistent with individuals' self-reported physical health. More than half of the adults who were languishing evaluated their physical health as either poor or fair. In contrast, fewer than 15% of completely mentally healthy individuals reported that their physical health was either poor or fair. However, 28.7% of moderately mentally healthy adults and 33.3% of adults with at least one mental disorder saw their physical health as either poor or fair. Sixty-two percent (62%) of the completely mentally healthy individuals felt that their physical health was either very good or excellent. In contrast, none of the pure languishing or languishing individuals, or those who were languishing and had at least one mental disorder, said their emotional health was excellent.

Participants reported their *mental or emotional health* on a scale from *poor*, *fair*, *very good*, to *excellent*. Figure 5.4 reveals that the diagnosis of complete mental health matches the individuals' self-reported mental or emotional health. More than half of the adults who were languishing evaluated their emotional health as either poor or fair. In contrast, fewer than 4% of completely mentally healthy individuals said their emotional health was either poor or fair. However, 26.3% of moderately mentally healthy adults and 29.3% of adults with at least one mental disorder saw

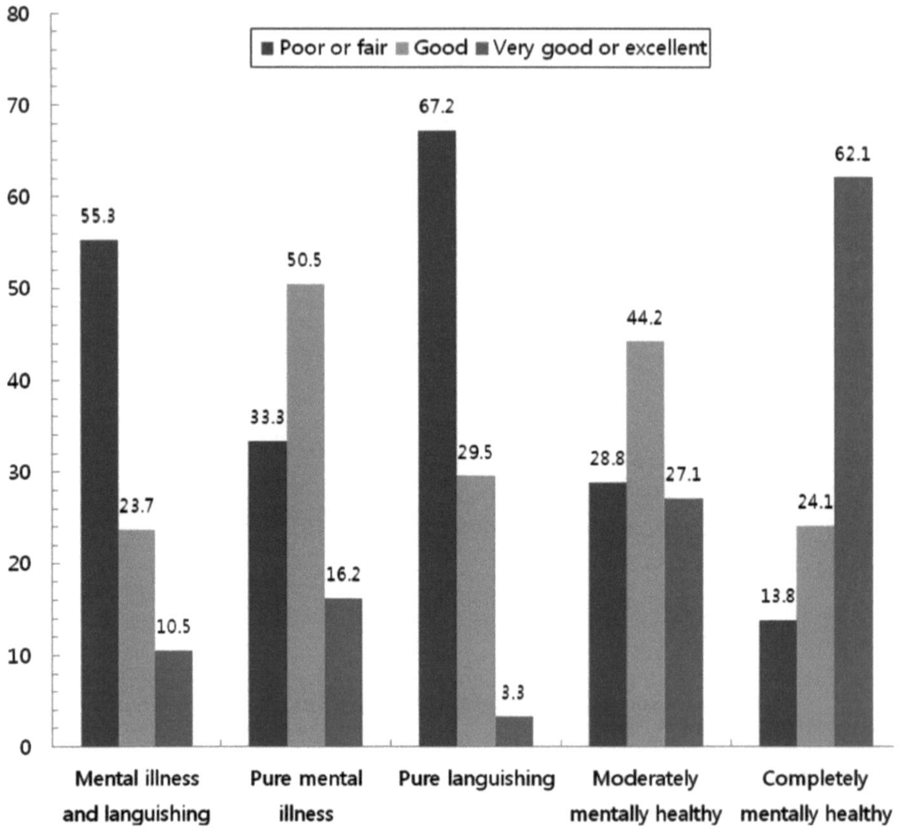

Fig. 5.3 Self-rated physical health by mental illness and mental health status

their emotional health as either poor or fair. Almost 80% of the completely mentally healthy individuals felt that their emotional health was either very good or excellent. In contrast, only 6.5% of pure languishing individuals and 10.5% of the adults who were languishing and had at least one mental disorder said that their emotional health was either very good or excellent.

Adults were also asked whether they agreed or disagreed with the following statements about helplessness: "I often feel helpless in dealing with the problems of life" and "There is little I can do to change the important things in my life." To measure goal formation, we asked respondents whether the statements "I know what I want out of life" and "I find it helpful to set goals for the near future" described them *a lot*, *some*, *a little*, or *not at all*. Two additional statements were used to measure respondents' resilience: "When faced with a bad situation, I do what I can to change it for the better" and "I find I usually learn something meaningful from a difficult situation." Participants responded as to whether each statement described them *a lot*, *some*, *a little*, or *not at all*. Finally, intimacy was measured by asking respondents to

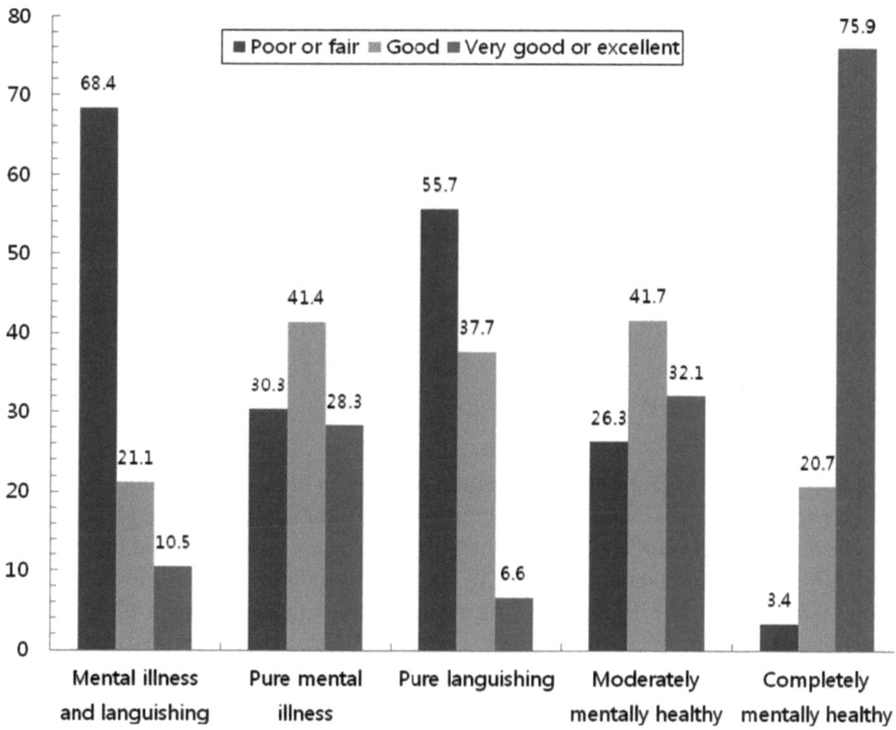

Fig. 5.4 Self-rated mental, emotional health by mental illness and mental health status

Table 5.2 Psychosocial functioning by categorical diagnosis of complete mental health (*N*=467)

	Mental illness and languishing	Pure mental illness	Pure languishing	Moderate mentally healthy	Completely mentally healthy
N	38	99	61	240	29
%	8.1	21.2	13.1	51.4	6.2
Resilience	4.71(1.35)	5.34(1.06)	4.80(1.09)	5.40(1.13)	6.31(1.07)
Goals	4.92(1.40)	5.76(1.01)	4.90(1.31)	5.67(1.27)	6.51(1.02)
Helplessness	5.18(1.43)	4.32(1.46)	4.14(1.47)	3.86(1.26)	3.72(1.66)
Intimacy	3.76(1.19)	5.03(1.41)	4.31(1.45)	5.27(1.26)	5.75(1.27)

indicate whether their (a) spouse or partner (or other family members) and (b) friends "really care(s) about them." Again, respondents were asked whether each statement applied to them *a lot*, *some*, *a little*, or *not at all*.

Table 5.2 presents the mean level of psychosocial assets (resilience, goal formation, helplessness, and intimacy) by level of mental health. Completely mentally healthy individuals had higher scores on resilience and goal formation than any other group.

They also scored higher on intimacy than purely languishing individuals. In addition, resilience, goal formation, and intimacy were higher among adults with pure mental illness than in adults with pure languishing.

In summary, completely mentally healthy adults reported higher levels of psychosocial functioning than those with pure languishing. Languishing with at least one mental disorder was associated with the worst outcomes and the most psychosocial impairment when compared with all diagnoses of complete mental health. Pure languishing, or the absence of mental health, appears to be more onerous to psychosocial functioning than the presence of at least one mental disorder.

Mental Health: Sociodemographic Correlates

Household Income

Regarding the reported monthly household income level of the respondents, 28.0% of the respondents had a household income of less than KW 2,500,000 (US$2,037), 56.6% of the respondents had a household income between KW 2,500,000 and KW 5,000,000 (US$2,037–4,074), and 15.4% had a household income of more than KW 5,000,000 (US$4,074). Figure 5.5 illustrates the association between the total and sub-domain scores of the MHC–SF and participants' self-reported household income level. Adults with a monthly income of more than KW 5,000,000 had higher scores on the PWB subscale ($M=14.88$, $SD=6.55$) than people earning between KW 2,500,000 and KW 5,000,000.

Education Level

In terms of reported educational attainment, more than two-fifths of the respondents (44.6%) had a college education, 12.7% of participants had a primary or middle school education, and more than two-fifths (42.6%) had a high school education. Figure 5.6 shows the relationship between the total and subscale scores on the MHC–SF and respondents' self-reported education level. Adults with a primary or middle school education had lower scores on the total scale and on the SWB and PWB subscales than any other groups. In addition, participants with a college education had higher scores on the EWB and PWB subscale of MHC–SF than any other group.

Type of Community

In terms of type of community, 25.5% came from metropolitan cities (more than 1,000,000 residents), 21.3% from Seoul (the capital of South Korea), and 53.2% from smaller cities or from towns and rural areas. Participants from different communities

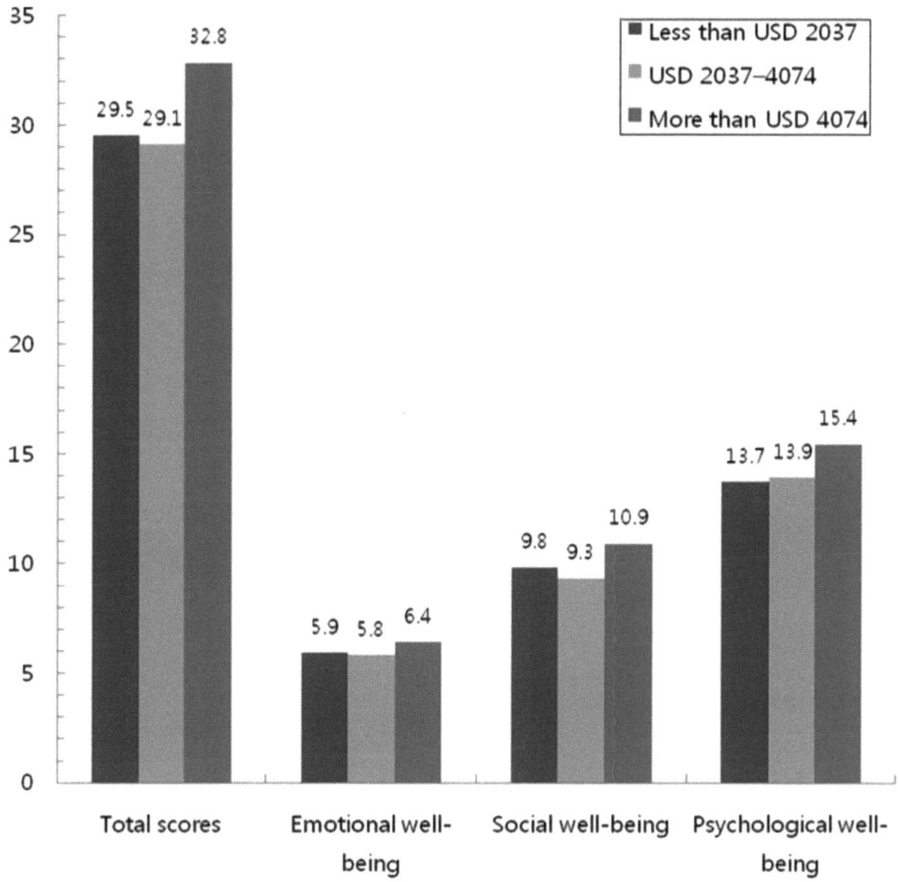

Fig. 5.5 The MHC–SF subscales and total MHC–SF score by household income per month

exhibited significantly different scores on the MHC–SF. Adults in Seoul ($n = 212$) had lower EWB subscale scores than did individuals from metropolitan cities ($n = 255$) and smaller cities, towns, and rural areas ($n = 528$). In addition, residents in Seoul had lower total and PWB subscale scores than did individuals from smaller cities, towns, and rural areas.

With regard to community differences in PWB, our study has also uncovered an important interaction effect of community × monthly household income on PWB. Adults in Seoul with a monthly income of more than KW 4,000,000 (US$3,259) reported lower PWB in comparison with individuals in smaller cities, towns, and rural areas with a monthly income of more than KW 4,000,000 (US$3,259). However, participants who dwell in Seoul with a monthly income of less than KW 4,000,000 (US$3,259) reported PWB comparable with that of adults in smaller cities, towns, and rural areas with a monthly income of less than KW 4,000,000 (US$3,259; Fig. 5.7).

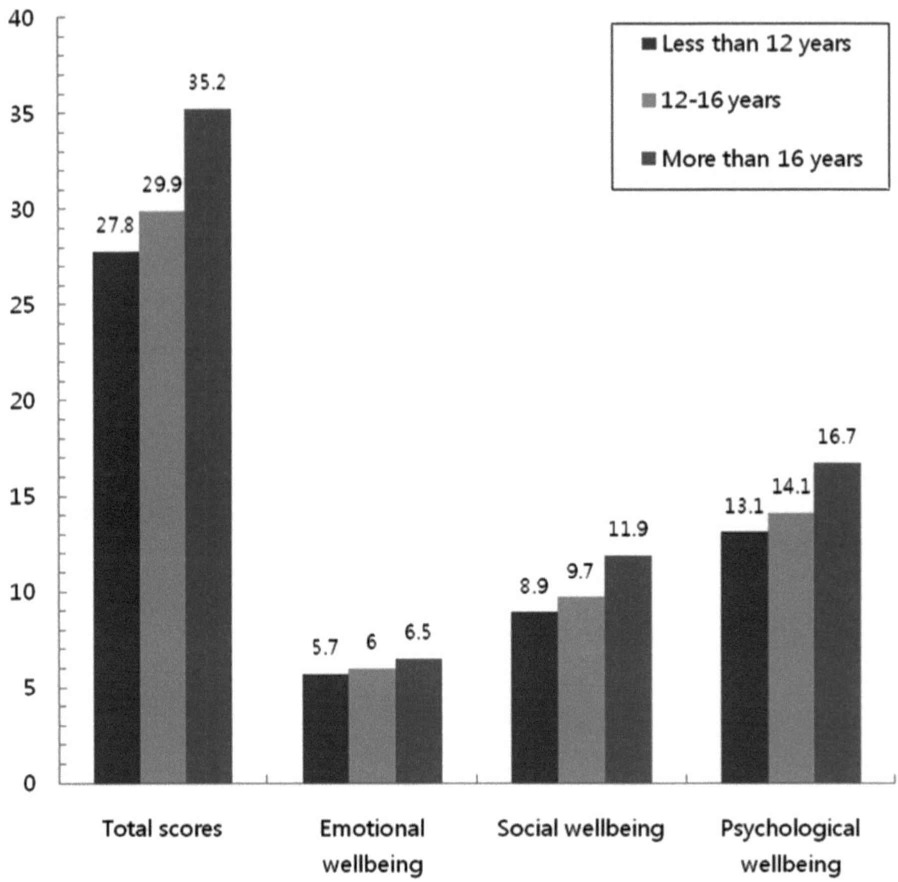

Fig. 5.6 The MHC–SF subscales and total MHC–SF score by education level

Age

The age breakdown of these respondents was 20.0% aged 19–29 years, 21.5% aged 30–39 years, 22.7% aged 40–49 years, 16.7% aged 50–59 years, and 19.1% aged 60 years and above. Participants from the different age groups exhibited significantly different scores on the total scale of the MHC–SF. More specifically, adults who were aged 60 and above ($n=189$) had lower total scale scores than did (a) individuals who were aged 19–29 years, (b) individuals who were aged 40–49 years ($n=227$), and (c) individuals who were aged 50–59 years ($n=167$).

Moreover, participants in the different age groups showed different scores on the PWB subscale of the MHC–SF. More specifically, adults who were aged 60 and above ($n=189$) had lower PWB subscale scores than did (a) individuals who were aged 19–29 years ($n=199$), (b) individuals who were aged 30–39 years ($n=213$), and (c) individuals who were aged 40–49 years ($n=227$).

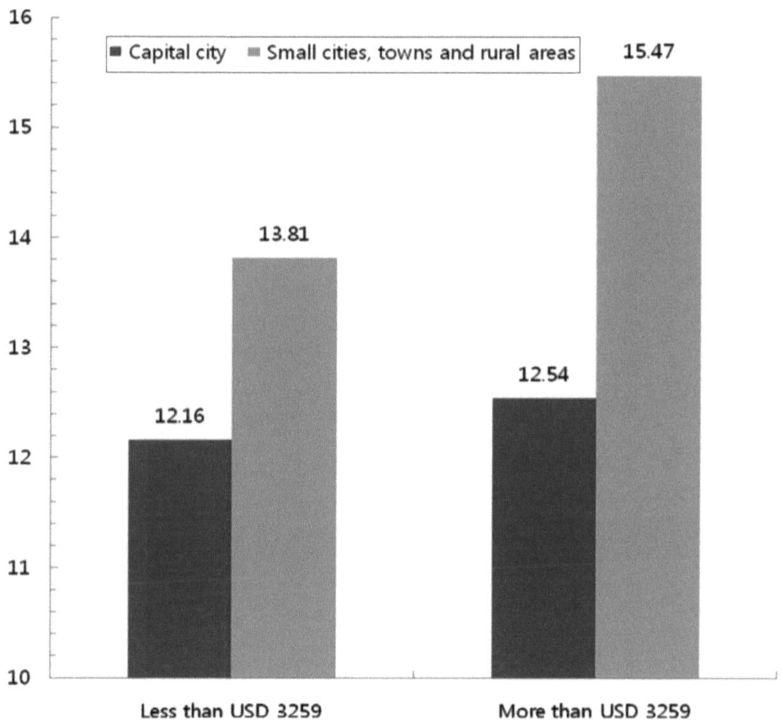

Fig. 5.7 The psychological well-being scores by household income per month and type of community

We conducted additional analyses to investigate whether these differences in the total and the PWB subscale scores of the MHC–SF were due to education level rather than age. We suspected there could be education-based differences because education levels in South Korea vary according to age group. In fact, this is reflected in our sample's education distribution for the following age groups: 77% of those aged 19–29 years were college graduates or undergraduates, whereas only 6.8% of those aged 60 and above were college graduates or undergraduates. Additionally, as we reported earlier, there was a difference in the total scores of the MHC–SF between the participants with a primary or middle school education and those with a college education. When we conducted an ANOVA in which we controlled for the effects of education, we found that the differences in the total and the PWB subscale scores of the MHC–SF between adults who were aged 60 and above and other age groups were no longer significant.

Number of Children

Adults with two or less children at home ($n = 600$) had significantly lower total scale and SWB and PWB subscale scores on the MHC–SF than did individuals with three or more children at home ($n = 149$). We conducted an additional analysis to examine

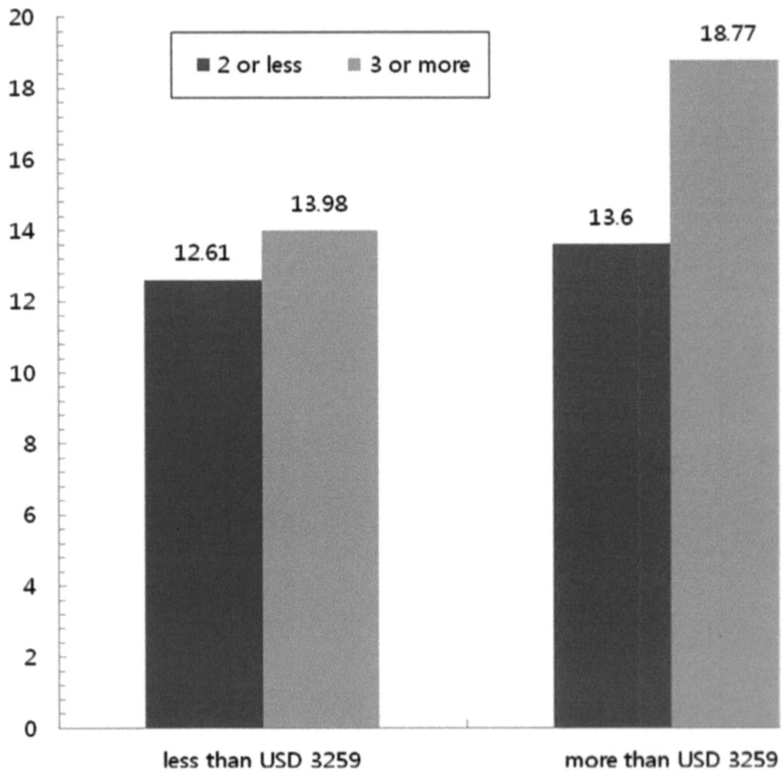

Fig. 5.8 The psychological well-being scores of women by number of children and monthly house income

whether monthly household income moderates the relation between number of children and the total scores on the MHC–SF for the female participants. The results revealed a significant interaction with the number of children and monthly household income. Females with a monthly income of more than KW 4,000,000 (US$3,259) and three or more children at home reported greater PWB when compared with female participants with a monthly income of more than KW 4,000,000 (US$3,259) and two or less children. However, female adults with a monthly income of less than KW 4,000,000 (US$3,259) and three or more children at home reported levels of PWB, which were similar to female participants with a monthly income of less than KW 4,000,000 (US$3,259) and two or less children (Fig. 5.8).

Occupation Type

Of the male participants, 32.8% owned their private businesses, 36.6% were blue-collar workers, and 30.6% were white-collar workers. There were no differences in the total and subscale scores on the MHC–SF among these three groups for males.

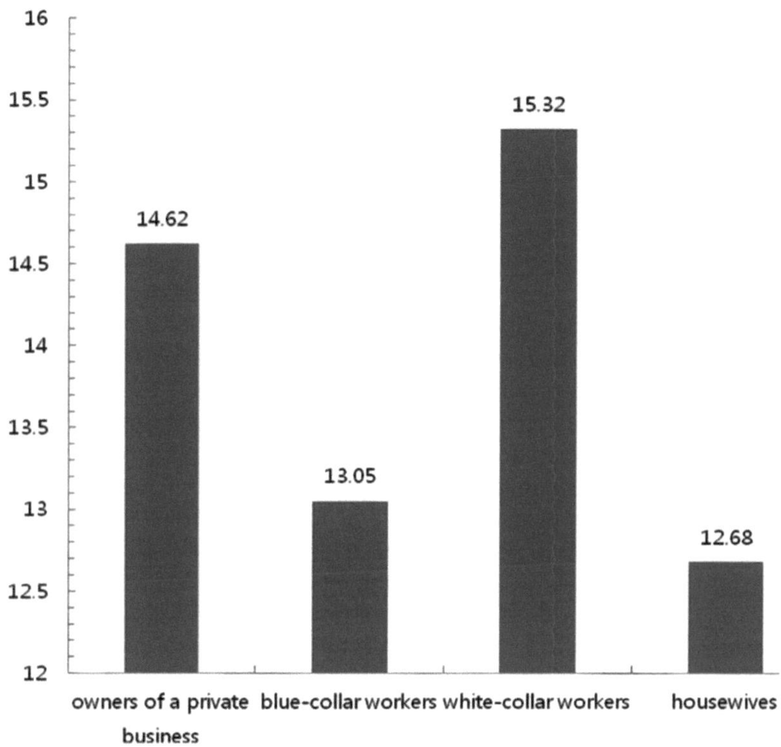

Fig. 5.9 The psychological well-being scores of women by occupation type

However, the findings were different for the females, of whom 18.2% owned private businesses, 22.8% were blue-collar workers, 16.4% were white-collar workers, and 42.5% were housewives. Female housewives ($n = 189$) had lower PWB subscale scores on the MHC–SF than did the female white-collar workers ($n = 45$). When we conducted an additional analysis to control for the effects of education and monthly income, this difference remained significant (Fig. 5.9).

Gender

There were no differences between males and females on either the total or subscale scores of the MHC–SF. We conducted an additional analysis to investigate whether monthly household income moderates the relation between gender and the total and subscale scores of the MHC–SF. Results indicated a significant interaction between gender and monthly house income on the EWB scale. Female adults with a monthly income of more than KW 4,000,000 (US$3,259) reported greater EWB when compared with males who had a monthly income of more than KW 4,000,000 (US$3,259). However, there were no differences in EWB between males and females with a monthly house income of less than KW 4,000,000 (US$3,259).

Conclusion

As mentioned earlier, South Korea has experienced political, social, and economic upheavals since the 1980s. The democratic transition from authoritarian rule in 1987 enabled South Korean people to achieve increased political rights and civil liberties. An increase in budgetary support for social welfare plans pushed South Korea toward a welfare state. Moreover, having fully recovered from the 1997 economic and financial disaster, South Korea is becoming a competitive market economy. People must wonder how these transformations might have affected the subjective well-being of the South Korean people.

The analysis reveals that, despite economic and technological advancements, fewer South Koreans are mentally healthy or flourishing (about 8% less) than would be expected on the basis of the previous survey on the mental disorder in Korea (i.e., Cho et al. 2010), which would suggest that nearly 85% of adults have no mental disorder and are therefore mentally healthy. Using diagnostic criteria of positive mental health, estimates of the prevalence of mental health in South Korea have revealed differences from those found in the United States: 8% flourishing (18% in the USA), 71% with moderate mental health (65% in the USA), and 21% languishing (17% in the USA). In short, over 70% of South Koreans were moderately mentally healthy, and one in five adults was mentally unhealthy or met the criteria for languishing.

These findings suggest that the South Korean people have not yet fully acquired subjective well-being. The analysis reveals that socioeconomic progress has failed to ensure that every South Korean will achieve positive mental health. At present, only small minority of South Koreans report experiencing lives of complete mental health, and the degrees of subjective quality of life or positive mental health found for South Korean people, in general, do not match the objective circumstances in which they dwell. Furthermore, our findings suggest that, in terms of the measures of SWB, although South Korea today is a developing democracy, the residents of South Korea tend not to believe that society can evolve positively and tend not to feel that society is logical, predictable, and meaningful. In spite of the economic, political, and social transformations which South Korea has achieved since the 1980s, South Korean citizens still believe that there is plenty of room for improvement in their SWB.

It is possible that cultural factors may account for some of the low level of positive mental health reported by South Koreans. Previous research which examined emotional expression in East Asian cultures has consistently found that South Koreans are reluctant to express their positive emotions (e.g., happiness) to another person. This suggests that the levels of EWB reported by Koreans could be underestimated.

Another possible reason for the low level of subjective well-being arises due to a difference in the value systems of Koreans and Western people. Koreans are more future oriented and place less value on present satisfactions than do Westerners. Because of this, in comparison with Westerners, they tend to underestimate satisfactions with present experiences and overestimate those from future successes. Responses to items on the MHC–SF could be affected by this difference in value systems. For example, on one item, subjects were asked how frequently they felt satisfied. In responding to this, the more future-focused South Korean might think, "I am pleased with the progress I've made, but I'm not satisfied."

Finally, the self-construal of Koreans is different from that of Westerners. The Korean people consider the self as context dependent, whereas Western people think of the self as context independent. Thus, some items in the MHC–SF (e.g., "confident to think or express your own ideas and opinions") might not be seen as relevant by Korean adults.

The present results support the hypotheses that flourishing individuals function better psychosocially than moderately mentally healthy adults and those adults with moderate mental health have better psychosocial functioning than those adults who are languishing. Completely mentally healthy adults reported the highest levels of mental, emotional, and physical health and the highest levels of resilience, goal formation, and intimacy. South Korean adults with the comorbid condition of languishing with at least one mental disorder had the lowest levels of mental, emotional, and physical health and the lowest levels of resilience, goal formation, and intimacy. Thus, the validity of the MHC model is confirmed for South Koreans in terms of their psychosocial assets.

The analysis of determinants of mental health indicates that family income and education level influence positive mental health. However, family income and education did not have an effect on EWB. Socioeconomic factors, such as family income and education, therefore appear to exert effects on the *function* rather than the *emotion* of people. Also, the effects of family income and education on positive mental health were found only at the high end of the variables.

The effect of age on positive mental health was shown at the high end of the age range. Adults aged 60 or over reported the lowest level of subjective well-being among all age groups. Since there were differences in household income and education level between adults aged 60 or over and adults aged less than 60, we conducted an additional analysis to control for household income and education level. When this was done, there was no difference between the two age groups in terms of positive mental health. However, it may be premature to conclude that there was no age effect on positive mental health because the present study used a cross-sectional design and, as such, is subject to cohort effects where age differences may reflect some specific shared temporal life experience rather than a true developmental change.

The present findings indicate that community type plays an important role in explaining variations in positive mental health. High-income adults in Seoul, the capital of South Korea, showed a lower level of PWB than did high-income residents outside of Seoul. In addition, there was no difference in PWB between the high-income and low-income adults in Seoul, suggesting that household income has no impact on PWB for Koreans living in Seoul.

As was the case in studies on adults in the United States, flourishing or moderately mentally healthy South Koreans reported lower levels of psychopathology than did languishing individuals. However, unlike findings in the United States

(Keyes 2005), there was no difference in the prevalence of a diagnosis of major depressive disorder between flourishing South Korean adults and those who were languishing. The latter result may be associated with differences in the measures of psychopathology which were used. The tool used in the United States study (Keyes 2005) was an interview-based instrument, whereas the PHQ used in the present study was an online self-report measure. It is recommended that in any future research, in order to further test the applicability of the MHC model, a comprehensive, fully structured interview is included for the diagnosis of mental disorders.

In summary, we believe the present results are encouraging in terms of the potential applicability of the MHC model in various East Asian cultures including Japan, Singapore, and China. The application of the MHC model in East Asian countries could help the study and promotion of mental health as well as the study and treatment of mental illness in East Asia. Mental health is clearly more than the absence of mental illness, and anyone who is less than flourishing is unlikely to reach an acceptable level of optimal functioning in life.

References

Cho, M., Chang, S., Lee, Y., Bae, A., Ahn, J., Son, J., Hong, J., Bae, J., Lee, D., Cho, S., Park, J., Lee, J., Kim, J., Jeon, H., Sohn, J., & Kim, B. (2010). Prevalence of DSM-IV major mental disorders among Korean adults: A 2006 National Epidemiologic Survey (KECA-R). *Asian Journal of Psychiatry, 3*, 26–30.

Diener, E., & Emmons, R. A. (1985). The independence of positive and negative affect. *Journal of Personality and Social Psychology, 47*, 1105–1117.

Diener, E., Emmons, R. A., Larsen, R. J., & Griffin, S. (1985). The satisfaction with life scale. *Journal of Personality Assessment, 49*, 71–75.

Diener, E., Oishi, S., & Lucas, R. E. (2003). Personality, culture, and subjective well-being: Emotional and cognitive evaluations of life. *Annual Review of Psychology, 54*, 403–425.

Freedom House. (2010). *Freedom in the world 2010*. Freedom House. Available at: http://www.freedomhouse.org/template.cfm?page=439.

Kaufman, D., Kraay, A., & Mastruzzi, M. (2009). *Governance matters VIII aggregate and individual governance indicators 1996–2008*. World Bank Policy Research Working Paper No. 4978. Available at SSRN: http://ssrn.com/abstract=1424591.

Keyes, C. L. M. (1998). Social well-being. *Social Psychology Quarterly, 61*, 121–140.

Keyes, C. L. M. (2002). The mental health continuum: From languishing to flourishing in life. *Journal of Health and Social Behavior, 43*, 207–222.

Keyes, C. L. M. (2003). Complete mental health: An agenda for the 21st century. In C. L. M. Keyes & J. Haidt (Eds.), *Flourishing: Positive psychology and the life well-lived* (pp. 293–312). Washington, DC: American Psychological Association Press.

Keyes, C. L. M. (2005). Mental health and/or mental illness? Investigating axioms of the complete state model of health. *Journal of Consulting and Clinical Psychology, 73*, 539–548.

Keyes, C. L. M., & Lopez, S. J. (2002). Toward a science of mental health: Positive directions in diagnosis and interventions. In C. R. Snyder & S. J. Lopez (Eds.), *Handbook of positive psychology* (pp. 45–59). New York: Oxford University Press.

Keyes, C. L. M., Wissing, M., Potgieter, J., Temane, M., Kruger, A., & van Rooy, S. (2008). Evaluation of the Mental Health Continuum—Short Form (MHC-SF) in Swetsana-speaking South Africans. *Clinical Psychology & Psychotherapy, 15*, 181–192.

Lu, L., & Gilmour, R. (2004). Culture and conceptions of happiness: Individual oriented and social oriented SWB. *Journal of Happiness Studies, 5*, 269–291.
OECD Factbook. (2008). *Economic, Environmental and Social Statistics*. Available at: http://puck.sourceoecd.org/vl=764185/cl=11/nw=1/rpsv/fact2008.
Park, C. (2009). The quality of life in South Korea. *Social Indicators Research, 92*, 263–294.
Ryff, C. D. (1989). Happiness is everything, or is it? Explorations on the meaning of psychological well-being. *Journal of Personality and Social Psychology, 57*, 1069–1081.
Ryff, C. D., & Keyes, C. L. M. (1995). The structure of psychological well-being revisited. *Journal of Personality and Social Psychology, 69*, 719–727.
Ryff, C. D., & Singer, B. (1998). Human health: New directions for the next millennium. *Psychological Inquiry, 9*, 69–85.
Strümpfer, D. J. W., Hardy, A., De Villiers, J. S., & Rigby, S. (2009). Organisationally relevant variables and Keyes's Mental Health Continuum Scale: An exploratory study. *Journal of Industrial Psychology, 35*, 1–7.
United Nations Development Programme. (2010). *Human development report 2010*. New York: Palgrave Macmillan. Available at: http://www.beta.undp.org/content/dam/undp/library/corporate/HDR/HDR_2010_EN_Complete_reprint-1.pdf.
Westerhof, G. J., & Keyes, C. L. M. (2010). Mental illness and mental health: The two continua model across the lifespan. *Journal of Adult Development, 17*, 110–119.

Chapter 6
Positive Mental Health: Measurement, Prevalence, and Correlates in a Chinese Cultural Context

Ke Li Yin, Jia Mei He, and Yan Fen Fu

There is growing recognition of the importance of mental health and well-being in China. Recently, more researchers in China have been examining mental health according to the established literature, searching under keywords such as *mental health* in the Chinese Academic Journal full-text database. The number of articles that have been published on the subject of mental health was zero from 1979 to 1993. Since then, this number has increased: A total of 668 articles were published as of 1994, and from 1994 to 2011, there have been a whopping 63,002 articles published on mental health in China. However, the concept of well-being in China has been limited to *physical* but not *mental health,* while mental health has referred to the presence or absence of psychopathology.

The reason that the measurement, diagnosis, and promotion of mental health have become an important issue in psychological and pedagogical research in China is due to the introduction and prevalence of western ideology, theory, and research in China and because of the desire to increase psychological knowledge in correspondence to the social revolution and development in China.

During the reforms of the past 30 years, the Chinese people have experienced many different pressures, trials, and tribulations and have had to confront the types of mental health issues that normally accompany social renovations. And even though these renovations have brought great improvements to the Chinese economy, policies, society, and culture, their effects—especially with regard to mental health—have not always been positive. For example, although the economy has

K.L. Yin (✉)
School of Education and Management, Yunnan Normal University, Yunnan, China
e-mail: yayasles@163.com

J.M. He
School of Education, Liaoning Normal University, Liaoning, China
e-mail: hejiamei998@gmail.com

Y.F. Fu
School of Nursing, Dali University, Dali, China
e-mail: yanfen1998@hotmail.com

C.L.M. Keyes (ed.), *Mental Well-Being: International Contributions to the Study of Positive Mental Health*, DOI 10.1007/978-94-007-5195-8_6,

experienced a boom, basic survival costs have been heavily increasing, thereby increasing stress in everyday life in China. Therefore, given this situation, *subjective well-being* and *satisfaction with life* have become issues which have become quite important in China (Sun et al. 2010).

It is popular among Chinese psychologists to view the concept and operation of mental health from a traditional Chinese cultural perspective. Moreover, a number of discussions and studies have taken place on the standards of mental health and on mental health improvement within a Chinese cultural context (Jing and Guo 1998; Jing 2002; Deng and Dai 2010; Yang and Zhang 2007). However, Chinese psychologists still cannot agree upon a general concept, standard, or measure of mental health, even after so much research and discussion on the topic. Indeed, as Keyes (2005) has pointed out, there really is no standard by which to measure, diagnose, and research the presence of mental health, regardless of the culture under examination.

Although there is no doubt that a gap exists between western and eastern cultures, there is also no doubt that modern Chinese people have been affected by the value system used in the western world. Therefore, because the eastern and western cultural exchange has been taking place more frequently and much more easily than in the past, within China it has become more acceptable to simply revise western mental health scales and to use these scales on the Chinese people as an important way to measure and diagnose Chinese mental health. However, there is a desire for mental health scales to fit Chinese culture, which has driven Chinese psychologists to develop their own kinds of questionnaires of mental health. And although the mental health measurement in practice has mostly consisted of the diagnosis of psychopathological symptom, more recently in China, the trend has been to start to explore the measurement of positive mental health in ordinary populations.

Mental Health Measures Focused on Psychopathological Symptoms

The view of psychopathology is both familiar and accepted by Chinese people, and diagnosis and assessment of psychopathological symptom have been expected in clinical practice. In fact, the tools that are frequently used to define, diagnose, and intervene in mental health issues have focused on symptoms, with the majority of these tools consisting of revisions of mental health measurements in the west. In particular, the most frequently used mental health scale in China is the *Symptom Check List 90* (SCL-90), which was developed by Derogatis in 1975 and consists of nine factors, such as somatization, obsessive symptoms, interpersonal sensitivity, depression, anxiety, hostility, terror, crankiness, and psychosis (Li 2007; Liao et al. 2007). The current meta-analytic reports on mental health measures published in Chinese journals consist almost entirely of results from operating the SCL-90 on different populations in China, such as the Chinese military (Feng and Dai 2008), policemen (Meng et al. 2010), primary and middle school students (Fan and Zhang

2005; Xin and Zhang 2009), college students (Hu and Zhang 2009), college students among ethnic minority groups (Luo et al. 2010), and rail workers (Yi et al. 2010). These applications of the SCL-90 on extensively different populations have thus far supplied sufficient data for meta-analysis.

In addition to the SCL-90, there have been other scales that have been adapted and used by Chinese psychologists to measure Chinese populations, such as *Achenbach's Child Behavior Checklist* (CBCL), the *Minnesota Multiphasic Personality Inventory* (MMPI), the *16 Personality Factor Scale*, and the *Eysenck Personality Questionnaire* (EPQ). Moreover, in measuring certain symptoms of mental health in China, some questionnaires that have been used frequently include *Beck's Depression Inventory* (BDI), the *Hamilton Rating Scale for Depression* (HRSD), and the *Hamilton Rating Scale for Anxiety* (HRSA). And finally, in diagnosing mental disorders in clinics and hospitals in China, the *Diagnostic and Statistical Manual of Mental Disorders IV* (DSM-IV) by the American Psychiatric Association and the *International Classification of Disease* (ICD-10) by the World Health Organization have been most frequently used as a facility reference guide.

In the meantime, Chinese research psychologists have been actively working on developing a mental disorder diagnostic tool within a Chinese cultural context. For example, the *Chinese Diagnostic Criteria for Mental Disorder* (*CCMD-3*) and the *Treatment and Nursing of Mental Disorder Related to CCMD-3* were published by the Chinese CCMD-3 working group, using ICD-10 and DSM-IV as references and by combining the results from spot tests and random tests within a Chinese cultural context. However, it is important to note that these publications borrowed heavily from the clinical descriptions and diagnoses of the ICD-10, particularly when describing the symptoms of mental illness, and that the research standards from both the ICD-10 and DSM-IV were involved in developing diagnosis criteria (Song et al. 2008).

The criticism of these kinds of tools has been that they were not appropriate for mental health assessment on normal populations or on populations with few symptoms of mental disorder because they aimed to differentiate diagnoses based on illness symptoms. Such measures have nonetheless been used by Chinese scholar psychologists and mental health practitioners for some time now; Chinese researchers and mental health practitioners continue to introduce western scales into their work in order to meet the needs of their research and practice. For example, Chinese researchers recently revised the *Kessler 10* scale and used it to assess the mental health of older Chinese people in order to simply and easily assess mental health on a large population (Zhou et al. 2009). Although the Kessler 10 is specifically designed for large populations, it actually focuses on predicting the occurrence of mental illness based on the frequency of the occurrence of a nonspecific mental health symptom, such as anxiety and stress level.

The idea of creating an indigenous tool for the assessment of mental health has been gaining attention from Chinese psychologists who would like to do more than simply introduce and revise alien mental health assessment tools. In fact, since the twentieth century, Chinese researchers have been claiming that it is necessary to develop mental health scales specifically for Chinese populations. And indeed, there have been a few mental health scales that have been developed for different populations in China as of now. For example, a mental health scale with three dimensions (learning, personal relations, and the self) was developed for pupils (Yu et al. 1999): Its learning subscale consists of five dimensions, such as self-satisfaction and body brain coordination; its personal relations subscale consists of five dimension, such as intimacy and confidence; and its self subscale consists of five dimension, such as social self and family self, and so on. Additionally, a scale consisting of five dimensions—cognitive normality, feeling coordination, volitional health, perfect personality, and adaptability (Liu 2003; Tan 1998)—has been created for middle school students. Also, a college mental health scale has been created, consisting of 96 questions in 12 dimensions, such as somatization, anxiety, and depression (Zheng et al. 2005). As well, there is now an adult mental health scale which consists of 80 questions, including tense and sensitive interpersonal relations, weak psychological withstanding ability, and weak adaptation (Wang et al. 2006). Finally, there are also scales that have been developed for more general populations; for example, the scale built by Xu and Gong (2004) consists of 104 items including three secondary factors (psychological problem and mental disorder, positive moods, and cognitive attention to health) and 13 first-class factors, such as happiness and health attention.

Recently, hundreds of mental health assessment tools have been developed within a wide range of content; however, their quality is low and a lot of repeated work is present. Up till now, not many scales have been prevalently accepted, and those that have been accepted have been used more for special research projects and not in clinical practice.

The Mental Health Scales on Positive Mental Function

Mental health is not merely the absence of mental illness; mental health should include and focus on positive states of being. The definition by the World Health Organization (WHO) recently reflects this kind of positive view of mental health. The WHO pointed out that in mental health, a status of well-being is one whereby individuals are able to recognize their abilities, cope with the normal stresses of life, work productively and fruitfully, and make a contribution to their communities (WHO 2001). In 2003, the WHO produced a developed definition of mental health that was not simply lacking in mental disorder but which also included subjective well-being, self perceived self-efficacy, autonomy, competence, intergenerational dependence, and the ability to realize one's intellectual and emotional potential (WHO 2003). The definition of mental health by the WHO describes mental health as a status that is not simply lacking of mental illness, but that has some positive mental functioning as well. Therefore, the knowledge of positive mental health causes people to think about the necessity to assess mental health from the viewpoint of positive mental functions.

In recent years, some Chinese researchers have started to question the process of assessing mental health using psychopathological symptoms as criteria. In their opinions, the tools created and used in China, which aim at measuring symptoms, can only be used to assess negative outcomes resulting from mental illness and not to assess the integral mental health level from positive states, such as when measuring social activities range, satisfaction with life, self-esteem, social support, and subjective well-being. Therefore, it is hard to capture and reflect an individual's mental health with the tools created and used in China (Song et al. 2008).

Since constructing the mental health scale, Chinese researchers have been noticing more positive mental health issues. At present, the best Chinese representation of positive mental health is the construct of the *healthy personality* described by Huang et al. (2006). There are different levels of mental health within a healthy personality, as claimed by Huang and colleagues. They include mental disorder, normal mental functioning, and healthy personality, with mental disorder considered to be unhealthy. The lower level of normal mental health is also known as *negative mental health*. Individuals who are at the level of normal mental functioning maintain their internal balance by eliminating excessive nervousness, being submissive, having no internal conflict, and being ingratiating toward other people. However, having internal balance is not the only motivation for humans who seek to embrace living; there are other motivations in addition, such as the pursuit of new stimulation and persistent growth, which humans desire in their pursuit toward better living. Therefore, a higher level of mental health must also be conceptualized, which can be called *positive mental health*.

Having a healthy personality and positive mental health is the highest level of mental health, and its representation can be seen in individuals who are at the level of healthy personality and who have and pursue excellent interpersonal relationships. Additionally, these are people who produce creative work that benefits the community, aspire to meet challenges, and search for stability and meaning in life (Huang et al. 2006).

Under the guidance of healthy personality theory, some mental health scales have been developed for different populations in China. The mental health scale for middle school students was created by Su and Huang (2007), and it has been used to assess the adaptation of students in middle school. This scale has five dimensions, such as being happy in life, being willing to study, being calm when taking exams, having interpersonal concordance, and having stabilization of feelings (Su and Huang 2007). Chen and Huang (2009) invented a mental health scale for college students, since these students are not just good at adapting but also tend to naturally pursue a healthy personality. There are six positive dimensions in this scale, which include the experience of happiness, interpersonal concordance, willingness to study, mediation of emotion, pursuit of goals, and braveness when facing challenge (Cheng and Huang 2009). Another scale on college student mental health style was invented within a Chinese cultural context, and adaptability, way of life, attitude, and personality were involved in its design. Its seven subscales, including harmoniousness, optimism, happiness, assiduity, perseverance, sagaciousness, and conservation, compose the integrated assessment of positive mental health for Chinese college students (Tong et al. 2010).

Nonetheless, the positive mental health scales invented by Chinese researchers within a Chinese cultural context have neither been sufficient nor have they played a role in clinical practice. Even worse, some scales are not suitable for clinic diagnosis, such as the college student mental health style scale (269 items), because the inventors did not take its clinical adaptation into consideration when attempting to display the completeness of the assessment of mental health within a Chinese cultural context.

Chinese researchers have used both negative mental symptoms and positive mental functioning when inventing scales. For example, the five dimensions of normality of cognitive function, stability and positivity of emotion, appropriation of self-evaluation, concordance of interpersonal relations, and excellent adaptability were all taken into consideration when the aged Chinese mental health scale was invented (Li et al. 2009). The teacher mental health scale, which consists of four subscales (self, society, work, and life), assesses whether teachers have problems with professional development and interpersonal adaptation (Yu et al. 2010). The problem is that the invention of this type of mental health scale does not differentiate negative psychological pathology symptoms from positive mental health status, which results in a lack of exploration of the relationship between the two statuses or in considering them as identical factors.

So far, there is still a lot of work to be done in developing indigenous measurements of mental health in China. Although plenty of mental health scales have been revised and adapted clinically in China, it has been a rare occurrence to compare the research that has been done between these assessments; still, Chinese researchers have begun to contribute to international mental health assessments. Unfortunately, few of their findings are currently available within Chinese journals.

How Many Chinese Participants Are Flourishing? Application of Keyes' Model of Mental Health Continuum-Short Form in Chinese Adults

Subjective well-being is seldom used directly as a measure of mental health in China but is taken as a variable related to mental health. In recent years, psychological well-being (Zhang and Zuo 2007) and social well-being (Miao et al. 2008) were introduced in several Chinese articles, and the knowledge of Keyes' theory on social well-being and two-factor mental health theory have helped people to understand the concept of happiness much more clearly, extending the application of the field of happiness and building a bridge to connect the concepts of subjective well-being and positive mental health (Miao and Zhao 2009). However, the results of revising Keyes' mental health continuum have not been published in China as of yet.

The study of mental health as a complete state offers new directions for research on subjective well-being (Keyes 2006b). Keyes suggested that mental health should be operationally defined as a syndrome of symptoms of an individual's subjective well-being in which the mental health state should be reflected. Two compatible traditions have been integrated into the operational definition of mental health, such as the tradition that focuses on feelings toward life (hedonic well-being) and the tradition that focuses on functioning in life (eudaemonic well-being; Keyes et al. 2008). The mental health continuum model by Keyes is composed of emotional well-being, social well-being, and psychological well-being (Keyes 2002), which gained support from studies on American adults (Keyes 2005), adolescence (Keyes 2006a), and university students (Robitschek and Keyes 2009), and from the studies on Setswana-speaking adults in the North West province of South Africa (Keyes et al. 2008). It can be concluded that there might be huge costs to improve the health in society if we do not first distinguish between these three types of happiness, namely, emotional well-being (EWB), psychological well-being (PWB), and social well-being (SWB) (Keyes and Annas 2009).

Keyes adopted the approach used to diagnose major depression as a theoretical guide for the diagnosis of mental health, which classifies mental health status based on responses to 3 items of emotional well-being and 11 items of positive functioning. This approach has provided a standard to assess and classify the levels of positive mental health and has provided an opportunity for researchers from different countries to compare their study results and to promote the mental health of their own people. Keyes' *Mental Health Continuum Scale* (MHC) has both a long form (MHC-LF) and short form (MHC-SF). We have attempted to test the validity of MHC-SF (which has 14 questions derived from the long form) in China for its distinct advantages of category diagnosis of positive mental health status, time savings, and ease of use in practice.

This chapter presents the results of the cross-cultural application of the MHC-SF in Chinese adults, with three purposes of the study. The purposes were (a) to test the psychometric properties of the MHC-SF satisfactorily in terms of factor structure (including EWB, PWB, and SWB) and internal consistency and validity, (b) to estimate the prevalence of mental health and depression among adult participants from six provinces in China, and (c) to investigate the prevalence of positive mental health and depression by selecting sociodemographic characteristics.

Methods

Sample

We conducted a pre-investigation before we conducted our formal investigation. A total of 125 questionnaires were distributed to primary and secondary school teachers who were accepted within training programs in a university in Yunnan, China, with 109 valid questionnaires having been returned for use in this study. Another 45 questionnaires were given to elderly college students in Yunnan, and of these, 35 valid questionnaires were returned. Additionally, 200 questionnaires were given to teachers who were present at a kindergarten seminar in Chongqing, with 182 valid questionnaires returned. Altogether, a total of 326 valid questionnaires were received from March to May in 2009. Participants consisted of 109 males and 215 females. Of these participants, 113 were aged 20–30 years, 133 were aged 31–40 years, 60 were aged of 41–50 years, and 14 were over the age of 51. As far as education is concerned, 296 had up to 16 years of education, and 39 had between 6 and 12 years of education. Any disparity in numbers is due to missing data.

Stratified cluster sampling was used to investigate adults from Yunnan, Chongqing, Shanxi, Hubei, Beijing, and Guangdong in formal investigations from September 2009 to October 2010. The sociodemographic characteristics of participants were planned in advance: (a) age upward of 20 years, (b) nonstudents, and (c) counterbalancing of participants' gender, age, district, education, employer, and earnings.

Kindergartens, elementary schools, middle schools, and high schools were commissioned to ask the parents of their students to voluntarily complete the questionnaire in a major research project called *Mental Health Service System Countermeasures in China* as a formal investigation by the China Ministry of Education, Philosophy, and Social Sciences. To ensure that questionnaires were completed by parents, the following approaches were employed: (a) special questionnaire instructions were designed to explain the organizer of the investigation, the purpose of the survey, the reason the questionnaire should be finished by parents, and the process of finishing the survey; (b) students were informed to send the questionnaire to their father or mother (or to a grandfather or grandmother) and were instructed to have only one of their parents fill out the questionnaire, and the instructions emphasized that students were not to finish it by themselves; (c) completed questionnaires were inspected strictly during the data entry process, and questionnaires were deleted where three or more items on five demographic data (e.g., not including district data) were not responded to, where responses were filled out with a certain methodological way of answering, or where similar answers were given within a same class.

In addition, in order to completely capture the elder participants over 50 and the younger participants between 20 and 30, we recruited 112 elder students from an elder college to finish the questionnaire (95 questionnaires were valid), and the same method was employed to recruit 120 new staff members from a job training class (112 questionnaires were valid). We also received 27 valid questionnaires by email from adults who lived in Shanghai and Tianjin.

In total, we distributed 2,250 questionnaires and received 2,021 valid questionnaires in return, which is a response rate of 89.82%. According to the responses on the MHC-SF, we removed some questionnaires from the 2,021 received because of missing values, and in the end, 1,981 valid questionnaires were used. Participants consisted of 815 males and 1,142 females. Altogether, 267 participants were between 20 and 30 years of age, 978 were between 31 and 40 years of age, 536 were between 41 and 50 years of age, 82 were between 51 and 60 years of age, and 70 were over the age of 60. Also, 964 participants had completed 16 years of education, 472 had completed 12 years of education, 395 had 9 years of education, and 110 had 6 years of education. As far as employers were concerned, 139 worked in government jobs, 536 worked in public institutions, 463 worked in enterprises, 445 were self-employed, 148 were farmers, and 176 were in other vocations. As far as earnings are concerned, 556 participants' income was less than 1,500 yuan per month, 789 participants' income was between 1,501 and 3,000 yuan per month, 336 participants' income was between 3,001 and 5,000 yuan per month, and 232 participants were earning over 5,001 yuan per month. Geographically, 520 were from Yunnan, 230 were from Chongqing, 309 were from Guangdong, 459 were from Beijing, 166 were from Hubei, 265 were from Shanxi, and 27 were from other provinces in China. Any disparity in numbers is due to missing data.

Measures

Mental Health Continuum-Short Form

The Mental Health Continuum-Short Form (MHC-SF) was translated into Chinese, discussed in a research group, and back translated. During this process, we recruited 12 adults to finish the Chinese version of MHC-SF and asked them to report their views on the items of the questionnaire. According to the results of this small sample investigation, we modified the expression of two items of social well-being (social contribution and social acceptance). The MHC-SF consists of 14 items and measures the degree of (a) EWB (items 1–3, including positive affection/satisfaction with life), (b) SWB (items 4–8, including social acceptance, social actualization, social contribution, social coherence, and social integration), and (c) PWB (items 9–14, including autonomy, environmental mastery, personal growth, positive relations with others, purpose in life, and self-acceptance). Participants were asked to report the frequency of the occurrence of the symptoms described in the 14 items of the MHC-SF from the time period between past 2 weeks to the past 1 month. The response option included *never, once or twice, about once a week, about 2 or 3 times a week, almost every day*, and *every day* and were scored from 0 to 5 (Keyes 2009).

Center for Epidemiological Studies Depression Scale

Radloff developed the *Center for Epidemiological Studies Depression Scale* (CES-D) in 1997 (Radolff 1977). The CES-D consists of 20 items, and participants were asked to respond to questions concerning the frequency with which they felt depression symptoms during the past week. The scale is scored from 0 to 3, and higher scores indicate higher levels of depression (Robinson and Wrightsman 1990, p286). A large sample study showed that the Chinese version of CES-D had good reliability and validity across all ages in urban populations. Cronbach's alpha was 0.90 on the scale, and the correlation of test-retest in the 8-week interval was 0.49. Nineteen points corresponded with the 75th percentile, and 22 points corresponded with the 80th percentile. Radloff reported that 16 points corresponded with the 80th percentile so that using 16 points as the demarcation point may be low in China

Table 6.1 Maximum likelihood estimation of confirmatory factor models of theories of the latent structure of the MHC-SF items (N = 1,981)

Latent model	x^2	df	RMSEA	GFI	AGFI	AIC	CN	χ^2different/df different
1. Independence	18240.197	91						
2. Single factor	3628.047	77	0.153	0.754	0.665	3684.047	60	1043.725 1–2*
3. Two factor	1579.952	76	0.100	0.880	0.835	1637.952	135	2048.095 2–3*
4. Three factor	975.624	74	0.078	0.930	0.901	1037.624	214	302.164 3–4*

*$P < 0.001$

(Zhang et al. 2010). In this study, Cronbach's alpha was 0.88 on CES-D; 50.9 % participants scored less than 16 point, and 25 points corresponded with the 80th percentile. Considering the general demarcation point that was recommended by Radloff, the findings of the large sample study in China, and the findings of this study, we set 22 points as the general demarcation point and defined the people who scored greater than or equal to 22 points as having depressive symptoms.

Subjective Well-Being Face Scale

Andrews and Withey compiled the *Subjective Well-being Face Scale* (SWB-FS) in 1976. This scale provided a method to estimate the degree of subjective well-being using face pictures (Robinson and Wrightsman 1990, p109).

Results

Structure and Psychometrics of Subjective Well-Being

Confirmatory factor analyses were computed to explore the factor structure of the MHC-SF. The results of our pre-investigation initially confirmed three factors (i.e., emotional, psychological, and social well-being), just like the construction proposed by Keyes (2002, 2005). A three-factor model fit the experiment data very well, χ^2 = 166.646, df = 71, χ^2/ df = 2.347, RMSEA = 0.063, GFI = 0.935, AGFI = 0.904. The Chinese version of MHC-SF was slightly modified according to this result.

Table 6.1 shows the results of confirmatory factor analyses on the formal investigation data. According to the methods of Keyes, a two-factor model measure of emotional well-being loaded on one factor, and the measures of psychological and social well-being loaded on the second (Keyes et al. 2008). A single-factor model and a two-factor model were compared with a three-factor model. Both single- and two-factor models indicated poor fit, yielding a root mean square error of approximation (RMSEA) above the threshold of 0.08 adopted by Wu (2009). The RMSEA measure indicated a good fit of the three-factor model, as suggested by the criteria.

Table 6.2 Descriptive statistics of the MHC-SF subscales and total MHC-SF score and validity measures

Mental health dimensions	Internal reliability	Correlations			Validity measures	
		1	2	3	Face scale	CES-D
1. Emotional well-being	0.92				0.46***	–0.48***
2. Social well-being	0.83	0.66***			0.37***	–0.36***
3. Psychological well-being	0.91	0.63***	0.74***		0.43***	–0.41***
4. Total MHC-SF	0.94	0.81***	0.91***	0.92***	0.46***	–0.46***

*$P<0.001$

Both goodness of fit index (GFI) and adjusted goodness of fit index (AGFI) for the three-factor model indicated good fit, but the GFI and AGFI for single- and two-factor models indicated poor fit. The chi-squared statistic of both the single- and two-factor models were significantly higher than the one yielded from the fit of the three-factor model. Hoelter's Critical *N* (CN) for the three-factor model is higher than the recommended cutoff point of 200. Akaike information criterion (AIC) for the three-factor model is lower than AIC for single- and two- factor models. The smaller value of AIC for the model showed better fit (Wu 2009). Thus, the three-factor model was the best-fitting model to these data; its descriptive fit indices suggest it is an excellent fit to the data, and this model replicates the proposed latent structure of positive mental health by Keyes. The chi-squared statistic is susceptible to sample size so that the other indices are also needed for model estimation. The sample size was relatively large ($n=1,981$), and the chi-squared statistic of the three-factor model was also large. However, the overall model fit was good, as indicated by the model index recommended by Wu (2009), so no further amendments to the model were needed.

Table 6.2 presents the internal consistency of the total MHC-SF and three subscales. Wu suggested that Cronbach's alphas should be greater than 0.90 and should not be less than 0.70 to indicate good internal consistency (Wu 2010). The total MHC-SF had high internal consistency ($\alpha=0.94$). The EWB subscale had the highest internal consistency ($\alpha=0.92$), and the PWB had the second highest internal consistency ($\alpha=0.91$). Although the SWB subscale had relatively lower internal consistency ($\alpha=0.83$) in the three subscales, it was also above the recommended cutoff point of 0.80 (Wu 2010, p238). The total MHC-SF scale and its three subscales had good criterion validity. The pairwise correlations between each of the other three subscales were moderate, and all the three correlations were lower than the correlations between the subscales and the total MHC-SF. The correlation of the three subscales to SWB-FS and the correlation of total MHC-SF to SWB-FS were between 0.37 and 0.46 and the total MHC-SF and the three subscales correlated to CES-D between –0.36 and –0.48, where the correlations were significant. The SWB correlated with CES-D and SWB-FS less than with the other two subscales, and the PWB subscale correlated to CES-D and SWB-FS more strongly than the other two subscales.

Table 6.3 Descriptive statistics of the MHC-SF score of pre- and formal investigations and the population prevalence of the positive mental health categories

Descriptive statistics	Emotional well-being mean (St. Dev)	Social well-being mean (St. Dev)	Psychological well-being mean (St. Dev)	Total mean (St. Dev)
Pre-investigation	3.09 (1.21)	3.19 (1.05)	3.39 (0.95)	3.23 (0.92)
Formal investigation	3.21 (1.23)	3.11 (1.15)	3.38 (1.12)	3.24 (1.03)
Population prevalence	Flourishing *N* (%)	Moderately mentally healthy *N* (%)	Languishing *N* (%)	Total *N* (%)
Pre-investigation	124 (38)	187 (57.4)	15 (4.6)	326 (100)
Formal investigation	862 (43.5)	980 (49.5)	139 (7.0)	1,981 (100)

Note: Pre-investigation sample = 326; Formal investigation sample = 1,981

Categories of Positive Mental Health on the Chinese Adult Population

Our pre-investigation and formal investigation showed roughly the same results. In our formal investigation, the total mean score of 1,981 Chinese adult participants was 3.24 on the mental health continuum. The categorical diagnosis with the MHC-SF by Keyes (2009) was applied to the data to obtain estimates of the prevalence of the mental health categories for the population. If individuals reported that they experienced at least seven of the symptoms *every day* or *almost every day*, where one of the symptoms was from the hedonic (i.e., EWB) cluster (i.e., happy, interested in life, or satisfied), they were flourishing. If individuals reported that they *never* or *once or twice* experienced at least seven of the symptoms, where one of the symptoms was from the hedonic (i.e., EWB) cluster (i.e., happy, interested in life, or satisfied), they were languishing. Individuals who did not fit the criteria of flourishing or languishing were categorized as moderately mentally healthy. Based on these diagnostic criteria, the formal investigation revealed that 7.0% of the sample was languishing, 49.5% was moderately mentally healthy, and 43.5% was flourishing. These estimates were similar to those found in our pre-investigation (Table 6.3).

The Prevalence of Mental Health and Depression

Table 6.4 reveals the prevalence estimates of depression episodes and mental health status, as well as the cross-classification of mental health status with depression. Among 1,961 Chinese adults, 43.4% of the participants were flourishing, and 49.5% were in moderate mental health. In the last week before the investigation, most adults (72.2%) did not have depression, whereas 27.8% of adult participants had an episode of depression. Among the adults who did not have depression during

Table 6.4 The prevalence of mental health and depression among 1,961 Chinese adults

	Mental health status							
CES-D score	Languishing		Moderately mentally healthy		Flourishing		Total	
≥22	*N*	(%)	*N*	(%)	*N*	(%)	*N*	(%)
No	56	(2.9)	617	(31.5)	743	(37.9)	1,416	(72.2)
Yes	83	(4.2)	354	(18.1)	108	(5.5)	545	(27.8)
Total	139	(7.1)	971	(49.5)	851	(43.4)	1,961	(100)

the prior week, 37.9% were flourishing in life, 31.5% were moderately mentally healthy, and only 2.9% were languishing. Among the 27.8% of adults who had a depression episode, 5.5% of these depressed adults were flourishing, 18.1% were moderately mentally healthy, and 4.2% were languishing.

In all, 59.7% of languishing adults had an episode of depression, while 36.5% of moderately mentally healthy adults and 12.7% of flourishing adults had a depressive episode during the week before the investigation. Thus, moderately mentally healthy adults were 2.87 times more likely to suffer from depression than were flourishing adults, while this number was 4.7 for languishing adults who suffered from depression compared to flourishing adults. The findings suggest that languishing adults more likely may suffer depression than do flourishing adults.

The Prevalence of Mental Health and Depression by Select Sociodemographics Characteristics

Table 6.5 presents the descriptive epidemiology of the mental health diagnosis on gender, age, education, type of work place, and monthly income. The study did not find a significant difference of the prevalence of mental health and depression between males and females, nor was there a significant difference between ages. However, the study found a significant difference of the prevalence of mental health and depression among participants with different levels of education, among participants with different types of employers, and among participants with different monthly incomes. The most dysfunctional category of languishing with an episode of depression was more prevalent among individuals with 6 years of education, among the self-employed, among adults whose monthly income was less than 1,500 yuan, and among adults whose monthly income was between 3,001 and 5,000 yuan. Pure languishing was more prevalent among individuals with 6 years of education, among self-employed individuals, and among adults whose monthly income was less than 1,500 yuan. Pure flourishing was more prevalent among adults who worked in government agencies, among individuals who worked in public institutions, among adults whose monthly income was more than 5,000 yuan, and among individuals whose monthly income was between 1,501 and 3,000 yuan.

Table 6.5 The prevalence of mental health and depression by select sociodemographic characteristics (N=1,961)

	Mental health status and depression						
	Languishing and depression	Pure languishing	Moderate mental health and depression	Pure moderate mental health	Flourishing and depression	Pure flourishing	Total
Sociodemographics	*N* (%)	*N* (%)	*N* (%)	*N* (%)	*N* (%)	*N* (%)	χ^2
Gender							
Males	33 (4.1)	25 (3.1)	144 (17.9)	259 (32.1)	42 (5.2)	303 (37.6)	0.72 df=5
Females	49 (4.3)	30 (2.7)	205 (18.1)	351 (31)	61 (5.4)	435 (38.5)	
Age							
20–30	12 (4.5)	2 (0.8)	53 (19.9)	95 (35.7)	11 (4.1)	93 (35)	20.77 df=20
31–40	37 (3.8)	35 (3.6)	155 (15.9)	313 (32.2)	52 (5.3)	381 (39.2)	
41–50	26 (4.9)	12 (2.3)	100 (18.9)	157 (29.7)	25 (14.7)	209 (39.5)	
51–60	3 (3.8)	2 (2.5)	17 (21.2)	27 (33.8)	7 (8.8)	24 (30.0)	
61 and over	2 (3.1)	2 (3.1)	12 (18.5)	17 (26.2)	5 (7.7)	27 (41.5)	
Education							
16 or more	39 (4.1)	23 (2.4)	159 (16.6)	297 (31.1)	36 (3.8)	402 (42.1)	37.17** df=15
12 years	21 (4.5)	11 (2.3)	94 (20.0)	132 (28.1)	34 (7.2)	178 (37.9)	
9 years	15 (3.9)	15 (3.9)	69 (17.8)	144 (37.1)	23 (5.9)	122 (31.4)	
6 years	7 (6.5)	6 (5.6)	21 (19.4)	37 (34.3)	9 (8.3)	28 (25.9)	

Workplace type							
Government	1 (0.7)	0 (0)	22 (15.9)	33 (23.9)	11 (8.0)	71 (51.4)	59.57*** df=25
Public institution	19 (3.6)	15 (2.8)	101 (19.1)	149 (28.1)	25 (4.7)	221 (41.7)	
Enterprises	19 (4.1)	10 (2.2)	77 (16.7)	158 (34.3)	26 (5.6)	171 (37.1)	
Self-employed	25 (5.6)	18 (4.1)	73 (16.4)	133 (30.0)	30 (6.8)	165 (37.2)	
Farmer	5 (3.5)	5 (3.5)	32 (22.2)	59 (40.0)	5 (3.5)	38 (26.4)	
Others	13 (7.6)	7 (4.1)	30 (17.4)	67 (39.0)	4 (2.3)	51 (29.7)	
Monthly income							
0–1,500 ¥	24 (4.4)	19 (3.5)	99 (18.1)	194 (35.4)	37 (6.8)	175 (31.9)	31.81** df=15
1,501–3,000 ¥	27 (3.5)	26 (3.3)	127 (16.3)	239 (30.7)	37 (4.7)	323 (41.5)	
3,001–5,000 ¥	17 (5.1)	5 (1.5)	61 (18.2)	104 (31.0)	16 (4.8)	132 (39.4)	
5,001 ¥ and more	9 (3.9)	3 (1.3)	57 (24.6)	56 (24.1)	14 (6.0)	93 (40.1)	

Note: *$p<0.05$ **; $p<0.01$ ***; $p<0.001$ (two tailed)

Conclusion

The mental health continuum (MHC) by Keyes provides a classification for assessing positive mental health status. There are 40 items in the long form of the mental health continuum; of these, 14 of the most representative items were selected from the original subscales in 14 dimensions to form the short form of the mental health continuum for convenient use in clinical assessments. Anchor selection was changed from *agree* and *disagree* (seven score scale from weak to strong) to *never* and *every day* (Keyes et al. 2008). The result from operating the long MHC on American adults (Keyes 2005) and American college students (Robitschek and Keyes 2009) and the results from operating MHC-SF on teenagers showed the long and short form of the mental health continuum fit the American population very well. The potential cross-cultural applicability was shown by the result of operating the MHC-SF on South Africa adults, which also provided support for the mental health continuum model consisting of three factors, as determined by Keyes (Keyes et al. 2008).

The confirmatory factor analysis on the data from operating the MHC-SF on Chinese adults showed the three-factor model was consistent with the data, and the items in the three subscales showed the three factors (emotional well-being, social well-being, and psychological well-being) were three distinguished potential variables which were also related to each other. The results from our research were consistent with those from operating the MHC-SF on American and South Africa adults. Internal consistency reliability (greater than 0.80) was good, as reported by Keyes (2009), and the retest reliability after 2 weeks was 0.64 for EWB, 0.71 for SWB, and 0.71 for PWB. The internal consistency α factor was 0.74 for South Africa participants; particularly, Cronbach's α was 0.73 for emotional well-being, 0.59 for social well-being, and 0.67 for psychological well-being (Keyes et al. 2008). However, Cronbach's α was 0.94 for Chinese adults; particularly, Cronbach's α was 0.92 for EWB, 0.83 for SWB, and 0.91 for PWB. High reliability was shown in operating this questionnaire on Chinese adults, which was consistent with the reliability (0.81–0.91) from operating the long questionnaire on American adults.

That the reliability was consistent for two different populations suggests the Chinese version of the MHC-SF is suitable for Chinese adults and possesses cross-cultural applicability. However, some Chinese participants reported that it was hard for them to account for the frequency of occurrence of the things described in the 14 items for temporal distance from the period between the past 2 weeks to the past 1 month (e.g., the anchors *about once a week* and *about 2 or 3 times a week*) when completing the survey. Moreover, the anchors *almost every day* and *every day* were vague in meaning and often interpreted as "almost once or twice every day," or "a whole 24-hour day."

Based on the above information, the result from operating the MHC-SF on Chinese adults may not reflect the exact frequency, but just a vague estimation, of the occurrence of the three mental health symptoms. It was pointed out by Yang and Zhao (1987) that "twice or three times" does not exactly mean between two or three separate occasions but could mean "seldom" when Chinese people say "I have been there twice or three times." On the contrary, the meaning of these frequency adverbs is more exact when they are spoken by western people; it *really* means twice or three times. Chinese participants do not classified frequency into detailed classes, which is what western participants usually do when discussing the concept of frequency. Therefore, the item occasionally could have meant seldom, similar to what the item twice or three times means (Yang and Zhao 1987).

Keyes chose item of frequency instead of *agree* or *disagree* to evaluate the occurrence of symptoms in the long from in order to keep consistent with the same frequency evaluation used in major depression episodes (Keyes et al. 2008). However, for Chinese people, the items *almost every day* and *every day* are just a general estimation and mean "a lot of the time" or "plenty of times." Additionally, the items *never, once or twice, about once a week*, and *about twice or three times a week* probably mean "never happen," "rarely," and "seldom happen," respectively. In short, the selections of frequency items made by Chinese participants on the MHC-SF were not exact estimations but rather a kind of generally estimated result.

The results from the investigation and pre-investigation were consistent with each other. The second investigation, which provided confirmation with the first, showed that the percentage of participants in poor mental health (i.e., were languishing) was below ten. Forty percent of participants were in good mental health and were flourishing, and about 50–60 % of participants were moderately mentally healthy. It should be emphasized that the sample used in our research may have impacted the results. The investigation was conducted in kindergartens, primary schools, and middle schools, where administrators at these institutions asked their students' parents to complete the questionnaire. Therefore, although the age distribution of adults was included in the consideration of the sample, as were the district, employer, education, and income distribution, the selection of participants was not randomly sampled. According to the sociodemographic characteristics of participants, our research could be used to display the mental health of participants in government, public institutions, enterprises, and the self- employed in large, medium, and small cities within China. The percentage of participants who were farmers was so low in the investigation that this research could not be used to show the mental health of farmers, which is a large percentage of the Chinese population.

The different results of the three mental health statuses between the two investigations on Chinese adults and the two investigations in American and South African samples by Keyes have been displayed. The result from the investigation on American adults was similar to the result from the investigation on South Africa adults in mental health classification. Eighteen percent of the American adults who took part in the investigation by Keyes were flourishing, 65 % of these adults had moderate mental health, and the last 17 % of adults were languishing (Keyes 2005). The average scores of South African adult participants in the EWB and SWB were below three, and the score was 3.3 in psychological well-being, which showed that 20 % of the South African adults who took part in the investigation were flourishing,

68 % of these adults had moderate mental health, and the last 12 % of adults were languishing (Keyes et al. 2008). In previous research, it was found that Chinese adults scored lower than American adults in six dimensions of psychological well-being; American adults scored from 82 to 97 (Ryff 1995), the Chinese adults scored from 70 to 90. The lower score of Chinese adults on PWB might be caused by the traditional Chinese cultural context (Xu et al. 2003).

The doctrine of the golden mean had such a powerful effect on Chinese people's lives that extreme selections were rarely chosen, such as *quite agree* or *quite disagree*. In this research, Chinese adults scored 3.38 on PWB, similar to the scores of South African adults on PWB. A question remains as to whether the higher score that Chinese participants received in six dimensions of PWB was due to Chinese adults having developed autonomy, environmental mastery, personal growth, positive relations with others, purpose in life, and self-acceptance or whether it was simply easier for Chinese participants to make positive responses on the six representative items selected by Keyes for PWB. More research is needed to identify the real reason for this. Through perspective research, we would like to use MHC-LF to investigate this issue further.

Previous research on PWB has found that eastern people had lower happiness feelings than had western people (Diener et al. 1995); however, the reason for lower happiness feelings found in eastern people was that there was a cultural preference of eastern people for low emotional arousal (i.e., to not include "quite" and "excitement") and modest emotional expression, which reduced the degree of distinction on these emotion scales (since they were ignored in the subjective well-being questionnaire—a questionnaire constructed with positive emotion, negative emotion, and life satisfaction; Wu et al. 2009).

The three items of the emotional well-being subscales *happy*, *interested in life*, and *satisfied* were not representative of highly aroused emotion, and it was not easy to arouse modest emotional expression in the MHC-SF. Therefore, the perspective contained in the 14 dimensions of these three subscales tends to be much more suitable to the view of mental health in modern Chinese people. *Relation* and *harmony* were taken as the standard to assess mental health in a traditional Chinese cultural context (Jing and Guo 1998). The view of Chinese mental health included the harmony of the individual self, the harmony of humans to society, and the harmony of humans with a meaningful world (Yang and Zhang 2007). The harmony of body and thoughts, self-acceptance, the unity of knowledge and action, and complete personality were emphasized in the harmony of the individual self; the harmony of humans with a meaningful world referred to pursuing the value of life and having an aim in life. The harmony of the individual self and the harmony of humans with a meaningful world were certainly consistent with the content of psychological well-being and emotional well-being in the MHC-SF. Moreover, the sense of belonging the individual feels to the group, the harmony of interpersonal relationships, the development of personal status, the adaptation of social roles, and the feeling of circumstantial security, which were included in the harmony of humans to society, were consistent with the content of social well-being.

In short, the three-factor mental health continuum model is suitable to measure the mental health of Chinese people, which may explain why a larger percentage of Chinese participants were flourishing. The fact that there were few languishing people may be a reflection of the way Chinese people think. In a sense, the way of thinking represents a cultural characteristic, which is the core of Chinese national culture (Hou 2007). Nisbett and colleagues said that easterners and westerners have different ways of thinking based on their different historical traditions and regional cultures (Nisbett et al. 2001). In their opinion, the way of thinking in the east is holistic: this way of thinking emphasizes the relation of things to one another, the harmony of subjects and circumstance, and the impact of the environment on subjects and acknowledges contradiction and viewing the world from a point of contradiction. Instead, the way of thinking in the west is more analytical: it emphasizes the characteristics of things, seeing and analyzing questions from a point of logic, and noncontradiction.

Three axioms have been included in the Chinese dialect: change, contradiction, and neutrality. The world is in change, and there is no eternal validity and falseness according to the axiom of change. It is said, in contradiction, that all things are composed of a paradox from the opposite spectrum. And neutrality embodies the doctrine of the mean, where modest reasonability is suitable for all things (Peng and Nisbett 1999). The Chinese dialect does not look at problems in any extreme way, and it rarely considers a situation as the worst it could ever be, which may be the reason for why few Chinese participants were languishing.

The result found in this research that indicating that depression symptoms were produced in mentally unhealthy Chinese adults was consistent with the result found by Keyes (2002). Significant differences of mental health status of Chinese adult participants and the prevalence rate of depression on population variables were found with factors such as education, employer, and income, but no significant differences were found for gender and age.

Previous research has pointed out that the satisfaction with life included in Chinese happiness is highly related to their economic status. The research on life satisfaction for Chinese people born at different times showed that the overall life satisfaction decreased from 1990 to 2001 and then increased beginning in 2007. Life satisfaction can be predicted from economic satisfaction and sense of control; economic satisfaction had powerful predictability, especially when in an economic crisis mode (Sun et al. 2010). The income of urban and rural residents has increased distinctively after constant economic development over many years. The panel study of 21 counties and cities in China from 2004 to 2010 showed that there was a significant positive relation between the average family income and the average level of life satisfaction in these counties and cities (Zheng et al. 2010). These situations described above have had a strong relationship with Chinese national conditions. Generally speaking, government and institutions are nationally owned units in China, their staffs have higher education, and the occupational stability, steady income source, and above-average welfare have caused people to develop a deep sense of belonging. However, the majority of the adults had lower education levels, were self-employed or freelancers, and had lower incomes. Their welfare, social status, and sense of belonging were lower than the staff in government and other institutions. Therefore, the percentage of mentally unhealthy participants was higher in this population than in other populations.

Score on the CSE-D was used as an indicator when studying mental illness. Previous research in China has shown that there was a significant statistical difference between the patients with mental illness and the normal population on the score of the CES-D Chinese version. Moreover, the patients with depression and dysthymic disorder had the highest score on the CES-D Chinese version (Zhang et al. 2010). However, the CES-D is not clinical diagnostic criteria or an assessment of disease severity in a therapeutic process (Robinson and Wrightsman 1990, p286) but a scale measuring the frequency of the occurrence of depression symptoms, which emphasizes depressive emotions and mood.

Roughly 12.7 % of flourishing Chinese adults scored more than 22 on the CES-D. Although their score of depression symptoms was higher than the recommended 16, they still were flourishing in positive mental health status, which might show that depression symptoms are not abnormal for Chinese people. Because slightly unhealthy was normal, it could be concluded that *life is full of trouble*—as the Chinese saying goes. It might to be a distinct characteristic of adult mental health in a Chinese cultural context that the score of positive mental health is high as well as the score on the CES-D. Considering current perspective research, more scales, such as the *General Health Questionnaire*, should be used to investigate Chinese mental health problems with the MHC-SF.

References

Cheng, K., & Huang, X. T. (2009). A preliminary research on the structure of college students mental health with a healthy personality orientation. *Psychological Science, 32*, 514–516.

Deng, Y. L., & Dai, J. (2010). A tentative interpretation of mental health criterion with Chinese traditional cultural. *Chinese Journal of Clinical Psychology, 18*, 125–126.

Diener, E., Suh, E. M., Smith, H., & Shao, L. (1995). National differences in reported subjective well-being: Why do they occur? *Social Indicators Research, 34*, 7–32.

Fan, H. Y., & Zhang, J. F. (2005). A meta-analysis of reports concerning SCL-90 and Chinese middle school students during the past10 years. *Psychological Science, 2005*(28), 1424–1426.

Feng, Z. Z., & Dai, Q. (2008). A meta-analysis concerning the mental health status of members of the Chinese army. *Acta Psychologica Sinica, 40*, 358–367.

Hou, Y. B. (2007). Research progress in thinking styles from the perspective of cultural psychology. *Advances in Psychological Science, 15*, 211–216.

Hu, F. J., & Zhang, Q. L. (2009). A meta-analysis of reports concerning SCL-90 of university freshmen. *Journal of Southwest University (Natural Science Edition), 31*, 152–155.

Huang, X. T., Zheng, Y., & Li, H. H. (2006). Nurturance and education of students' healthy personality: A psychological perspective. *Journal of Guangxi Normal University: Philosophy and Social Sciences Edition, 42*, 90–94.

Jing, H. B. (2002). Three approaches to mental health in traditional Chinese culture. *Acta Psychologica Sinica, 34*, 327–332.

Jing, Y., & Guo, I. P. (1998). Historical development of the view of mental health. *Psychological Science, 21*, 465–466.

Keyes, C. L. M. (2002). The mental health continuum: From languishing to flourishing in life. *Journal of Health and Social Behavior, 43*, 207–222.

Keyes, C. L. M. (2005). Mental illness and/or mental health? Investigating axioms of the complete state model of health. *Journal of Consulting and Clinical Psychology, 73*(3), 539–548.

Keyes, C. L. M. (2006a). Mental health in adolescence: Is America's youth flourishing? *The American Journal of Orthopsychiatry, 76*(3), 395–402.

Keyes, C. L. M. (2006b). Subjective well-being in mental health and human development research worldwide: An introduction. *Social Indicators Research, 77*, 1–10.

Keyes, C. L. M. (2009). *Atlanta: Brief description of the mental health continuum short form (MHC-SF)*. Available: http://www.sociology.emory.edu/ckeyes/

Keyes, C. L. M., & Annas, J. (2009). Feeling good and functioning well: Distinctive concepts in ancient philosophy and contemporary science. *The Journal of Positive Psychology, 4*(3), 197–201.

Keyes, C. L. M., Wissing, M., Potgieter, J. P., Temane, M., Kruger, A., & Rooy, S. V. (2008). Research article evaluation of the mental health continuum-short form (MHC-SF) in Setswana-speaking South Africans. *Clinical Psychology & Psychotherapy, 15*(3), 181–192.

Li, J. (2007). An analysis of use frequency of psychological health measurement tools and suggestions. *Journal of South China Normal University (Social Science Edition), 3*, 119–123.

Li, J., Wu, Z. Y., & Han, B. X. (2009). Development of mental health inventory for the elderly (Urban Version). *Chinese Mental Health Journal, 23*, 656–660.

Liao, Q. M., Su, D., & Huang, X. T. (2007). Ordinary questionnaires of mental health in China: Retrospection and reflection. *Psychological Exploration, 27*, 74–77.

Liu, Y. R. (2003). Compiling mental health self scales for primary and middle school students. *Psychological Science, 26*, 515–516.

Luo, M. C., Huang, X. T., Yan, J. H., Fu, Y. F., & Yin, K. L. (2010). A meta- analysis of the mental health status of Chinese minority college students. *Psychological Science, 33*, 779–783.

Meng, W., Yang, Z. N., & Wang, X. M. (2010). A meta–analysis concerning the mental health status of Chinese police. *Psychological Research, 3*, 78–81.

Miao, Y. J., & Zhao, S. (2009). From social well-being to positive mental health model: Introduction and assessment on Keyes. *Psychological Research, 2*, 13–16.

Miao, Y. J., Chen, H. B., & Bai, S. Y. (2008). A new viewing angle on well-being: A description of social well-being. *Social Psychological Science, 23*, 17–21.

Nisbett, R. E., Peng, K., Choi, I., & Norenzeyan, A. (2001). Culture and system of thought: Analytic and holistic cognition. *Psychological Review, 108*, 291–310.

Peng, K. P., & Nisbett, R. E. (1999). Culture, dialectics, and reasoning about contradiction. *American Psychologist, 54*(9), 741–754.

Radolff, L. S. (1977). The CES-D scale: A self- report depression scale for research in the general population. *Applied Psychological Measurement, 1*, 385–401.

Robinson, J. P., & Wrightsman, L. S. (1990). *Measures of personality and social psychological attitudes*. (Yuyin Yan & Xuezhi Zhang (1997), Trans.). Taibei: Yuan-liou publishing co., Ltd.

Robitschek, C., & Keyes, C. L. M. (2009). Keyes's model of mental health with personal growth initiative as a parsimonious predictor. *Journal of Counseling Psychology, 56*(2), 321–329.

Ryff, C. D. (1995). Psychological well-being in adult life. *Current Directions in Psychological Science, 8*(4), 99–104.

Song, Y., Fang, J., & Sun, L. N. (2008). A new general-purpose system of psychological well-being scales: Integrating functions, symptoms and psychogenic analysis. *Psychological Science, 31*, 1195–1197.

Su, D., & Huang, X. T. (2007). A preliminary research on the structure of secondary school students' mental health with an adaptive orientation. *Psychological Science, 30*, 1290–1294.

Sun, R. C., Liu, W. J., & Xu, Y. (2010). Change of life satisfaction of Chinese in different years of birth. *Advances in Psychological Science, 18*, 1147–1154.

Tan, H. P. (1998). Compiling mental health scales for middle school students. *Psychological Science, 21*, 429–432.

Tong, H. J., Yang, Y. J., Li, L. H., Yan, Y. X., & Lv, H. (2010). Development of the mental health style questionnaire and the test of double constructs hypothesis. *Chinese Mental Health Journal, 24*, 473–477.

Wang, J. S., Wei, W. Q., & Din, X. H. (2006). Compiling mental health scales for Chinese adults. *China Public Health, 22*, 137–138.

WHO. (2001). *The world health report: 2001. Mental health: New understanding, new hope*. Retrieved from http://www.who.int/whr/2001/en/

WHO. (2003). *Investing in mental health*. Geneva: World Health Organization. Retrieved from http://bpp.wharton.upenn.edu/betseys/papers/Happiness.pdf

Wu, M. L. (2009). *Structural equation model: AMOS operation and application*. Chongqing: Chongqing University Press.

Wu, M. L. (2010). *Statistical analysis of questionnaire: SPSS operation and application*. Chongqing: Chongqing University Press.

Wu, S. T., Wang, L., Zhou, M. J., Wang, W. Z., & Zhang, J. X. (2009). Belief in a just world and subjective well-being: Comparing disaster sites with normal areas. *Advances in Psychological Science, 17*, 579–587.

Xin, Z. Q., & Zhang, M. (2009). Changes in Chinese middle school students' mental health (1992–2005): A cross temporal meta analysis. *Acta Psychologica Sinica, 41*, 69–78.

Xu, M. Z., & Gong, Y. X. (2004). Development of mental health scale. *Chinese Journal of Clinical Psychology, 12*, 111–115.

Xu, S. L., Wu, Z. P., Wu, Z. Y., Sun, C. H., & Zhang, Y. (2003). Age differences of psychological well-being of Chinese adults. *Chinese Mental Health Journal, 17*, 167–170.

Yang, Z., & Zhang, X. K. (2007). The theoretical construct of mental health conceptions of the modern Chinese. *Psychological Science, 30*, 629–631.

Yang, Z. F., & Zhao, Z. Y. (1987). Contradictory dilemma of Chinese participants: Reflecting on over-reliance on west scale. *Journal of Chinese Psychology, 29*, 113–132.

Yi, X. F., Liu, Y., Liao, J. Q., Dou, D. H., & Peng, K. P. (2010). Changes in Chinese railwaymans mental health (1988–2009): A cross temporal meta analysis. *Journal of Beijing Jiaotong University (Social Sciences Edition), 9*, 47–53.

Yu, G. L., Lin, C. D., & Wang, Y. (1999). Developing mental health scale for students. *Psychological Development and Education, 3*, 49–53.

Yu, G. L., Jin, D. X., & Zheng, J. J. (2010). A study on development of teachers' mental health scale and its status. *Psychological Development and Education, 5*, 295–301.

Zhang, L., & Zuo, B. (2007). Eudaimonic well-being: A review on psychological well-being. *Advances in Psychological Science, 15*, 134–139.

Zhang, J., Wu, Z. Y., Fang, G., Li, J., Han, B. X., & Chen, Z. Y. (2010). Development of the Chinese age norms of CES-D in urban area. *Chinese Mental Health Journal, 24*, 139–142.

Zheng, R. C., Deng, L. F., Zhang, Z. H., & Guo, Z. L. (2005). Development of Chinese college student mental health scale. *Studies of Psychology and Behavior, 3*, 102–108.

Zheng, Y., Zhao, N., & Wang, E. P. (2010). The dynamic relationship between family income and life satisfaction: Based on a panel study about 21 cities and counties from 2004 to 2010. *Advances in Psychological Science, 18*, 1155–1160.

Zhou, C. C., He, J. J., & Xu, L. Z. (2009). First application of Kessler 10 scale to mental health status of the aged in China. *Chinese Journal of Clinical Psychology, 17*, 761–776.

Chapter 7
The Warwick-Edinburgh Mental Well-Being Scale (WEMWBS): Performance in Different Cultural and Geographical Groups

Sarah Stewart-Brown

Public health policy and practice has traditionally focused on the causes of disease rather than the determinants of well-being and has concerned itself more with physical than mental disease. In the United Kingdom and in Europe, this situation is now beginning to change, as evidenced by the publication of the World Health Organization's Action Plan for Europe (2005), the European Commission's European Pact for Mental Health and Well-being (2008), and the mental health and well-being strategies of both Scottish and English governments (Scottish Government 2009; Department of Health 2011). In England at least, the general public and National Health Service patients have played a part in bringing about this change. It seems that they have a clearer concept of the holistic nature of health and of the importance of mental well-being in this context. And with the advent of policy relating to patient and public voices, they now have a greater chance of having their views heard (HM Government 2006). The change has also been supported by a growing body of research which suggests that mental well-being predicts future physical health and longevity (Chida and Steptoe 2008; Pressman and Cohen 2005), with studies providing the evidence for possible neurological and neuroendocrine mechanisms that underpin these observations (Davidson 2004) and with an emerging understanding of the role of mental health and well-being in the management of the increasing burden of chronic disease (DiMatteo et al. 2000).

The concept of mental well-being has been debated within the context of the UK public health (Freidli 2006; Huppert and Whittington 2004; Huppert 2008), as it has elsewhere. In the context of policy making in the UK, it is now conceived eclectically (Parkinson 2007; HM Government 2009), encompassing both subjective and psychological well-being (Keyes et al. 2002; Ryan and Deci 2001). There has been debate in the UK, as well as internationally, over the relationship of mental well-

---

S. Stewart-Brown (✉)
Warwick Medical School, University of Warwick,
Coventry, UK
e-mail: Sarah.Stewart-Brown@warwick.ac.uk

C.L.M. Keyes (ed.), *Mental Well-Being: International Contributions to the Study of Positive Mental Health*, DOI 10.1007/978-94-007-5195-8_7,

being to mental illness (Tudor 1996; Keyes 2007). Most now see this relationship as more complicated than a single continuum, and the term mental health has come to cover the range of continua envisaged within the field. This is different from the past, in which the term *mental health* was used almost exclusively to cover mental illness and mental illness services, and almost all epidemiologically accepted measures of mental health aimed to measure levels of mental illness.

The Development of the Warwick-Edinburgh Mental Well-Being Scale (WEMWBS)

In this evidence-based day and age, policies need outcomes and outcomes need to be measurable. Interventions and approaches developed to implement these policies need to be evaluated. The lack of measures of mental well-being was, therefore, seen to be a problem (Stewart-Brown 2002). It was with these needs in mind that the Warwick-Edinburgh Mental Well-Being Scale (WEMWBS) was developed (Tennant et al. 2007a) on funding provided by the Scottish Government as part of the development of their new mental health policies. Working with colleagues from many different disciplines while developing this scale, the aim was to provide a short instrument which was easily understood, accepted by the public as a measure of mental health, practical, and inexpensive, to be included in large-scale health surveys. The central tenet of development was that the instrument would focus both on positive aspects of mental health and the key attributes of mental well-being discussed in the literature. It aimed to combine both eudemonic and hedonic principles and aspects of both psychological and subjective well-being (Ryff and Keyes 1995; Diener et al. 1985).

The final instrument includes 14 items, all of which are positively worded and all of which cover positive aspects of mental health. The instrument has five levels of response to be assessed over a 2-week period, from none of the time to all of the time. Close scrutiny of the items evokes an echo of familiar and very well-established mental health scales, such as the General Health Questionnaire (Goldberg and Williams 1988). Indeed, the only difference between some of the items is in the negative: "I've been losing confidence in myself" in contrast to the positive "I've been feeling confident." While this could beg the question of what WEMWBS adds to the current knowledge, those working in mental health promotion and public mental health more generally perceive there to be an important difference. Practitioners in the UK say that they used to feel very ambivalent about evaluating their mental-health-promoting projects and programs with existing scales, with items focused on, for example, feeling "down in the dumps." WEMWBS proclaims the purpose of the project with the implicit statement: "This is what we want for you." Such practitioners have intuitively recognized that which the discipline of positive psychology has demonstrated (Linley and Joseph 2004), that is, what you pay attention to is what you get more of, and that when promoting the positive, it is essential to focus on the positive. At some level, the use of positive scales like WEMWBS, in both surveys and evaluations, has thus become a mental-health-promoting intervention in its own right. Since the

The Warwick-Edinburgh Mental Well-Being Scale (WEMWBS), Below are some statements about feelings and thoughts

Please tick the box that best describes your experience of each over the last 2 weeks Statements	None of the time	Rarely	Some of the time	Often	All of the time
I've been feeling optimistic about the future	1	2	3	4	5
I've been feeling useful	1	2	3	4	5
I've been feeling relaxed	I	2	3	4	5
I've been feeling interested in other people	1	2	3	4	5
I've had energy to spare	1	2	3	4	5
I've been dealing with problems well	1	2	3	4	5
I've been thinking clearly	1	2	3	4	5
I've been feeling good about myself	1	2	3	4	5
I've been feeling close to other people	1	2	3	4	5
I've been feeling confident	1	2	3	4	5
I've been able to make up my own mind about things	1	2	3	4	5
I've been feeling loved	1	2	3	4	5
I've been interested in new things	1	2	3	4	5
I've been feeling cheerful	1	2	3	4	5

Warwick-Edinburgh Mental Well-Being Scale (WEMWBS)

publication of the validation of this instrument, it has been incorporated into key national health surveys in Scotland and England as well as into a host of other large surveys and cohort studies. In Scotland, a reduction in WEMWBS score is now one of seven health targets for the Scottish Government and in England WEMWBS is recommended for monitoring mental well-being at national level as part of the new Public Health Outcomes Framework (Department of Health 2012)

The original validation of WEMWBS was undertaken in a large representative population in Scotland, with a group of students at Scottish and English universities and with focus groups in both countries (Tennant et al. 2007a). While the student sample, in particular, and Scottish and English populations more generally are multicultural, white British responses were predominant in the validation. Culture is self-evidently important to the interpretation of concepts of well-being, and while concepts dating back to ancient Greece have informed current thinking, the latter has arisen predominantly in modern, western capitalist societies (Christopher and Hickinbottom 2008). In order for WEMWBS to be used to monitor positive mental health at the national level, and in order to discriminate and investigate social inequalities in health (which may be culturally determined), it is critically important to know that the instrument works for all sectors of the population.

Cross-Cultural Validation of WEMWBS

The National Institutes for Mental Health in England provided a small grant to begin to embark on the process of cross-cultural validation of WEMWBS in England. After deliberation, we chose to focus on two distinct cultural groups: Muslims from Pakistan and the Chinese. We were influenced in this decision by a recent report from Scotland in which a review of the literature relating to concepts of mental well-being had been undertaken, focusing on these two groups (Newbiggging et al. 2008) which allowed our limited resources to be devoted to data gathering and analysis. At the same time, we recognized that both groups represented relatively distinct cultures, influenced by specific spiritual and philosophical traditions, which were therefore likely to reveal diversity in the conceptualization of mental well-being. However, neither group is homogeneous. While both have been established in the UK for many decades, they include recent and long-term immigrants who live in a variety of socio-economic circumstances, university students, young people who have been born and educated in the UK, and elderly who socialize almost exclusively within their own community. The Chinese community in the UK includes a high proportion of students and encompasses Chinese from both Hong Kong and mainland China. While we were limited by the resources available for the project, to working with members of these minority groups who spoke English to complete the WEMWBS in English (the group most relevant from the point of view of large-scale population surveys with English questionnaires), We worked with two community workers who were able to translate for participants when this was requested or seemed appropriate.

Measures of positive mental health are in demand from diverse parts of the world. We have now given permission for WEMWBS to be used in Australia, Canada, the United States, Italy, Spain, Germany, France, the Netherlands, Belgium, Iceland, India, Pakistan, Malaysia, and South Africa. So far, two of these research groups have completed formal quantitative evaluations of WEMWBS. Both Paola Gremigni in Italy and Marie Wissing in South Africa (with the Setswana community) have given permission for their results to be included in this chapter. These studies add much to the current topic due to their valuable translations of WEMWBS into other languages and therefore begin to provide a picture of how the instrument might work with black African cultures.

Methods Involved in Validating WEMWBS with Pakistani and Chinese Communities in the UK

We undertook both quantitative and qualitative investigations of WEMWBS in two minority ethnic English communities. We worked with one of the Primary Care Trusts (the organizations which manage primary care and public health services in England) and a local charity in Birmingham, a city with a high proportion of minority ethnic inhabitants and a high level of social inequalities. The Trust employed community workers for both of the communities we were interested in and gave invaluable help in designing the study. Neither of these communities had been known to be typically easy to access. Few people, especially in the Pakistani community, were familiar with or interested in university research, and many were reluctant to give personal details to strangers. In both groups and among Chinese men in particular, there is reluctance to discuss mental health. With the help of the community workers, we developed an approach that was tailored to each community and involved door-to-door assessment in streets with high proportions of Pakistani residents, most of whom knew each other having immigrated from one community in Pakistan; direct contact with people through fitness gyms, access to which was at that time being provided free of charge in deprived communities; and contact through taxi bases, sewing groups, youth groups, and from social network groups. The Chinese community members were approached by the community worker at places where they typically gathered on Sundays or at Chinese restaurants, supermarkets, travel agencies, hairdressers, local colleges, local housing associations, and by word of mouth. We offered £20 to focus group participants to cover their expenses and a mobile phone voucher worth £2.00 to those who completed the questionnaires. For the quantitative evaluation, we were able to supplement the data we had collected with data derived from a representative population survey undertaken in Coventry, a smaller, multiculturally deprived city close to Birmingham. Public health practitioners in this locality had undertaken a general population survey, which included WEMWBS alongside 44 other health-related questions, in a survey that took 15 min to complete. The data collection team used a quota sampling method to achieve a representative population and undertook interviews on doorsteps and on the street using computer-assisted technology. Overall, the respondents were representative of the population of the city in terms of demographic characteristics, with 44 % engaged in paid work, nearly half of which were male (48 %), and with a good spread across age range. Out of a total population of 3,750 (from a sampling frame of 8,500—a response rate of 44 %), data were collected on 43 Chinese and 94 Pakistani respondents, and these were included in the quantitative evaluation.

For the Birmingham study, a booklet containing WEMWBS together with two comparator scales—the General Health Questionnaire (GHQ-12; Goldberg et al. 1997) and the WHO-5 Well-Being Index (Bech 2004) with demographic details—was designed by the research team at Warwick University and approved by representatives of the Chinese and Pakistani community in Birmingham, by public health practitioners working in the Primary Care Trust, and by the University Ethics Committee. The latter involved considerable negotiation because committee members felt that in order to get effective consent, participants should be offered a week between first contact and taking part in the study, an approach which was not considered practical or necessary by community workers. Letters of invitation for door-to-door and on-the-spot recruitment, information sheets, thank you cards, and consent forms for both the survey and the focus groups were also approved.

Community workers distributed 120 questionnaires in each community using a quota sampling method so that equal numbers of men and women were represented and so that the age mix reflected that of the UK population. Many people who were approached declined to complete the questionnaire. Most participants answered the questionnaire on the spot, but some preferred to take it away to complete at home.

Of those who agreed to take a questionnaire, for the Pakistani group, 107 out of 120 (89%) questionnaires were returned, while for the Chinese group, 116 out of 120 (97%) were returned. The mean age of respondents was 48 (SD 9.0) for the Pakistani community, with a preponderance of young and middle-aged respondents. In the Chinese community, the mean age for men was 47 (SD 9.3), and for the women, the mean age was 50 (SD 11.2); there was a good spread across the age range. In both groups, even though just over half of the participants had been born in the UK, three quarters were less confident in English than they were in their first language. Half of those in the Pakistani community and two thirds of those in the Chinese community were engaged in paid work. Furthermore, all participants in the Pakistani group reported their religion to be Islam, and three quarters of the Chinese reported no religion.

Five age- and gender-specific focus groups were held in the Pakistani community: men aged 16–24 years, men aged 25–49 years, men aged 50–75 years, women aged 16–24 years, and women aged 25–49 years. Three age-specific groups were held in the Chinese community: ages 16–24 years, ages 25–49 years, and ages 50–75 years. Ten people were invited to each group. Participants were all able to speak English, with the exception of one older Chinese woman and three middle-aged Pakistani women for whom the community worker or other young women interpreted, respectively. We defined English speaking as the capacity to complete the questionnaire since this is how it would be defined in any population survey.

Quantitative Findings

We undertook an evaluation of content, construct, and criterion validity, as well as an assessment of internal consistency, with data on a total of 159 Chinese and 211 Pakistani participants (using data from both Birmingham and Coventry). Tim Friede, in Germany, undertook the main statistical analysis and Alan Tennant, from Leeds University, undertook a Rasch analysis.

WEMWBS' content validity in these two communities was good. There were no significant floor or ceiling effects, and all level of response categories were checked for all items by at least one respondent in each community (see Fig. 7.1). Some block responding was evident at a mean of 42, which meant that respondents were likely to have checked the middle level for all 14 items; this problem was not marked. Pakistani respondents were more likely to miss individual items than Chinese respondents; they were most likely to miss item 1 "I've been feeling optimistic about the future" and item 14 "I've been feeling cheerful."

Among the Pakistani community, several items were rarely scored as *none of the time*. These items were 2, 3, 7, 8, and 9 (feeling useful, relaxed, thinking clearly, feeling good about oneself, and feeling close to others). For the Chinese community, the only item which was rarely scored as *none of the time* was item 12 (feeling loved).

The results of the latent variable confirmatory factor analyses for a single factor solution are shown in Table 7.1. The goodness of fit index and adjusted goodness of fit index were acceptable for both communities and compare well with that achieved in the origi-

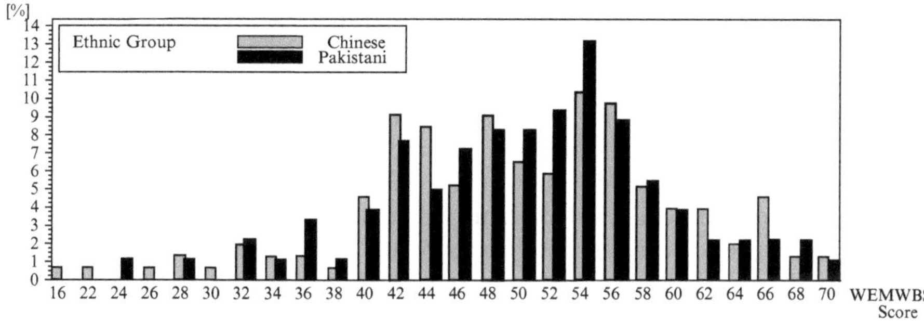

Fig. 7.1 Score distributions for WEMWBS in Chinese and Pakistani samples

Table 7.1 Confirmatory factor analysis of WEMWBS in Chinese and Pakistani groups and the majority of the UK population

Measure	Chinese ($n=154$)	Pakistani ($n=183$)	Tennant et al. (2007a, b): gen population ($n=1,749$)	Tennant et al. (2007a, b): students ($n=348$)
Goodness of fit index (GFI)	1.00	1.00	0.91	0.93
Adjusted goodness of fit index (AGFI)	1.0	1.0	0.87	0.89
Root mean square error of approximation (RMSEA)	0.0464	0.0455	0.0502	0.0551
Chi-square statistic (df) *P* value	$p=0.035$	$p=0.025$	$p<0.05$	$p<0.01$

nal population. The root mean square error of approximation (RMSEA) was somewhat below the desirable level. Also, there was a significant lack of goodness of fit ($P=0.035$ for the Chinese and $P=0.025$ for the Pakistani group). These results are similar to those obtained with the original validation of WEMWBS in the general population. They are consistent with the Eigen values, which were 7.33 (Chinese) and 6.8 (Pakistani) for the first factor, below 1 for other factors in the Chinese group, and were just greater than 1 in the Pakistani group for a second (1.1) and third factor (1.01). The difference between the Eigen values for the strongest factor and the other factors in the two communities is reasonably strong evidence in favor of a one factor solution.

With regard to internal consistency, Cronbach's alphas were high: 0.92 in the Chinese and 0.91 in the Pakistani groups, suggesting there may be room to shorten the scale as we found in the main validation. With regard to item total correlation, which measures whether responses vary for each item in line with the total score, we found that item 1, "I've been feeling optimistic," had the lowest correlation in the Pakistani group. The next lowest was item 5; "I've had energy to spare." Among the Chinese, the lowest item correlation was found with item 4, "I've been feeling interested in other people," but the difference between items was not marked. In both groups, items 8 "I've been feeling confident" and 10 "I've been feeling good about myself" had the highest item correlation ($p > 0.70$).

Criterion validity could only be assessed in the Birmingham group because the relevant data were not collected in the Coventry Household Survey. Spearman correlation coefficients for WEMWBS with the GHQ-12 were as follows: −0.63 with the Chinese and −0.58 with the Pakistani community. Correlation with the WHO-5 general well-being scale was lower than we found in the original validation (0.77): among the Chinese, it was 0.62, and among the Pakistani is 0.64.

Rasch Model Analysis

Rasch modeling was developed to investigate the psychometric properties of scales and instruments. Based initially on examination data, it assumed a hierarchy among items with questions being more or less difficult to answer. It also assumed that each item retained its hierarchical order in all cases (or students). Instruments which meet Rasch criteria have the important property of numerical scaling, so the difference between 5 and 10 can be assumed to the same as the difference between 20 and 25. These assumptions are implicitly made about most instruments used to measure mental health, but they are not necessarily justifiable from a mathematical point of view. Lack of fit to the Rasch model does not invalidate a scale, but it does violate many of the assumptions of the statistical tests which are used to assess their significance and the implicit assumptions about the scores. Such scales can show respondents to be higher or lower on a scale than other respondents but are not clear as to how much better or worse they are.

The initial analysis of WEMWBS data from both minority ethnic groups in both cities, together and separately, showed a poor fit to Rasch model assumptions. This was no surprise, as WEMWBS data from the majority population in the UK also showed a poor fit with this model (Stewart-Brown et al. 2009). The latter analyses identified a seven-item scale, which we have called SWEMWBS (the shortened WEMWBS), that met Rasch criteria well. This shortened scale is now being used in many surveys where respondent burden is an issue.

The fit of SWEMWBS minority ethnic data to the Rasch model was much better than the fit of WEMWBS data. This was true both in individual minority groups and in the combined dataset. The results were characterized by chi-square fit, strict unidimensionality, and the absence of local dependency of data. Rasch analysis identifies items that show differential item functioning (DIF), that is, they seem to be answered in different ways by different groups relative to their overall responses or total scores. In the original analysis (Stewart-Brown et al. 2009), for example, we found that the item "I've been feeling confident" showed significant DIF for gender. At each level of WEMWBS' score, men were more likely to report more confidence. This finding seems to replicate past observations and, at some level, reassures that the scale is working well. At the mathematical level, however, it caused problems in

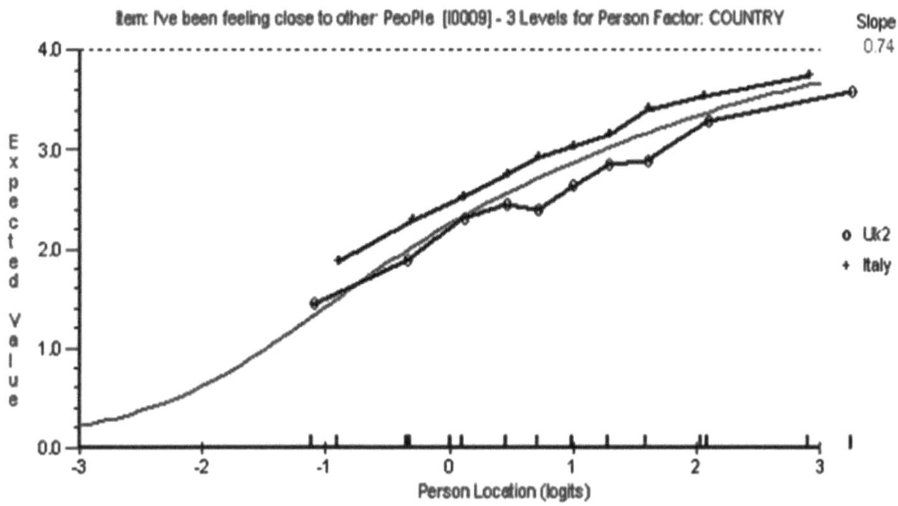

Fig. 7.2 Differential item functioning by nationality in samples from the UK and Italy

that the item needed to be abandoned. Among the Pakistani and Chinese communities, one item showed DIF in the SWEMWBS data at a marginal level that was corrected for in the analysis. This was item 7; "I have been thinking clearly." Interestingly, the DIF here was both minority group and community specific; the Birmingham Pakistanis and Coventry Chinese rated the item similarly with regard to their total scores, as did the Coventry Pakistanis and Birmingham Chinese. The latter rated the item higher at the same level of overall well-being or total score. This analysis also identified about 5 % of respondents who block responded, that is, who answered all questions at one level. We saw this in Fig. 7.1. It is inevitable that some respondents will answer in this way, aiming to complete the question rapidly rather than thoughtfully, but this can create problems with the data by reducing variability in response. The respondents who did this were mostly young. When block responders where removed from the analysis, the fit of the SWEMWBS data improved further in both the Chinese and Pakistani samples.

Validation in Italian and Setswana Communities

Paola Gremigni translated and back translated SWEMWBS and collected data from 325 people in Bologna, Italy, with a mean age of 39 years. She found that that the shortened instrument worked well in this context. Rasch modeling showed no local dependency of data, strict unidimensionality, and chi-square fit to the model. In the Italian sample, she found no differential item functioning, but when the data were pooled with a sample of similar size and age distribution from the UK, she found DIF for nationality on four items. Figure 7.2 illustrates this DIF with regard to item 9;

The Short Warwick-Edinburgh Mental Well-being Scale (SWEMWBS)

Below are some statements about feelings and thoughts.

Please tick the box that best describes your experience of each over the last 2 weeks

STATEMENTS	None of the time	Rarely	Some of the time	Often	All of the time
I've been feeling optimistic about the future	1	2	3	4	5
I've been feeling useful	1	2	3	4	5
I've been feeling relaxed	1	2	3	4	5
I've been dealing with problems well	1	2	3	4	5
I've been thinking clearly	1	2	3	4	5
I've been feeling close to other people	1	2	3	4	5
I've been able to make up my own mind about things	1	2	3	4	5

"I've been feeling close to other people." As we might have guessed, at each level of WEMWBS, Italian people scored this item higher than British. As with the excess of confidence in men identified above, this is entirely consistent with caricatures of national characteristics. When all four items were considered together in the combined populations, their effects canceled each other out, meaning that cross-national characteristics are valid (Gremigni and Stewart-Brown 2011).

Marie Wissing undertook a more sophisticated translation with sensitivity to cultural factors and use of a research committee to translated into Setswana. Setswana is one of the 11 official languages of southern Africa used by approximately four million people. This language has much in common with Sesotho and Sepedi, and together, these three languages are used by a quarter of the South African population. As part of a major epidemiological project in the northwest province of South Africa, she collected WEMWBS data on a randomly selected community sample of 581 adults (mean age 55.7 year) living in urban areas. Structured interview format was used for illiterate people. Preliminary analyses suggest that WEMWBS is working well in this population. Item total correlations ranged from 0.46 for item 1, "I've been feeling optimistic about the future," to 0.64 for item 8, "I've been feeling good about myself." In confirmatory factor analysis using the principal components method of factor extraction, all items loaded on a single factor, with loadings ranging from 0.53 for item 5, "I've had energy to spare," to 0.71 for item 9, "I've been feeling close to other people." Cronbach's alpha was 0.88.

Levels of Mental Well-Being in Minority Groups

These various quantitative validations have provided mean scores for WEMWBS, and they show significant differences between ethnic groups and geographical locations. In the UK, given their socioeconomic circumstances and the assumption that the latter are a key determinant of well-being, minority groups' scores were surprisingly higher (i.e., showed better mental well-being) than those of the general population in the UK. What was also notable was that those living in Coventry from either ethnic group reported higher levels of well-being than those living in Birmingham ($F = 5.92$, $p < 0.001$). The Italian population that took part in the Bologna validation recorded significantly lower scores on SWEMWBS than the UK population, and the Setswana community recorded the highest scores of all (i.e., best mental well-being of all). Given the response rates to some of the surveys in which the data were collected (42 % in Coventry overall and unknown but anecdotally well below 50 % in the minority ethnic communities in both cities), significant questions remain about the representativeness of some of the samples; we need to be cautious when interpreting these very interesting findings. However, they provide a fruitful area for further research with highly significant implications for our understanding of the determinants of mental well-being.

Qualitative Findings

In our Birmingham study, we had the opportunity to undertake qualitative research with a number of age and—in the Pakistani community—gender-specific focus groups. The groups were gender specific in the Pakistani community because the community worker advised that it would be unlikely that we would be able to persuade women to speak freely of these matters in the presence of their male relatives or neighbors. The purpose of this aspect of the research was to identify whether participants understood the instrument and the individual items and whether they found them acceptable. We also aimed to explore what participants understood by mental well-being and whether they thought the instrument addressed these perceptions. Groups were run by Frances Taggart, and all were also attended by a community worker from the relevant community. The researcher worked from a topic guide and recorded all group conversations. All the recordings were transcribed in full.

General Impressions of WEMWBS

Focus group members completed WEMWBS together with some basic demographic details before the discussions began. They were first asked to offer general comments about the instrument, and responses to this were positive. Group members described the questionnaire as easy to complete, easy to understand, and acceptable. Some commented that they positively enjoyed the opportunity it offered for self-reflection. A small number of people commented that the questions were a bit general and nonspecific. Some said that while they understood the questions themselves, the questions might be misunderstood by others who lacked the capacity for self-reflection. There was some concern that other people might be inclined just to check all items at the highest level. This comment, coming from a Chinese group, stands in contrast to what others have found about the Chinese that there is a cultural modesty which means that they are unlikely to say they are feeling wonderful even if they are (Christopher 1999). The comment was also made that the subjective responses collected in completing WEMWBS might not concur with an objective view of that individual's mental health.

Reflections of Individual Items

Half of the items (6, 7, 8, 9, 10, 12, and 14) posed no problems for either minority group. Discussions sometimes revealed a sophisticated understanding of the nature of well-being, for example, the reciprocal nature of cheerfulness (item 14: "If you were cheerful with others, they cheered up and could be more cheerful with you and vice versa"). Discussion about item 12, "I've been feeling loved," revealed the various levels on which this could be interpreted, including consideration by others, support, love for others because that was part of religious duty, the love of god, and the fact that some people found it easier to love than others because that was in their character. Some of these findings are consistent with the quantitative analyses. In particular, the items "I've been feeling good about myself" (item 8) and "I've been feeling confident" (item 10) were those with the highest item total correlation. However, it is interesting that only three out of these seven easily understood items (6, "I've been dealing with problems well"; 7, "I've been thinking clearly"; and 9, "I've been feeling close to other people") were retained in the Rasch modeling and are, therefore, represented in SWEMWBS.

Several items created discussion about context. Participants queried in what context they were meant to think about "feeling relaxed" (item 3), "feeling useful" (item 2), or "interested in new things" (item 13). Was this, they asked, intended to relate to work, home, or leisure? However, there was also some sophisticated discussion about "feeling useful" and how this related to self-confidence or (especially among the women from both communities) being busy and having no time for oneself or shouldering responsibility. Among the Chinese community, some respondents talked about being useful to themselves in the context of being able to prove themselves to others. Individuals made the connection between lack of "interest in new things" and fear of change, which was regarded as negative. Issues related to the use of drugs and alcohol were also raised in discussions about "feeling relaxed."

Two items were well understood but clearly interpreted differently from the UK population in both minority groups. In both communities, but especially the Pakistani community, there was discussion about the item "I've been able to make up my own mind about things" (item 11). While this was appropriately linked to self-confidence, group members also described how it was considered inappropriate, even arrogant, to not consult and take advice from elders and family members in their community. Discussions in the different groups revealed some age differences here, with the young showing more inclination to make their own decisions and expressing frustration at not being allowed to. The item "I've had energy to spare" revealed interesting cultural differences relating to the Chinese understanding of the importance of physical activity in raising energy levels.

Two items created discussion because they were not clearly understood by all group members. One of these was item 1, "I've been feeling optimistic about the future." There is no direct translation of the word *optimism* in Pashtun, the language of most Pakistani focus group members. The nearest group members came to this were *feeling good about the future*, but other group members said things like "I am not sure what that means" and "I don't like that question." The other item which created some confusion was item 13, "I've been feeling interested in other people." While the observation that people who are stressed tend to withdraw socially was made, together with comments about the need for self-confidence, others thought this item might be interpreted negatively as being *nosey* or *gossipy*. Some of the young men said they interpreted this in sexual terms: whether they were "interested" in girls.

A significant qualitative study was undertaken during the WEMWBS development project on another mental well-being instrument: the Affectometer 2 (Tennant et al. 2006). Validation of the latter instrument was the starting point for the development of WEMWBS. However, qualitative data relating to WEMWBS from the general UK population is limited to two focus groups undertaken in 2006 (Tennant et al. 2006). The latter studies showed that the UK general population finds WEMWBS easy to understand and acceptable to complete, but there is little in the way of qualitative data reviewing individual items. However, item 1 which states "I've been feeling optimistic" was one of the items that was spontaneously mentioned in these groups as causing difficulty because people were not sure of their response. This is rather different from saying that it was not understood. The other items that were spontaneously mentioned in this context were item 9, "I've been feeling close to other people," and item 4, "I've been feeling interested in other people." The context in which these items were mentioned was said to be "emotional," meaning that reflection on their responses brought feelings of sadness.

A much larger qualitative study was undertaken in the recent validation of WEMWBS among 13–15-year-old youth in schools (Clarke et al. 2011) and two items, where item 1, "I've been feeling optimistic," and item 4, "I've been feeling interested in other people," caused the most difficulty with this age group. Item 1 was also the item with the lowest item total correlation in quantitative analysis of Pakistani data, yet it was retained in the Rasch modeling and is therefore represented in SWEMWBS. Item 4 was the item with the lowest item total correlation among the Chinese; this item caused some problems with the Rasch modeling and is not represented in the shortened version, SWEMWBS.

Qualitative Findings Relating to Concepts of Mental Well-Being

In focus group discussions, members were also asked to talk about their general perceptions of mental well-being. Overall, this was not a concept that either community understood. All groups focused instead on mental illness and poor mental health. This finding is consistent with studies on the majority population (Tennant et al. 2006). With respect to mental illness, the key issues raised by both minority groups were those related to shame and stigma. In neither community was it acceptable to acknowledge mental health problems. Nor did either community find it acceptable to seek help for such problems from health services. Shame was powerfully felt by family members as well as the individual, so becoming mentally ill had wider ramifications than it might in the general population.

Among the Pakistani community, women talked of finding help in support from other women and in religion; men talked of hiding, of returning home to Pakistan, and of Islam. In both groups, the family was seen to be a key support. Pakistani groups identified unemployment, social isolation, poor physical health, and the rigors of cultural adaptation as causes of mental distress. Another specific and real cause was worry about other family members, particularly in the context of how others might judge how *well* they were doing.

Among the Chinese, conversation turned to the need for endurance and getting on with things, not in complaining or blaming. There was some discussion within the groups on the value of *denial* as the appropriate coping mechanism, with some feeling that this was an inappropriate strategy, especially among relatives; still, there was a sense that it was considered inappropriate and bad manners to burden others with one's own distress. Groups spoke of Chinese understanding of positive and negative energy. Negative thoughts create negative energy, which affects others and is bad for all. It was therefore important to find ways to lift one's spirit. Here again, the importance of physical activity was mentioned, as well as general outlook on life and family support. The family was identified as the place where children should learn how to live in the right way and that *right living* protected against mental health problems. However, it was said that not all families offer this to their children, and families were also mentioned as a place where bad things could be learned.

Qualitative Findings in the Context of the Wider Literature

These findings are broadly in line with the findings of Newbiggging (2008) in her review of the literature relating to cultural concepts of mental well-being and her qualitative study with community workers in Pakistani and Chinese communities in Scotland. She found that the Chinese understood the term happiness, but not mental well-being. Pakistanis equally did not understand mental well-being and talked more of peace of mind and contentment. Both groups understood and talked about the concept of feeling good about oneself, and freedom from worry came up as important for happiness/contentment. Both freedom for worry (feeling relaxed) and feeling good about oneself are represented in WEMWBS, but not contentment or peace of mind.

Both groups identified the need to achieve a balance in life for it to be healthy and rewarding. For the Chinese, a good life also included prosperity; for the Pakistanis, serenity. Both groups were also clear about the need for acceptance of the inevitable, bowing to fate, and fulfilling family and gender obligations. Living in harmony with the others was of preeminent importance, together with interdependence in family and community. The Chinese identified peaceful attitudes toward others; the Pakistanis identified the concept of collective shame. Both groups reported that the need for acceptance by others was strong, with the suggestion that this is more important than acceptance by self.

The Chinese identified endurance and hard work as protective. They believed that living a virtuous life, which required internal strength, leads to material abundance, status, and health. Pakistanis identified patience and fulfilling family and religious duties as protective.

While there are items relating to relationships with others in WEMWBS, these fall short of describing the preeminence of harmonious relationships described by these two communities. WEMWBS, reflecting western influences, does not cover balance in life, acceptance of fate, serenity, endurance, or fulfilling obligations or responsibilities.

Conclusions

So what does all this mean for the use of WEMWBS, and the shortened version SWEMWBS, in cultures and countries other than that in which they were developed? From a quantitative point of view, it would seem that both instruments perform better than could reasonably have been expected. There are very significant differences between the different cultures' views of mental health, and they have very different beliefs about its determinants. Nevertheless, these quantitative evaluations in diverse communities suggest WEMWBS and SWEMWBS perform as well as they do with the UK general population. It also seems that other cultural groups find the instrument acceptable and that, in general, people understand the items and enjoy filling them in.

With regard to the choice of WEMWBS or SWEMWBS, both continue to have their advantages. WEMWBS contains a number of items that are associated with concepts of positive mental health in other cultures that are not represented in SWEMWBS (feeling good about self and confident) and therefore may have greater face validity. SWEMWBS includes one of the items (optimism) that seems to cause most problems with all groups who have been asked for their views. The advantage of SWEMWBS' unidimensional scaling properties is great not only in monitoring general population health and well-being, but also for confidence in statistical assessment of the significance of differences attributed to interventions. SWEMWBS also represents half of the respondent burden. However, it is in the nature of mental well-being that different cultures and genders will respond to items differently and these differences may result in differential item functioning with regard to total score. So whether a strictly Rasch compatible instrument is practical in mental well-being remains to be seen. It would be satisfying if the items that seem to cause people problems in qualitative analysis were also those which cause problems in the quantitative analyses, but this does not often seem to be the case (Scott et al. 2010). One advantage of WEMWBS over SWEMWBS is that data is beginning to come in from empirical studies, both controlled and uncontrolled, showing that WEMWBS is sensitive to the changes that might be expected to occur in mental health promotion programs. To date, we do not have such data for SWEMWBS.

At the same time, it is clear that some items in WEMWBS and SWEMWBS cause difficulty in minority populations. Some of the offending items have been identified as causing difficulty with groups of the majority population, as well. Others, like items representing autonomy, though not creating difficulty, do carry different meanings with regard to mental health in minority groups. These do not necessarily seem to show differential item functioning as might be expected. Some concepts of importance to mental health in minority groups, for example, peace of mind and doing one's duty toward others, are not adequately represented in WEMWBS. While items reflecting relationships are featured in the instrument, the preeminent importance of social harmony in the family and community is not.

Instrument development is something of an art as well as a science, and in both respects, instruments can almost always be improved upon. It would be satisfying to improve the wording of problem items in WEMWBS. It would also be a good to add items reflecting missing concepts. However, both of these actions would invalidate trend-based data, which has now started to be collected internationally. WEMWBS is playing a part in developing the public mental health agenda and is helping to put mental well-being on the map, both at the level of policy making and in the general public. It seems sensible, therefore, to take the results of the studies described in this chapter at face value and conclude that WEMWBS and SWEMWBS perform well enough at present. In a few years, when understanding of mental well-being and its importance has moved on, there is likely to come a time when the instrument needs to be updated.

Acknowledgements This chapter could not have been written without the help and support of many individuals and organizations. The National Institute of Mental Health in England funded the study with Pakistani and Chinese communities in Birmingham. Gregor Henderson was instrumental in allocating this funding. Heart of Birmingham PCT, the public health practitioners and community workers (Michelle Chan and Ibrar Uddin) provided the support necessary to carry out studies in Birmingham. Coventry Primary Care Trust funded the survey of Coventry residents, and Peter Barker gave permission for us to use the data on Pakistani and Chinese groups in this study. Frances Taggart undertook all the fieldwork, including designing questionnaires for the Birmingham study and analyses of the quantitative and qualitative data. Tim Friede undertook the main statistical analyses, and Alan Tennant undertook the Rasch analysis. Rebecca Putz undertook the analysis of the Coventry Lifestyle Survey. Steve Platt, Scott Weich, and Aileen Clarke have made important contributions to this study as advisors and have contributed in many ways to the development and validation of WEMWBS, with the help and support of Jane Parkinson, and with funding from NHS Health Scotland. Paola Gremigni in Italy and Marie Wissing in South Africa undertook the validations of WEMWBS in those countries and have permitted their data to be included here.

References

Bech, P. (2004). Measuring the dimensions of psychological general well-being by the WHO- 5. *QoL Newsletter, 32*, 15–16.

Chida, Y., & Steptoe, A. (2008). Positive psychological wellbeing and mortality: A quantitative review of prospective observational studies. *Psychosomatic Medicine, 70*, 741–756.

Christopher, J. C. (1999). Situating psychological well-being; exploring the cultural routes of its theory and research. *Journal of Counseling and Development, 77*(1), 141–152.

Christopher, J. C., & Hickinbottom, S. (2008). Positive psychology, ethnocentrism and the disguised ideology of individualism. *Theory and Psychology, 18*(5), 563–589.

Clarke A, Friede T, Putz R, Ashdown J, Martin S, Blake A, Adi Y, Parkinson J, Flynn P, Platt S, Stewart-Brown S. Warwick-Edinburgh Mental Well-being Scale (WEMWBS): *Mixed methods assessment of validity and reliability in teenage school students in England and Scotland.* BMC Public Health 2011;487 http://www.biomedcentral.com/1471–2458/11/487

Davidson, R. J. (2004). Well-being and affective style: Neural substrates and biobehavioural correlates. In F. A. Huppert, N. Baylis, & B. Keverne (Eds.), *The science of well-being* (pp. 307–340). Oxford: Oxford University Press.

Department of Health. (2011). *No Health without mental health: A cross-government mental health outcomes strategy for people of all ages*. Available at http://www.dh.gov.uk/prod_consum_dh/groups/dh_digitalassets/documents/digitalasset/dh_124058.pdf. Last accessed 10 Aug 2011.

Department of Health (2012) Healthy Lives, Healthy People: Improving Outcomes and Supporting Transparency (http://www.dh.gov.uk/en/Publicationsandstatistics/Publications/PublicationsPolicyAndGuidance/DH_132358

Diener, E., Emmons, R. A., Larsen, R. J., & Griffin, S. (1985). The satisfaction with life scale. *Journal of Personality Assessment, 49*(1), 71–75.

DiMatteo, M. R., Lepper, H. S., & Croghan, T. W. (2000). Depression is a risk factor for noncompliance with medical treatment: Meta-analysis of the effects of anxiety and depression on patient adherence. *Annals of Internal Medicine, 160*(14), 2010–2107.

European Pact for Mental Health and Wellbeing. (2008). http://ec.europa.eu/health/ph_determinants/life_style/mental/docs/pact_en.pdf. Accessed 15 Nov 2009.

Freidli, L. (2006). *Mental health improvement: Concepts and definitions*. Briefing paper for the National Advisory Group Scottish Executive: National Programme for Improving Mental Health and Wellbeing. Edinburgh: Scottish Government.

Goldberg, D. P., & Williams, P. (1988). *A user's guide to the general health questionnaire*. Windsor: NFER-Nelson.

Goldberg, D. P., Gater, R., Sartorius, N., Ustun, T. B., Piccinelli, M., & Rutter, C. (1997). The validity of two versions of the GHQ in the WHO study of mental illness in general health care. *Psychological Medicine, 27*, 191–197.

Gremigni P, Stewart-Brown S. *Una Misura del Benessere mentale: Validazone Italiana Della Warwick-Edinburgh Mental Well-being Scale (WEMWBS)*. Giornale Italiano di Psicologia, 2011, 2: 543–563

HM Government. (2006). *Our health, our care, our say: A new direction for community health services*. http://www.dh.gov.uk/en/Publicationsandstatistics/Publications/PublicationsPolicyAndGuidance/DH_4127602

HM Government (2009) New Horizons: a shared vision for mental health http://www.dh.gov.uk/en/Publicationsandstatistics/Publications/PublicationsPolicyAndGuidance/DH_109705

Huppert, F.A. (2008). Psychological wellbeing. Evidence regarding its causes and consequences. *Foresight state-of science review SR –x2 government office for science*.

Huppert, F. A., & Wittington, J. E. (2004). Positive mental health in individuals and populations. In F. A. Huppert, N. Baylis, & B. Keverne (Eds.), *The science of well-being* (pp. 307–340). Oxford: Oxford University Press.

Keyes, C. L. M. (2007). Promoting and protecting mental health as flourishing: A complementary strategy for improving national mental health. *American Psychologist, 62*, 95–108.

Keyes, C. L. M., Shmotkin, D., & Ryff, C. D. (2002). Optimizing well-being: The empirical encounter of two traditions. *Journal of Personality and Social Psychology, 82*, 1007–1022.

Linley, P. A., & Joseph, J. (2004). *Positive psychology in practice*. Hoboken: Wiley.

Newbiggging, K., Bola, M., & Shah, A. (2008). *Scoping exercise with Black and minority ethnic groups on perceptions of mental wellbeing in Scotland*. Edinburgh: NHS Health Scotland. http://www.healthscotland.com/documents/2803.aspx

Parkinson, J. (2007). *Establishing a core set of national, sustainable mental health indicators for adults in Scotland*. Rationale paper, Scottish Government and NHS Health Scotland.

Pressman, D. P., & Cohen, S. (2005). Does positive affect influence health? *Psychological Bulletin, 15*(6), 925–971.

Ryan, R. M., & Deci, E. L. (2001). On happiness and human potential: A review of research on hedonic and eudaemonic well-being. *Annual Review of Psychology, 52*, 141–166.

Ryff, C. D., & Keyes, C. L. M. (1995). The structure of psychological well-being revisited. *Journal of Personality and Social Psychology, 69*, 719–727.

Scott, N. W., Fayers, P. M., Aaronson, N. K., Bottomley, A., de Graeff, A., Groenvold, M., Gundy, C., Koller, M., Petersen, M. A., & Spraners, M. A. G. (2010). Differential item functioning (DIF) analyses of health-related quality of life instruments using logistic regression. *Health and Quality of Life Outcomes, 8*(81). doi:10.1186/1477-7525-8-81.

Scottish Government. (2009). *Towards a mentally flourishing Scotland: 2009-2011 Policy and Action Plan*. Edinburgh: Scottish Government. www.scotland.gov.uk

Stewart-Brown, S. (2002). Measuring the parts most measures do not reach: A necessity for evaluation in mental health promotion, (guest editorial). *Journal of Mental Health Promotion, 1*, 4–9.

Stewart-Brown, S., Tennant, A., Tennant, R., Platt, S., Parkinson, J., & Weich, S. (2009). Internal and construct validity of the Warwick-Edinburgh Mental Well-Being Scale (WEMWBS): A Rasch analysis using data from the Scottish Health Education Population Survey. *Biomed Central Health and Quality of Life Outcome, 7*, 15, 63. http://www.hqlo.com/content/7/1/15. 19 February 2009.

Tennant, R., Fishwick, R., Platt, S., Joseph, S., & Stewart-Brown, S. (2006). *Monitoring positive mental health in Scotland: Validating the Affectometer 2 scale and developing the Warwick-Edinburgh Mental Well-Being Scale for the UK*. Edinburgh: NHS Health Scotland. http://www.healthscotland.com/documents/2327.aspx

Tennant, R., Hiller, L., Fishwick, R., Platt, S., Joseph, S., Weich, S., Parkinson, J., Secker, J., & Stewart-Brown, S. (2007a). The Warwick-Edinburgh Mental Well-Being Scale (WEMWBS): Development and UK validation. *Health and Quality of Life Outcome, 5*, 63. doi: 101186/1477-7252-5-63. http://www.hqlo.com/content/5/1/63

Tennant, R., Joseph, S., & Stewart-Brown, S. (2007b). The affectometer 2: A measure of positive mental health in UK populations. *Quality of Life Research, 16*(4), 687–695.

Tudor, K. (1996). *Mental health promotion: Paradigms and practice*. London: Routledge.

WHO. (2005). *World Health action plan for Europe*. http://www.euro.who.int/mentalhealth/publications/20061124_1. Accessed 15 Nov 2009.

Part II
Toward an Internationalized Understanding of Mechanisms of Positive Mental Health

Chapter 8
Universals and Cultural Differences in the Causes and Structure of Happiness: A Multilevel Review

Ed Diener, Shigehiro Oishi, and Katherine L. Ryan

Universals and Cultural Differences in the Causes of Happiness

Over the past four decades, the study of subjective well-being has grown rapidly from a nascent field of inquiry to a major research endeavor. In its most succinct definition, subjective well-being (SWB) constitutes the level of well-being experienced by people according to their own subjective evaluations of their lives. These evaluations include cognitive judgments about life satisfaction, affective reactions to life events, interest and engagement, and satisfaction with specific domains, such as work, relationships, health, recreation, and meaning and purpose.

Interest in cross-cultural topics has flourished, primarily during the past 15 years. Several works fostered interest in the cultural–psychological perspective, namely, Veenhoven and Ehrhardt (1995), Diener et al. (1995a), Diener and Diener (1995), and Diener and Suh (2000). A growing body of research has shown that while many people around the globe are relatively happy, distinct differences in subjective well-being exist between nations which can be explained, to some extent, by the effects of culture. While most people within industrialized societies score above neutral in surveys of well-being (Diener and Diener 1996), international surveys reveal significant differences in subjective well-being levels (see Diener and Suh 2000 for a review) that can be explained, to some degree, by the level of economic development of the countries surveyed. For example, Diener et al. (1995a) found that wealthier nations

E. Diener (✉)
Department of Psychology, University of Illinois, Chicago, IL, USA

The Gallup Organization, Washington, DC, USA
e-mail: ediener@cyrys.psych.illinois.edu

S. Oishi
Department of Psychology, University of Virginia, Charlottesville, VA, USA

K.L. Ryan
Department of English, University of California, Irvine, CA, USA

C.L.M. Keyes (ed.), *Mental Well-Being: International Contributions to the Study of Positive Mental Health*, DOI 10.1007/978-94-007-5195-8_8,

frequently reported higher SWB and that it is not merely coincidental that some of the unhappiest nations are also the poorest (see also Stevenson and Wolfers 2008).

However, evidence from some cultures suggests that material wealth is not solely responsible for happiness across the globe. For example, Biswas-Diener et al. (2005) found that the Maasai, Amish, and Inughuit cultures reported levels of subjective well-being that were above neutral despite their relatively impoverished living conditions. This finding is consistent with data gathered from those living in slum housing, sex workers, and homeless pavement dwellers in Calcutta, who reported levels of life satisfaction that were only slightly below neutral (Biswas-Diener and Diener 2001). In addition, evidence suggests that the effects of poverty are moderated, to some degree, by culture. For example, while well-being in the homeless is predictably low across cultures, pavement dwellers in Calcutta show higher levels of life satisfaction than homeless groups in the United States (Biswas-Diener and Diener 2006). Interestingly, this occurs despite the fact that the homeless in the United States have better access to food, clean water, medical care, opportunities for employment, and adequate shelter. In addition, Biswas-Diener et al. (2012) found that low-income respondents in the United States reported higher negative affect and lower life satisfaction than low-income respondents in Denmark. Thus, the effects of income depend partly on the cultural context.

It is also important to note that the social benefits produced by a nation's wealth may contribute to citizens' experience of high subjective well-being. Diener et al. (1995a) found that human rights and social equality, factors which are highly correlated with subjective well-being, were highly correlated with national income. In addition, recent research (Tay and Diener 2011) has shown that psychosocial resources, such as feeling respected and being able to count on someone in an emergency, contribute significantly to well-being and, in some cases, are more important than material circumstances. In the past decade, researchers have increasingly focused on this distinction in the causes of well-being and have discovered the importance of both affluence and psychosocial resources in subjective well-being across nations. Diener et al. (2010) found that income best predicts life satisfaction, whereas psychosocial resources best predict positive emotions. We now know that the happiest nations are wealthy and are able to meet the psychosocial needs of their citizenry, whereas the unhappiest nations are less wealthy and are unable to meet these needs. Despite this general conclusion, intriguing cultural universals and differences in the causes and structure of subjective well-being in nations remain, which we will discuss in this chapter.

Components and Structure of Subjective Well-Being

The validity of these cultural comparisons depends on how subjective well-being is conceptualized within individual cultures. For example, do all societies understand the idea of life satisfaction? Are there a set of universal emotions, or are most emotions culture-specific? And if differences in the conception of subjective well-being do exist between cultures, how do we reliably and validly measure SWB in order to make cross-cultural comparisons?

As mentioned above, the concept of subjective well-being includes several key components. We will primarily discuss three: life satisfaction, frequent positive affect (or pleasant emotions), and infrequent negative affect (or unpleasant emotions). These components have been researched most thoroughly across nations and provide broad descriptions of subjective well-being around the globe.

A growing body of evidence reveals that cultures tend to have similar perceptions of which emotions are perceived as positive or negative (Diener et al. 2004; Watson et al. 1984; Shaver et al. 1992). A core cluster of positive emotions, such as *pleasant* and *happy*, as well as a core cluster of negative emotions, such as *unpleasant*, *sad*, and *angry*, tend to consistently reappear despite some variations in how noncore emotions, such as *pride*, are clustered (Diener et al. 2004). Tay et al. (2011) found that certain emotions are experienced as pleasant across cultural regions of the world, and the same is true of certain negative feelings. Evidence also suggests the similarity of structure of life satisfaction across cultures (Vittersø et al. 2002), providing support for the idea that SWB has a consistent general structure across the globe. Thus, there is reason to believe that these aggregates can be compared cross-culturally to yield valid results about the levels of subjective well-being in different societies.

Although high positive affect, low negative affect, and high life satisfaction are all components of high subjective well-being across nations, it is important to note that there are some differences between cultures in the relation of these components. Suh et al. (1998) found that life satisfaction and affect balance (the difference in frequency of positive and negative affect) correlated positively across 40 countries. However, Suh et al. also found that the correlations were stronger in individualistic societies and weaker in collectivistic societies. In the second part of their study, when life satisfaction was predicted from emotions and perceived norms, emotions were most predictive in individualistic cultures while perceived norms were most predictive in collectivistic cultures. Perhaps this difference exists because emotional feelings are considered very important in individualistic cultures, which emphasize people's personal goals and feelings. In contrast, collectivistic cultures may produce a greater tendency to rely on normative standards as a guide for one's actions and judgment because there is a greater emphasis on group harmony.

Norms for Subjective Well-Being

When discussing the well-being of nations, it may be surprising to learn that, on average, most societies are fairly happy. Diener and Diener (1995) found that the majority of respondents in 31 nations reported above-neutral levels of life satisfaction, and Diener and Diener (1996) found that 86% of a total 43 sampled nations reported above-neutral levels of subjective well-being. Even impoverished or nonindustrialized societies, such as the Maasai of Africa, the Inughuit of Greenland, and the Amish in the United States, report above-neutral levels of well-being (Biswas-Diener et al. 2005). This is not to say that suffering no longer exists in the world; importantly, many of the poorest nations of the world were often absent from the early data sets. People may be dispositionally prone to positive emotions due to their adaptive advantages (Fredrickson 1998).

Importantly, the societal norms for emotions and life satisfaction, which differ from culture to culture, affect the experience of well-being. For example, East Asian respondents often report lower SWB than Europeans or Americans (Diener and Diener 1995). While this difference could be linked to economic factors, it is interesting to note that Japan often reports lower SWB than Latin American countries, despite its far greater purchasing power (Diener and Diener 1995; Diener and Oishi 2000; Diener and Suh 1999). Some have posited that this phenomenon occurs because the Japanese and other Asians are more accepting of negative emotions than are other countries (Diener and Suh 1999). In addition, Asian-Americans and Chinese participants have been found to value low-arousal positive affect (calmness) more so than do European-Americans, whereas European-Americans value high-arousal positive affect (excitement) more than do Chinese participants (Tsai et al. 2006). Tsai et al. (2006) posited that Asian cultures show greater acceptance of negative emotions and value low-arousal emotions because these attributes foster greater attention to the social context. In this way, a culture's perception of the desirability of certain emotions might influence people's frequency of experiencing those emotions and their subsequent reporting of well-being. While many of these differences in societal norms are intriguing, it is important to note that valuing positive emotions less, for example, does not mean that East Asian cultures are unhappy. Rather, they only report less happiness relative to other cultures, such as those in Latin America. Actually, East Asians score consistently above the midpoint in SWB, and it is possible that, for a culture rooted in balance and moderation, these modest levels of well-being might be viewed as most desirable (Kitayama and Markus 2000; Schimmack et al. 2002a).

Do People Around the Globe Find SWB Desirable?

An important issue in assessing cross-cultural subjective well-being is the degree to which different societies value it. Evidence shows that the desire to be happy is virtually universal, with respondents in 47 nations ranking happiness highly, and as more important than wealth or physical attractiveness (Diener 2000; Diener and Oishi 2004). While on average, happiness is rated as most important, there is some variance between cultures in the degree of importance. For example, Latin Americans place more importance on happiness than do East Asians. However, despite variations in the degree to which SWB is valued, its universal desirability provides ample evidence that SWB should be studied cross-culturally.

Units for Studying Cultural Differences

In examining culture, one can study various sizes of units that capture the phenomena in different ways. Because shared practices, beliefs, and feelings can occur in various groupings of people, and because each of these will nevertheless contain some amount of heterogeneity, discrete cultural units that are completely homogeneous, but different from all other groups, do not exist. In other words, culture can be regarded as a group average that operates in a hierarchy, as below:

1. Cultural dimensions—for example, individualism and collectivism
2. Geopolitical/sociocultural regions—for example, sub-Saharan Africa and East Asia
3. Nations—for example, Denmark and Japan
4. Small distinct relatively homogeneous cultural groups—for example, the Maasai and the Amish

Studying each one of these levels of culture has its own advantages and limitations. For example, the dimensional approach has the advantage of being able to compare all people but has the potential problem of oversimplifying. For instance, the popular individualism–collectivism dimension can be applied to any world region, but at the same time, the collectivism of different regions often varies to some degree (Brewer and Chen 2007; Oyserman et al. 2002). The small-group approach, which has been most extensively used by anthropologists, has the advantage of focusing on relatively homogeneous groups with distinct characteristics, but at the same time, it leaves us with a very long list of different cultures and often very small sample sizes (see Henrich et al. 2005 for an exemplary work). The nation and geopolitical units define geographical regions with some cultural homogeneity owing to common factors, such as history, language, and politics, but at the same time, there can be distinct groups within these regions. Lucas and Diener (2008) discuss the issues involved in comparing the subjective well-being of nations.

All four approaches capture some of the cultural differences between groups. In each type of unit, there are shared cultural characteristics that, on average, apply to individuals within them and that, on average, are to some degree different from other groups. In each case, we can also examine the degree to which the cultural unit used is associated with differences in the factors that are associated with well-being. Thus, we analyze the universals and differences in the causes of well-being across these four types of cultural units. If the results tend to be consistent, we will have more confidence in our conclusions. We also examine mean-level differences between cultural groups and whether the structure of subjective well-being is consistent across culture. An important issue that we do not address is the degree of heterogeneity in cultural units.

Cultural Universals in the Causes of Well-Being

Cultural Dimensions

On a dimensional level, individualism has shown a strong correlation with well-being. Diener et al. (1995a) found that income, individualism, and human rights all showed strong relations to SWB in a survey of 55 nations. However, it has thus far been difficult to disentangle these variables. Because a nation's economic development

Table 8.1 Correlations with two types of well-being

	Life evaluations			Positive feelings		
	Log income	Basic needs	Household conveniences	Respect	Mastery	Social support
World	0.42	0.33	0.39	0.41	0.30	0.30
Africa	0.25	0.23	0.24	0.45	0.26	0.30
East Asia	0.39	0.29	0.32	0.38	0.27	0.28
Eastern Europe	0.27	0.26	0.23	0.44	0.30	0.30
Latin America	0.25	0.21	0.27	0.42	0.33	0.22
Middle East	0.23	0.42	0.50	0.43	0.34	0.27
N. Europe/Anglo	0.23	0.17	0.08	0.27	0.22	0.24
S. and S.E. Asia	0.29	0.33	0.44	0.38	0.33	0.23
Southern Europe	0.32	0.22	0.26	0.31	0.26	0.27

Note: Household conveniences included electricity, running water, telephone, computer, and television

usually occurs in tandem with cultural changes, it can be challenging to ascribe heightened subjective well-being to a specific economic or social improvement. Despite greater social support in collectivistic societies, some have theorized that individualism may be a predictor of well-being because people have greater freedom in choosing the course of their lives in individualistic societies. People in these societies also may attribute their success to themselves rather than to the social network and, thus, feel greater personal satisfaction and fulfillment, at least if they are succeeding.

Sociocultural Regions

On a sociocultural region level, there is evidence not only that universal causes of well-being exist across cultures but that these universals exist in connections to specific types of SWB. Tay and Diener (2011) examined six types of needs (basic needs for food and shelter, safety and security, social support and love, respect and pride in activities, mastery, and self-direction and autonomy) in relation to three types of subjective well-being (life evaluations, positive feelings, and negative feelings) across eight sociocultural regions of the world in order to assess the association between needs and types of SWB. Life satisfaction was best predicted by the fulfillment of basic needs, whereas positive feelings were best predicted by the fulfillment of social needs. Importantly, the associations of needs with particular forms of SWB were consistent across all eight sociocultural regions.

New research consistently suggests that income, conveniences, and satisfaction with standard of living consistently predict evaluations of life satisfaction but that psychosocial factors more strongly influence the components of positive and negative feelings (Diener et al. 2009a). In Table 8.1, we present correlations from the Gallup World Poll Wave 1, between income, household conveniences, psychosocial resources, and life evaluations and positive feelings. As can be seen throughout the world and in all world sociocultural regions, life satisfaction was related to material aspects of life, that is, household income, the ownership of household conveniences, and the meeting of basic needs for food and shelter. Positive feelings, in contrast, were most related to respect, mastery, and social support, and these correlations tended to be consistent in all regions of the globe. The weakest associations were found in the Northern Europe/Anglo region, probably because of ceiling effects, with most individuals owning conveniences and having their basic needs met. The correlations of life satisfaction and psychosocial resources, and of positive feelings and national measures, were not as strong. Thus, across sociocultural regions, there are several commonalities in the causes of life satisfaction, positive feelings, and negative feelings.

Nations

While there are some universal societal factors, such as democratic governance, human rights, and longevity, which are related to SWB across nations (Diener et al. 1995a), there are also cross-national similarities in terms of personality characteristics and social bonds that are associated with happiness. For instance, Lucas et al. (2000) found that extroversion was related to positive feelings in all 39 nations examined. Kuppens et al. (2008) also found that, across nations, positive emotions were more strongly associated with life satisfaction than was the absence of negative emotions. Fulmer et al. (2010) found that there is a congruity effect such that people who have personality characteristics that match the dominant traits in that cultures tend to report higher levels of well-being.

In terms of social resources, longitudinal studies and studies of large representative samples reveal that married people are, on average, happier than non-married people (Glenn 1975; Lee et al. 1991; Lucas et al. 2003). This correlation holds true across nations. Diener et al. (2000) found that being married was associated with high SWB almost universally across cultures, although there were some cultural differences, such as lesser negative affect among divorced persons in collectivist cultures. Therefore, strong social bonds such as those provided by supportive marriages seem to be universally beneficial to SWB, along with extraversion and positive feelings. However, the issue of reverse causality—high well-being leading to marriage better relationships and extraversion—cannot be ruled out.

Small Homogeneous Groups

Even when examining small cultural units, some universal causes of happiness emerge. In a study of homeless individuals from Calcutta in India, and from both California and Oregon, Biswas-Diener and Diener (2006) found that all three groups reported high levels of negative affect and low satisfaction with material resources, such as income and housing. Likewise, all three groups reported similar levels of high satisfaction with domains related to the self (e.g., morality, intelligence, and physical appearance), which indicates the resiliency of self-appraisal despite the negative effects of poverty. In each locale, homelessness was predictably associated with lowered well-being, which suggests that having one's basic needs unmet is a strong predictor of lowered life satisfaction around the globe. These results were replicated in another Calcutta study that surveyed those living in slum housing, sex workers, and pavement dwellers and found that life satisfaction decreased incrementally as the fulfillment of basic needs diminished (Biswas-Diener and Diener 2001). Specifically, pavement dwellers (i.e., those who live without housing) had much lower life satisfaction than both sex workers and those living in the slums. Thus, even among impoverished groups, the fulfillment of a basic need such as housing can drastically affect the way individuals evaluate their lives. Thus, satisfaction with material resources is strongly linked to overall life satisfaction across diverse groups.

Similarly, strong social relationships have been shown to universally aid well-being. Homeless groups in Calcutta showed greater satisfaction with social relationships than did homeless groups in the United States. Moreover, sharing living quarters with others was also related to increased life satisfaction in Calcutta, whereas homeless respondents in the United States commonly showed a lack of trust in other homeless people around them (Biswas-Diener and Diener 2006). Interestingly, respondents in Calcutta also reported higher satisfaction with material domains and income, despite having better access to food, clean water, medical care, employment, and adequate shelter available to them in the two US locations (Biswas-Diener and Diener 2006). Although respondents in India may display higher levels of satisfaction because the country, in general, shows much more sympathy and less social stigma for the poor, social support seems to play a key role in the differences between the homeless groups surveyed. Because homelessness in Calcutta is associated less with pathology or personal fault and more with economic conditions, the homeless in Calcutta tend to stay close to their family units, whereas their counterparts in the United States are often estranged from relatives, children, and spouses. In this way, the social support provided to the Indian homeless may be the reason why they show levels of life satisfaction not only higher than their American counterpart but which fall in the positive range.

Cultural Differences in the Causes of Well-Being

Cultural Dimensions

Although there are similarities across cultures in terms of the causes of well-being, cultural differences also exist. A few of the areas where there are substantial differences are in the way certain emotions are valued across cultures, in how social

Table 8.2 Life satisfaction and positive feelings of marital status groups in four world regions

		Married	Single	Divorced	Widowed
Arab Middle East	LS	6.4	6.3	5.6	6.3
	PF	0.68	0.67	0.55	0.51
South America	LS	5.8	6.1	5.7	5.5
	PF	0.79	0.78	0.75	0.73
Sub-Saharan Africa	LS	4.3	4.5	4.3	4.1
	PF	0.70	0.69	0.64	0.61
Northern Europe	LS	7.5	7.1	6.8	7.0
	PF	0.76	0.73	0.71	0.69

Note: Ten nations per region with a sample of approximately 1,000 per nation

approval affects judgments of life satisfaction, and in the perceived importance of individual achievement versus communal harmony. For example, the value of self-esteem to SWB is moderated by individualism, as indicated by the fact that self-esteem is a strong predictor of life satisfaction in individualistic cultures, but not in collectivist cultures (Diener and Diener 1995). Similarly, satisfaction with one's freedom was more strongly associated with life satisfaction in individualistic cultures than in collectivistic cultures (Oishi et al. 1999).

In the area of emotion, Suh et al. (1998) found that emotional experiences were more strongly associated with life satisfaction in individualistic cultures than in collectivistic cultures. Suh et al. (2008) extended these findings by using a priming procedure. Specifically, American and Korean participants in their study were primed either with the concepts associated with individualism or collectivism before making their life satisfaction judgments. When participants were primed with individualism, their life satisfaction judgments were based primarily on their own emotional experiences. When they were primed with collectivism, however, their life satisfaction judgments were more strongly influenced by social appraisals (how parents and friends viewed participants' lives) than their own emotional experiences. These findings suggest that many cultural differences are not absolute but depend on the focus of attention and salience of information at the time of reporting (see Oyserman and Lee 2008 for review). Because people are more likely to attend to information that is seen as important in their culture, differences in the correlates of life satisfaction arise because of the differential accessibility of relevant information (Oishi et al. 2000).

Sociocultural Regions

We could not locate previously published findings on regional differences in the patterns associated with well-being. Thus, we analyzed Wave 3 of the Gallup World Poll for well-being of marital status groups across a few regions of the world. Table 8.2 shows the life evaluation scores (0–10 scale) and positive feelings scores (0–1.0 scale) for each region.

Several important conclusions emerge from our examination of the table. First, the patterns are different for the two types of well-being. These pattern differences point to the absolute necessity of measuring different types of well-being in cross-cultural research and of not making blanket statements about happiness. For instance, widows in the Middle East are relatively high in life evaluations but very low in positive feelings. Across marital groups, Northern Europe is clearly highest in life evaluations, but South America is highest in positive feelings.

In terms of specific marital categories, widows are the worst off in life evaluation in two of the regions, but the divorced are lowest in the two other regions. In terms of positive feelings, widows are the worst off in all regions, but this deficit is most dramatic in the Middle East, where widows are also relatively highly in life evaluation. In every region, the married are highest in positive feelings, but singles score highest on life evaluations in two other regions. The finding that unmarried individuals are relatively happy (DePaulo and Morris 2005) replicates across regions and measures, as does the finding that divorced individuals are low in well-being. At the same time, the findings reveal that the relative standing of marital groups can differ depending on cultural region as well as type of well-being. Thus, we need to take a more careful look at where and why patterns replicate. Clearly, the processes leading to life evaluation versus positive feelings are distinct.

Nations

As stated above, Lucas et al. (2000) showed that the association between positive affect and extraversion was similar across 39 nations. Schimmack et al. (2002b) replicated this finding, showing that the latent link between extraversion and hedonic balance (PA–NA) was positive and the link between neuroticism and hedonic balance was negative in all five nations examined, namely, the United States, Germany, Mexico, Japan, and Ghana. Interestingly, however, consistent with Suh et al. (1998), the latent association between hedonic balance and life satisfaction was larger among Americans and Germans than among Mexicans, Japanese, and Ghanaians.

When specific types of pleasant emotions were examined, several cross-national differences also emerged. For instance, happiness was strongly associated with interpersonally disengaging positive emotions (e.g., pride) among Americans, whereas it was strongly associated with interpersonally engaging positive emotions among Japanese (e.g., *fureai,* Kitayama et al. 2000, 2006). Similarly, pride loaded on the positive mood factor along with other positive emotions among European-Americans and Hispanic Americans, whereas it loaded on both positive and negative moods among Asian-Americans, Japanese, and Indians (Scollon et al. 2005). More recently, Tsai and colleagues found that the ideal positive emotion entailed high activation (e.g., excitement) among Americans, whereas it entailed low activation (e.g., calm, peaceful) among Chinese (Tsai et al. 2007a, b).

In a similar vein, relationship harmony was more strongly associated with life satisfaction in Hong Kong than in the United States (Kwan et al. 1997). Likewise, among Japanese and Filipinos, social support had a direct effect on subjective well-being above and beyond self-esteem, whereas social support did not predict subjective well-being among Americans beyond self-esteem (Uchida et al. 2008). Namely, social support was associated with subjective well-being among Americans to the extent that it was associated with self-esteem.

There are also cross-national differences in motivational processes involving subjective well-being. For instance, Americans are more motivated to view themselves as consistent across different roles and situations than Koreans (Suh 2002). Furthermore, self-concept consistency was more strongly associated with life satisfaction in the United States than in Korea. There are cross-national differences in terms of the relation between goal attainment and subjective well-being. For example, Japanese college students who were pursuing their goals to make their family and friends happy became more satisfied with their lives over time as they achieved their goals than did those Japanese who were not pursuing their goals to make their family and friends happy (Oishi and Diener 2001). In contrast, American college students who were pursuing their goals for themselves became more satisfied with their lives over time as they achieved their goals than did other Americans who were not pursuing their goals for themselves. Likewise, among Americans, pursuing goals with an avoidant mindset was negatively associated with life satisfaction, whereas it was not negatively associated with life satisfaction among Koreans and Russians, who view avoiding negative evaluations as important (Elliot et al. 2001).

Other studies have shown cross-national differences in the role of specific situations or life events in subjective well-being. For instance, Oishi et al. (2004) conducted a cross-national experience-sampling study in which participants were beeped at random moments and asked to record the situations they were in, and their moods, for 1 week. For instance, they found that both Americans and Japanese were happier when they were with friends and their romantic partners than when they were alone. However, this effect of friend and romantic partner, respectively, was significantly stronger among Japanese than among Americans. In the same study, they found that Indians felt more negative emotions when they were with strangers than they were alone. American participants did not feel any more negative emotions when they were with strangers than when they were alone. Overall, Japanese and Indian negative affective experiences varied, to a greater degree, across different interpersonal contexts than did Americans'. In another study, Oishi et al. (2007) conducted a 3-week daily diary study in the United States, Korea, and Japan, in which participants were asked to record their daily life events and well-being. On average, American participants experienced more positive events per day than Koreans and Japanese. Interestingly, it took Americans about two positive daily events to mitigate the effect of one negative event on their daily satisfaction. In contrast, it took about one positive event to counteract the effect of one negative event among Japanese and Koreans. Because American participants experienced more positive events (e.g., compliments) than Koreans and Japanese in general, the value of a positive event among Americans was lower than among Koreans and Japanese (see Diener et al. 2003; Tov and Diener 2007 for more comprehensive review on cross-national differences in well-being).

Small Homogeneous Groups

Biswas-Diener et al. (2005) found that the Kenyan Maasai, the US Amish, and the Greenlandic Inughuit all reported above-average levels of life satisfaction, domain satisfaction, and affect balance. However, the Amish reported lower satisfaction with self-related domains, whereas the Maasai and Inughuit reported lower satisfaction with material domains. While all three groups reported high satisfaction with social domains, the Maasai were the only group that reported frequently feeling substantial pride. Thus, subjective well-being may differ in a more intricate pattern, even when the overall level is similar across groups.

More recently, Cox (2009) examined the subjective well-being of sex workers, dump dwellers, urban poor, rural peasants, and university students in Nicaragua. Among urban poor, income was significantly positively associated with global life satisfaction. In contrast, however, among sex workers, dump dwellers, rural poor, and university students, income was unrelated to global life satisfaction. One important issue here is the measurement of material wealth or resources among these groups. While income may not affect well-being in cultures such as the Maasai, where money is hardly used, the ownership of cattle, for instance—which is an important material asset—is correlated with life satisfaction.

Cultural Universals in the Structure of Well-Being

Cultural Dimensions

Although there has been debate regarding the universality of emotions, research shows that while individual emotions and the situations that cause them may differ from culture to culture, positive and negative affect can be validly assessed across individualistic and collectivistic cultures. A number of studies show that countries around the world use emotion words that cluster into the two main categories of positive or negative emotions. Positive and negative affect clusters emerged from studies examining emotion words in Japan (Watson et al. 1984), as well as in the United States, Italy, and China (Shaver et al. 1992). These studies provide evidence that positive and negative feelings are perceived across nations and that emotions, such as joy, anger, and sadness, appear to be universally experienced as positive or negative.

In addition to positive and negative affect, there is also support for the similarity of life satisfaction across cultural dimensions. Vittersø et al. (2002) found that a one-factor model of the Satisfaction with Life Scale (SWLS; Diener et al. 1985) fit reported life satisfaction in 41 nations. This study not only suggests that the SWLS measures a single construct but also suggests that cultures around the world have similar notions of life satisfaction regardless of what conditions they think contribute to it.

Sociocultural Regions

Diener et al. (2004) studied the frequency of 12 emotions and found that they resulted in positive and negative clusters for all seven regions of the world, including Africa, Latin America, East Asia, Southeast Asia, West Asia, Eastern Europe, and Western Europe. Importantly, in virtually all regions, certain emotions were consistently placed into the positive or negative clusters: positive emotions included *pleasant*, *cheerful*, and *happy,* while negative emotions included *unpleasant*, *sad*, and *angry*.

Similarly, Tay et al. found that across six cultural–political regions of the world, emotions fell along a positive–negative valence continuum. Words such as cheerful, pleasant, happy, and love were viewed as positive in all regions, and words such as sad, worry, unpleasant, and anger were seen as negative in all regions.

Nations

Nation-level studies have provided much support for the validity of measuring positive and negative affect across cultures. Based on 9,300 respondents from 48 nations, Kuppens et al. (2006) concluded that there are two broad universal affect factors—pleasant and unpleasant feelings—that characterize people across the globe. In addition, Scollon et al. (2004) found that positive feelings and negative feelings each formed similar clusters across nations. In this study, it is noteworthy that emotions for which there are no equivalent English-language emotions, which they called indigenous emotions, also clustered as would be expected in the pleasant or unpleasant clusters. Moreover, these results also extend to the within-person level analysis, as evident by Scollon et al. (2005) finding that positive and negative emotions formed separate and strong factors in all of the five cultures they studied. In other words, the feelings of the same valence tend to be experienced together.

Small Homogeneous Groups

Russell (1983) asked Indians from the Gujarat region of India (who spoke Gujarati only) to sort 28 emotion terms in terms of similarity and dissimilarity. Much like the two-dimensional structure of emotions in English, the similarity judgments of emotions in Gujarati resulted in the two-dimensional circumplex of emotion with the pleasant/unpleasant and arousal as the major dimensions.

Cultural Differences in the Structure of Well-Being

Cultural Dimensions

Despite cultural universals, interesting structural differences in SWB originate from cultural–emotional norms, which play an important role in the frequency of reported emotions, and thus provide insight into the measurement of well-being across the globe. Emotions which conflict with societal norms may be deemphasized and, consequently, experienced less frequently. This, in turn, may explain why some cultures report certain emotions as negative which are normally viewed as positive in the majority of nations.

Cultural dimensions may affect the way the separate components of SWB are related to each other. Kuppens et al. (2008) found that individualism moderated the association of negative emotions with life satisfaction, with people in individualistic nations being more adversely affected by unpleasant feelings. In cultures that value self-expression, positive feelings had a stronger relation with life satisfaction.

Kuppens et al. (2006) found that beyond the individual pleasant and unpleasant factors that strongly describe people's feelings across cultures, there were two nation-level factors that described less, but non-negligible, amounts of variance in the reports of feelings: positivity and interpersonal emotions. One nation factor consisted of feelings related to other people rather to than unpleasant feelings. This factor included high loadings on *guilt*, *shame*, *gratitude*, and *jealousy*. The positive-nation factor was related to the life satisfaction of nations and to the cultural appropriateness of expressing positive emotions. Importantly, the interpersonal dimension was inversely related to the individualism of nations, suggesting that in collectivistic nations, people pay more attention to interpersonal feelings. This attention to the collective may be explained by Kitayama et al. (2009) finding that individualistic cultures tend to favor emotions associated with independence, whereas collectivistic cultures tend to favor emotions associated with interdependence.

Sociocultural Regions

Schimmack et al. (2002a) found that pleasant and unpleasant emotions were inversely correlated in many sociocultural regions (e.g., Europe, Latin America). However, pleasant and unpleasant emotions were not inversely related in the East Asian region. Tay et al. (2011) used latent class analysis to examine the structure of affect in persons in greater detail. Using the Gallup World Poll, they did find a class with low levels of positive affect and high levels of several types of positive affect. Conversely, they found another class with moderate levels of positive affect and relatively low level of negative affect but also high stress. These two classes represent the positive–negative dimension that characterized most structural work on the emotions, with the exception of stress, which went with the positive emotions for the second latent class. However, there was also a class reporting relatively high negative and positive emotions found frequently in Latin America. Finally, there was a class with relatively light positive emotions, except pride, and very low levels of sadness and worry. Thus, a valence dimension was somewhat universal across the globe, but the patterns were, in fact, more intricate than values alone would suggest.

Although the Tay et al. study cited earlier found a positive–negative valence dimension in all regions of the world, there were certain terms that were more ambiguous in specific regions. The positive terms *pride* and *gratitude* and the negative terms *jealousy* and *guilt* did not have a clearly delineated valence value in some cultures, suggesting some experienced ambiguity in low positive versus negative valence dimensions.

Nations

Eid and Diener (2001) examined the desirability and appropriateness of pleasant and unpleasant affect in the United States, Australia, Taiwan, and China. Roughly 83% of Americans and Australians belonged to the latent class, in which all positive emotions *joy*, *affection*, *pride*, and *contentment* were perceived as appropriate. In contrast, China and Taiwan proved to be very heterogeneous, with people falling more evenly across several latent classes based on the desirability of various combinations of emotions. Pride was the outlier emotion in this study, with 57% of Taiwanese having mixed feelings about this emotion and 32% of Chinese feeling that pride was clearly inappropriate. Although it is important to recognize cross-national differences in emotional norms, it is also important to note that emotional norms might not always strongly influence emotional experience. For instance, Tsai et al. (2006) found that the emotions people value are not necessarily the emotions they experience most often.

For life satisfaction, Oishi (2006) used item response theory (IRT) to examine measurement equivalence of the Satisfaction with Life Scale (SWLS) between the United States and China. Item 2, "The conditions of my life are excellent," was equivalent across the two nations, whereas items 1, 3, 4, and 5 were significantly different (significant DIF). In particular, item 4, "So far I have gotten the important things I want in my life," and item 5, "If I could live my life over, I would change almost nothing," showed large DIF. These items did not measure life satisfaction of Chinese very well. In other words, Chinese who endorsed item 2, "The conditions of my life are excellent," did not necessarily endorse items 4 or 5. In contrast, Americans who endorsed item 2 also endorsed items 4 and 5. This differential item functioning (DIF) is disconcerting in interpreting the mean differences of life satisfaction across nations. Interestingly, however, the latent life satisfaction scores that were estimated based on the differential item functioning (more equivalent items get more weights than less equivalent items) did not substantially change the estimation of mean differences in the SWLS between the USA and China. With the raw scores, Cohen's D was 1.18, whereas with the IRT-based score, it was 0.71

(still the large effect). Thus, although life satisfaction has some common core across societies, there can also be culture-specific item differences at the national level, as well as reliability differences.

Small Homogeneous Groups

Although we were unable to find the studies that directly test the structure of emotions in small homogenous groups, there are many pieces of evidence that suggest cultural variations in the structure of well-being. Russell (1991), for instance, identified cultures that do not have the corresponding words for so-called basic emotions. There is no word for disgust in Polish, Ifaluk, and Chewong. Additionally, there is no word for sadness in Tahitian and Chewong, no word for fear in Ifaluk, Utku, and Pintupi, and no word for surprise in Fore, Dani, Malay, and Ifaluk.

In addition, anthropologists have identified many indigenous concepts associated with well-being. For example, Menon and Shweder (1994) identified the indigenous concept, "lajya," in the Orissa region of India. The best English translation of lajya is shame, though it also means shyness and embarrassment. Oriyas believe that lajya (shame) is a feminine virtue that is both powerful and good. Menon and Shweder asked participants in Orissa and the United States to pick one emotion that is most different from the rest. The target emotions were *raga* (anger), *sukha* (happy), and *lajya* (shame). Indians in the Orissa region viewed anger as the most different from shame and happy, whereas many Americans viewed happy as most different from anger and shame. For Oriyas, shame is instrumental to maintaining harmonious relationships with others, whereas anger is detrimental to harmonious relationships. Anger is detrimental to social relationships in the United States, as well. The critical difference, however, was that the instrumental value of emotion in social relationships did not come to mind naturally among Americans whereas that was the first dimension that came to mind among Oriyas. Instead, the pleasant versus unpleasant dimension was the first to come to mind for many Americans.

Mean Levels of Subjective Well-Being Around the World

Diener and Diener (1996) suggested that most people in the world are happy because humans are predisposed to experience mild positive emotions when they are in positive or neutral circumstances. Research has shown that in neutral, ambiguous, and positive circumstances, people show a slight positive offset, which engenders more sociable, approach-oriented, and optimistic behavior (Ito et al. 1998). This is consistent with the Pollyanna Principle advanced by Matlin and Stang (1978). Studies show that people are prone to dampen negative emotions quickly (Taylor 1991). Importantly, this pattern may be adaptive in that it causes most people to experience low-intensity positive feelings of well-being the majority of the time, as long as nothing bad is happening. These feelings of well-being yield a state in which individuals confidently explore their environment, approach new goals, and gain important personal resources (Fredrickson 1998). However, negative events can quickly draw people's attention to dangers. The person reacts quickly to the negative event, and thereafter, the unpleasant emotions are dampened and the person returns to a positive state.

Diener and Diener (1996) reviewed evidence from around the world and found support for the idea that most people *are*, in fact, happy, but since that time, the emerging picture has grown more intricate. For example, Diener et al. (2009) reported that although virtually all nations reported more positive feelings than negative feelings (or a positive affect balance), in a large number of nations, respondents reported average life satisfaction that was below neutral.

In this chapter, we have examined the first three waves of the Gallup World Poll, which included about 360,000 respondents representatively sampled from 146 nations. The results were compelling in showing a positive offset for feelings, but not for life evaluations. At the individual level, 54% of respondents were at or below neutral in life evaluations, and in 39% of nations, the average respondent was at or below neutrality on evaluations of life. In contrast, 62% of respondents felt more enjoyment than sadness, and in every one of the 146 nations, the average respondent felt more enjoyment than sadness. Thus, the positive offset applies to feelings, but apparently not to evaluations of life. Apparently, people can be dissatisfied in terms of having what they desire but nevertheless be prone to feel somewhat positive feelings. Thus, people might have, on average, a positive set point in their emotional lives yet be capable of judgments of their lives that are below the midpoint of the scale. Clearly, this is a very important question for future research.

The general predisposition to positivity offset does not mean, however, that all cultures are the same when it comes to livability and high SWB. There are pronounced differences between societies in each type of subjective well-being. For example, in the Gallup World Poll, life satisfaction on a 0–10 scale varied from an average of 3.1 in Togo to 7.9 in Denmark. Having frequently felt enjoyment yesterday varied from 89% of respondents (Canada, Denmark, and New Zealand) to 56 % in Georgia. Affect balance between enjoyment and sadness varied from a high of 87 in Laos, meaning 87% more people felt much enjoyment than felt much sadness, to a low of 49 in Armenia, where approximately the same number of people felt sadness and enjoyment.

The mean levels of SWB in cultures are related to circumstances such as income and lack of corruption (Diener et al. 2009) and also to cultural dimensions such as femininity, power distance, and uncertainty avoidance (Basabe et al. 2000). Basabe et al. (2002) found that the Human Development Index of the United Nations (assessing the income, education, and life expectancy of nations) correlated substantially with the life satisfaction of nations but only weakly with affect. In contrast, cultural dimensions such as masculinity, power distance, and individualism were substantially associated with affect balance.

Diener and Lucas (2000) presented evaluation theory to integrate the diverse findings on the causes of SWB and found that relative standards, cultural differences, and the fulfillment of *both* needs and goals can all influence SWB. They suggest that culture can direct people's attention toward certain factors, just as inborn needs can, and that this focus can lead to a greater impact for the factor receiving attention.

Integrating the Insights

Several broad conclusions are now clear regarding culture and the experiences of well-being. One finding is that variation exists in the causes of different types of SWB across cultures, for example, life satisfaction versus positive affect. Money is an important goal in the modern world, and obtaining it correlates with life satisfaction around the world. For cultures that rarely use money, such as the traditional Maasai, a proxy for money which gives access to resources (e.g., the ownership of cattle) can be associated with well-being. In contrast, positive affect, unlike life satisfaction, is strongly related to social support cross-culturally, supporting the notion that the positive affect system and social relationships are intimately tied.

Another important conclusion is that there are several cultural universals in the structure of SWB, for example, that positive emotions tend to be frequently experienced by the same individuals, as do negative emotions. Furthermore, there is much agreement about the values of most of the major emotions. However, there is variability across cultures in the desirability of high-arousal emotions, as well as specific emotions, such as pride. Therefore, researchers can compare cultures on pleasant and unpleasant feelings but need to be cautious about the meaning of specific feelings, such as pride, which can differ in their valence. Some caution is also needed in aggregating emotions of the same valence because there can be latent classes of individuals who experience different ensembles of emotions. Moreover, researchers should also pay careful attention to the ways in which the associations between positive and negative emotions can differ across cultures.

In general, our review gives reason for optimism in terms of our ability to study SWB across cultures. Data show that SWB generally can be validly measured across cultures. There are similarities in the structure of feelings so that comparisons across cultures are possible. Even where individuals within groups differ in the structure of their SWB, latent class analysis provides a method for comparing similar groups across cultures (Eid and Diener 2001). Tay et al. (2011) show how latent class analysis can be used to identify similar classes of people in each culture and then compare the frequency of these latent classes across cultures.

There is reason to believe that we can, to some degree, describe desirable societies in terms of certain universals that produce high SWB, for example, those with adequate material and social resources. At the same time, cultures, to some degree, also must be judged based on their own criteria, as some causes of happiness differ across cultures. In some cases, there are differences between cultures at the specific and concrete causes of well-being but consistency at a more abstract level.

For example, Oishi and Diener (2001) found that different types of goals most enhanced SWB in different cultures. However, it is likely that achieving goals leads to well-being in all cultures but that the specific goals can differ to some extent.

Future Directions

Despite the growing amount of data across cultures gathered at the dimensional, sociocultural, regional, national, and small homogenous group levels, our review indicates important future directions for research. One of the most important is the study of the outcomes of well-being across various groups and cultures. A growing body of evidence suggests that high levels of SWB provide benefits of effective functioning not only at the individual level but on the societal level as well. For example, happy people tend to engage more frequently than unhappy people in altruistic, prosocial activities such as volunteering, (Tov and Diener 2008); happy people tend to have better relationships, better health and longevity, and higher incomes (Pressman and Cohen 2005; Diener and Biswas-Diener 2008; Lyubomirsky et al. 2005). In addition, happy people report higher levels of trust, cooperation, and propeace attitudes, and they are generally more confident in the government and more democratic and less intolerant of immigrants or other racial groups (Tov and Diener 2008; Diener and Tov 2007). Similarly, Tov et al. (2009) found that high SWB led to greater societal trust and more confidence in parliament. Importantly, these patterns of association were stronger in societies that were objectively better, that is, in nations higher in equality and income and lower in war-related deaths. Thus, although happy people tend to perceive societal conditions in a more positive light, they did so most in the desirable conditions that justified these positive evaluations.

Despite the promising findings on the benefit of high subjective well-being, little research has been conducted comparing the majority of these outcomes across cultures. The finding of Diener et al. (2002) that happy students later earned higher income was replicated by Graham and her colleagues in Russia (Graham et al. 2004),, but there have been few longitudinal studies replicating results on the outcomes of well-being. The important question is whether the benefits of well-being generalize across cultures or are restricted to the westernized nations where most of the research has been conducted.

One area where more research is required is on measurement artifacts. To avoid these effects, multiple measures should be utilized in more studies. Diener et al. (1995b) found little evidence that measurement artifacts caused cross-nation differences in SWB. However, Scollon et al. (2004) found that the cultural groups they studied did not differ in negative emotions when online recording of emotions was used to measure them but that they did differ in retrospective global reports of emotions. Similarly, Oishi (2002) found that European-Americans and Asian-Americans did not differ in online positive emotions but did differ when they retrospectively recalled their emotions for the period of the online recordings. These findings indicate that online experience-sampling methods ought to be used more frequently, and careful attention ought to be paid to the patterns produced by online measures versus retrospective measures of feelings. Although some researchers might perceive differences between measurement methods as a threat to the field, in fact, they are a golden opportunity for understanding the origin of cultural differences.

Finally, the effects of language should be studied further in order to refine surveys of well-being used across cultures. Boroditsky (2001) demonstrated how language influences the way we think, and therefore, the connotation of words—the most frequent medium of measurement of SWB—could vary across cultures. In addition, it could be that for bilingual speakers, the language of the measure could prime different thoughts. For bicultural individuals, they can switch between different cultural frames. For example, we performed an initial analysis of language with a large cross-national college student sample and did not find strong effects. Namely, individuals within a nation using different languages appeared similar, whereas individuals in different nations who used a common language did not appear similar. However, this initial examination was far from definitive, and much more research is needed. For example, people may report different levels of life satisfaction depending on the language used or the measurement setting, for example, if the measure is administered at home versus at work. Thus, although we have made substantial progress in our understanding of subjective well-being across cultures, there are still many exciting and promising topics for future research.

References

Basabe, N., Paez, D., Valencia, J., Rime, B., Pennebaker, J., Diener, E., & Gonzalez, J. L. (2000). Sociocultural factors predicting subjective experience of emotion: A collective level analysis. *Psicothema, 12*, 55–69.

Basabe, N., Paez, D., Valencia, J., Gonzalez, J. L., Rimé, B., & Diener, E. (2002). Cultural dimensions, socioeconomic development, climate, and emotional hedonic level. *Cognition and Emotion, 16*, 103–125.

Biswas-Diener, R., & Diener, E. (2001). Making the best of a bad situation: Satisfaction in the slums of Calcutta. *Social Indicators Research, 55*, 329–352.

Biswas-Diener, R., & Diener, E. (2006). The subjective well-being of the homeless, and lessons for happiness. *Social Indicators Research, 76*, 185–205.

Biswas-Diener, R., Vittersø, J., & Diener, E. (2005). Most people are pretty happy, but there is cultural variation: The Inughuit, the Amish, and the Maasai. *Journal of Happiness Studies: An Interdisciplinary Periodical on Subjective Well-Being, 6*, 205–226.

Biswas-Diener, R., Vitterso, J., & Diener, E. (2012). The Danish effect: Beginning to explore high well-being in Denmark. *Social Indicators Research, 97*, 229–246.

Boroditsky, L. (2001). Does language shape thought?: Mandarin and English speakers' conceptions of time. *Cognitive Psychology, 43*, 1–22.

Brewer, M. B., & Chen, Y.-R. (2007). Where (who) are collectives in collectivism? Toward conceptual clarification of individualism and collectivism. *Psychological Review, 114*, 133–151.

Cox, K. (2009). *Happiness and unhappiness in the developing world: Life satisfaction among sex workers, dump-dwellers, urban poor, and rural peasants in Nigaragua.* Evanston: Northwestern University. A paper under review. *Journal of Happiness Studies, 13*, 103–128.

DePaulo, B. M., & Morris, W. L. (2005). Singles in society and in science. *Psychological Inquiry, 16*, 57–83.

Diener, E. (2000). Subjective well-being: The science of happiness, and a proposal for a national index. *American Psychologist, 55*, 34–43.
Diener, E., & Biswas-Diener, R. (2008). *Happiness: Unlocking the mysteries of psychological wealth*. Malden: Wiley-Blackwell.
Diener, E., & Diener, M. (1995). Cross-cultural correlates of life satisfaction and self-esteem. *Journal of Personality and Social Psychology, 68*, 653–663.
Diener, E., & Diener, C. (1996). Most people are happy. *Psychological Science, 7*, 181–185.
Diener, E., & Lucas, R. (2000). Explaining differences in societal levels of happiness: Relative standards, need fulfillment, culture, and evaluation theory. *Journal of Happiness Studies: An Interdisciplinary Periodical on Subjective Well-Being, 1*, 41–78.
Diener, E., & Oishi, S. (2000). Money and happiness: Income and subjective well-being across nations. In E. Diener & E. M. Suh (Eds.), *Culture and subjective well-being* (pp. 185–218). Cambridge, MA: MIT Press.
Diener, E., & Oishi, S. (2004). Are Scandinavians happier than Asians? Issues in comparing nations on subjective well-being. In F. Columbus (Ed.), *Asian economic and political issues* (Vol. 10, pp. 1–25). Hauppauge: Nova Science.
Diener, E., & Suh, E. (1999). National differences in subjective well-being. In D. Kahneman, E. Diener, & N. Schwarz (Eds.), *Well-being: The foundations of hedonic psychology* (pp. 434–450). New York: Sage.
Diener, E., & Suh, E. M. (Eds.). (2000). *Culture and subjective well-being*. Cambridge, MA: MIT Press.
Diener, E., & Tov, W. (2007). Subjective well-being and peace. *Journal of Social Issues, 63*, 421–440.
Diener, E., Emmons, R. A., Larsen, R. J., & Griffin, S. (1985). The satisfaction with life scale. *Journal of Personality Assessment, 49*, 71–75.
Diener, E., Diener, M., & Diener, C. (1995a). Factors predicting the subjective well-being of nations. *Journal of Personality and Social Psychology, 69*, 851–864.
Diener, E., Suh, E., Smith, H., & Shao, L. (1995b). National differences in reported subjective well-being: Why do they occur? *Social Indicators Research, 34*, 7–32.
Diener, E., Gohm, C., Suh, E., & Oishi, S. (2000). Similarity of the relations between marital status and subjective well-being across cultures. *Journal of Cross-Cultural Psychology, 31*, 419–436.
Diener, E., Nickerson, C., Lucas, R. E., & Sandvik, E. (2002). Dispositional affect and job outcomes. *Social Indicators Research, 59*, 229–259.
Diener, E., Oishi, S., & Lucas, R. E. (2003). Personality, culture, and subjective well-being: Emotional and cognitive evaluations of life. *Annual Review of Psychology, 54*, 403–425.
Diener, M. L., Fujita, F., Kim-Prieto, C., & Diener, E. (2004). *Culture and emotional experience*. Unpublished manuscript, University of Utah.
Diener, E., Kahneman, D., Tov, W., & Arora, R. (2009a). Income's association with judgments of life versus feelings. In E. Diener, D. Kahneman, & J. Helliwell (Eds.), *International differences in well-being*. New York: Oxford University Press.
Diener, E., Ng, W., & Tov, W. (2009b). Balance in life and declining marginal utility of diverse resources. *Applied Research in Quality of Life, 3*, 277–291.
Diener, E., Ng, W., Harter, J., & Arora, R. (2010). Wealth and happiness across the world: Material prosperity predicts life evaluation, while psychosocial prosperity predicts positive feeling. *Journal of Personality and Social Psychology, 97*, 143–156.
Eid, M., & Diener, E. (2001). Norms for experiencing emotions in different cultures: Inter- and intranational differences. *Journal of Personality and Social Psychology, 81*, 869–885.
Elliot, A. J., Chirkov, V. I., Kim, Y., & Sheldon, K. M. (2001). A Cross-Cultural Analysis of Avoidance (Relative to Approach). *Personal Goals Psychological Science, 12*, 505–510.
Fredrickson, B. L. (1998). What good are positive emotions? *Review of General Psychology, 2*, 300–319.
Fulmer, A., Gelfand, M., Kruglanski, C. K.-P., Diener, E., Pierro, A., & Higgins, T. (2010). On "feeling right" in cultural contexts: How person-culture match affects self esteem and subjective well-being. *Psychological Science, 21*, 1563–1569.
Glenn, N. D. (1975). The contribution of marriage to the psychological well-being of males and females. *Journal of Marriage and the Family, 37*, 594–600.

Graham, C., Eggers, A., & Sukhtankar, S. (2004). Does happiness pay? An exploration based on panel data from Russia. *Journal of Economic Behavior and Organization, 55*, 319–342.
Henrich, J., Boyd, R., Bowles, S., Gintis, H., Fehr, E., Camerer, C., McElreath, R., Gurven, M., Hill, K., Barr, A., Ensminger, J., Tracer, D., Marlow, F., Patton, J., Alvard, M., Gil-White, F., & Henrich, N. (2005). 'Economic Man' in cross-cultural perspective: Ethnography and experiments from 15 small-scale societies. *The Behavioral and Brain Sciences, 28*, 795–855.
Ito, T. A., Cacioppo, J. T., & Lang, P. J. (1998). Eliciting affect using the international affective picture system: Trajectories through evaluative space. *Personality and Social Psychology Bulletin, 24*, 855–879.
Kitayama, S., & Markus, H. R. (2000). The pursuit of happiness and the realization of sympathy: Cultural patterns of self, social relations, and well-being. In E. Diener & E. M. Suh (Eds.), *Culture and subjective well-being* (pp. 113–161). Cambridge, MA: MIT Press.
Kitayama, S., Markus, H. R., & Kurokawa, M. (2000). Culture, emotion, and well-being: Good feelings in Japan and the United States. *Cognition and Emotion, 14*, 93–124.
Kitayama, S., Mesquita, B., & Karasawa, M. (2006). Cultural affordances and emotional experience: Socially engaging and disengaging emotions in Japan and the United States. *Journal of Personality and Social Psychology, 91*, 890–903.
Kitayama, S., Park, H., Sevincer, A. T., Karasawa, M., & Uskul, A. K. (2009). A cultural task analysis of implicit independence: Comparing North America, Western Europe, and East Asia. *Journal of Personality and Social Psychology, 97*, 236–255.
Kuppens, P., Ceulemans, E., Timmerman, M. E., Diener, E., & Kim-Prieto, C. (2006). Universal intracultural and intercultural dimensions of the recalled frequency of emotional experience. *Journal of Cross-Cultural Psychology, 37*, 491–515.
Kuppens, P., Realo, A., & Diener, E. (2008). The role of positive and negative emotions in life satisfaction judgment across nations. *Journal of Personality and Social Psychology, 95*, 66–75.
Kwan, V. S. Y., Bond, M. H., & Singelis, T. M. (1997). Pancultural explanations for life satisfaction: Adding relationship harmony to self-esteem. *Journal of Personality and Social Psychology, 73*, 1038–1051.
Lee, G. R., Seccombe, K., & Shehan, C. L. (1991). Marital status and personal happiness: An analysis of trend data. *Journal of Marriage and the Family, 53*, 839–844.
Lucas, R. E., & Diener, E. (2008). Multilevel modeling of well-being across nations. In F. J. R. van de Vijver, D. A. van Hemert, & Y. H. Poortinja (Eds.), *Multilevel analysis of individuals and cultures* (pp. 223–248). New York: Lawrence Erlbaum Associates.
Lucas, R. E., Diener, E., Grob, A., Suh, E. M., & Shao, L. (2000). Cross-cultural evidence for the fundamental features of extraversion. *Journal of Personality and Social Psychology, 79*, 452–468.
Lucas, R. E., Clark, A. E., Georgellis, Y., & Diener, E. (2003). Reexamining adaptation and the set point model of happiness: Reactions to changes in marital status. *Journal of Personality and Social Psychology, 84*, 527–539.
Lyubomirsky, S., King, L., & Diener, E. (2005). The benefits of frequent positive affect: Does happiness lead to success? *Psychological Bulletin, 131*, 803–855.
Matlin, M. W., & Stang, D. J. (1978). *The Pollyanna principle: Selectivity in language, memory, and thought*. Rochester: Schenkman Pub. Co.
Menon, U., & Schweder, R. A. (1994). Kali's tongue: Cultural psychology and the power of shame in Orissa, India. In S. Kitayama & H. R. Markus (Eds.), *Emotion and culture: Empirical studies of mutual influence* (pp. 241–284). Washington, DC: American Psychological Association.
Oishi, S. (2002). Experiencing and remembering of well-being: A cross-cultural analysis. *Personality and Social Psychology Bulletin, 28*, 1398–1406.
Oishi, S. (2006). The concept of life satisfaction across cultures: An IRT analysis. *Journal of Research in Personality, 41*, 411–423.
Oishi, S., & Diener, E. (2001). Goals, culture, and subjective well-being. *Personality and Social Psychology Bulletin, 27*, 1674–1682.
Oishi, S., Diener, E., Lucas, R. E., & Suh, E. (1999). Cross-cultural variations in predictors of life satisfaction: Perspectives from needs and values. *Personality and Social Psychology Bulletin, 25*, 980–990.

Oishi, S., Wyer, R. S., Jr., & Colcombe, S. (2000). Cultural variation in the use of current life satisfaction to predict the future. *Journal of Personality and Social Psychology, 78*, 434–445.
Oishi, S., Diener, E., Scollon, C. N., & Biswas-Diener, R. (2004). Cross-situational consistency of affective experiences across cultures. *Journal of Personality and Social Psychology, 86*, 460–472.
Oishi, S., Diener, E., Choi, D. W., Kim-Prieto, C., & Choi, I. (2007). The dynamics of daily events and well-being across cultures: When less is more. *Journal of Personality and Social Psychology, 93*, 685–698.
Oyserman, D., & Lee, S. W. S. (2008). Does culture influence what and how we think? Effects of priming individualism and collectivism. *Psychological Bulletin, 134*, 311–342.
Oyserman, D., Coon, H. M., & Kemmelmeier, M. (2002). Rethinking individualism and collectivism: Evaluation of theoretical assumptions and meta-analyses. *Psychological Bulletin, 128*, 3–72.
Pressman, S., & Cohen, S. (2005). Does positive affect influence health? *Psychological Bulletin, 131*, 925–971.
Russell, J. A. (1983). Pancultural aspects of the human conceptual organizations of emotions. *Journal of Personality and Social Psychology, 45*, 1281–1288.
Russell, J. A. (1991). Culture and the categorization of emotion. *Psychological Bulletin, 110*, 426–450.
Schimmack, U., Oishi, S., & Diener, E. (2002a). Cultural influences on the relation between pleasant emotions and unpleasant emotions: Asian dialectic philosophies or individualism-collectivism? *Cognition and Emotion, 16*, 705–719.
Schimmack, U., Radhakrishnan, P., Oishi, S., Dzokoto, V., & Ahadi, S. (2002b). Culture, personality, and subjective well-being: Integrating process models of life satisfaction. *Journal of Personality and Social Psychology, 82*, 582–593.
Scollon, C. N., Diener, E., Oishi, S., & Biswas-Diener, R. (2004). Emotions across cultures and methods. *Journal of Cross-Cultural Psychology, 35*, 304–326.
Scollon, C. N., Diener, E., Oishi, S., & Biswas-Diener, R. (2005). An experience sampling and cross-cultural investigation of the relation between pleasant and unpleasant affect. *Cognition and Emotion, 19*, 27–52.
Shaver, P. R., Wu, S., & Schwartz, J. C. (1992). Cross-cultural similarities and differences in emotion and representation: A prototype approach. *Review of Personality and Social Psychology, 13*, 175–212.
Stevenson, B., & Wolfers, J. (2008). Economic growth and subjective well-being: Reassessing the Easterlin Paradox. *Brookings Papers on Economic Activity, 39*(Spring), 1–102.
Suh, E. M. (2002). Culture, identity consistency, and subjective well-being. *Journal of Personality and Social Psychology, 83*, 1378–1391.
Suh, E., Diener, E., Oishi, S., & Triandis, H. C. (1998). The shifting basis of life satisfaction judgments across cultures: Emotions versus norms. *Journal of Personality and Social Psychology, 74*, 482–493.
Suh, E. M., Diener, E., & Updegraff, J. A. (2008). From culture to priming conditions – Self-construal influences on life satisfaction judgments. *Journal of Cross-Cultural Psychology, 39*, 3–15.
Tay, L., & Diener, E. (2011). Needs and subjective well-being around the world. *Journal of Personality and Social Psychology, 101*(2), 354–365.
Tay, L., Diener, E., Drasgow, F., & Vermunt, J. K. (2011). Multilevel mixed-measurement IRT analysis: An explication and application to self-reported emotions around the world. *Organizational Research Methods, 14*, 177–207.
Taylor, S. E. (1991). Asymmetrical effects of positive and negative events: The mobilization-minimization hypothesis. *Psychological Bulletin, 110*, 67–85.
Tov, W., & Diener, E. (2007). Culture and subjective well-being. In S. Kitayama & D. Cohen (Eds.), *Handbook of cultural psychology* (pp. 691–713). New York: Guilford.
Tov, W., & Diener, E. (2008). The well-being of nations: Linking together trust, cooperation, and democracy. In B. A. Sullivan, M. Snyder, & J. L. Sullivan (Eds.), *Cooperation: The political psychology of effective human interaction* (pp. 323–342). Malden: Blackwell Publishing.

Tov, W., Diener, E., Ng, W., Kesebir, P., & Harter, J. (2009). The social and economic context of peace and happiness. In R. S. Wyer, C.- Chiu, & Y.- Hong (Eds.), *Understanding culture: Theory, research, and application*. New York: Taylor & Francis Group.
Tsai, J. L., Knutson, B., & Fung, H. H. (2006). Cultural variation in affect valuation. *Journal of Personality and Social Psychology, 90*, 288–307.
Tsai, J. L., Louie, J., Chen, E. E., & Uchida, Y. (2007a). Learning what feelings to desire: Socialization of ideal affect through children's storybooks. *Personality and Social Psychology Bulletin, 33*, 17–30.
Tsai, J. L., Miao, F., & Seppala, E. (2007b). Good feelings in Christianity and Buddhism: Religious differences in ideal affect. *Personality and Social Psychology Bulletin, 33*, 409–421.
Uchida, Y., Kitayama, S., Mesquita, B., Reyes, J. A. S., & Morling, B. (2008). Is perceived emotional support beneficial? Well-being and health in independent and interdependent cultures. *Personality and Social Psychology Bulletin, 34*, 741–754.
Veenhoven, R., & Ehrhardt, J. (1995). The cross-national pattern of happiness: Test of predictions implied in three theories of happiness. *Social Indicator Research, 34*, 33–68.
Vittersø, J., Røysamb, E., & Diener, E. (2002). The concept of life satisfaction across cultures: Exploring its diverse meaning and relation to economic wealth. In E. Gullone & R. Cummins (Eds.), *Social indicators research book series: The universality of subjective wellbeing indicators* (pp. 81–103). Dordrecht: Kluwer.
Watson, D., Clark, L. A., & Tellegen, A. (1984). Cross-cultural convergence in the structure of mood: A Japanese replication and a comparison with U.S. findings. *Journal of Social and Personality Psychology, 47*, 127–144.

Further Reading

Diener, E. (2009). *Culture and well-being: The collected works of Ed Diener* (Social Indicators Research Series, Vol. 38). Dordrecht: Springer.
Diener, E., Helliwell, J. F., & Kahneman, D. (Eds.). (2009). *International differences in well-being*. New York: Oxford University Press.
Diener, E., & Suh, E. M. (Eds.). (2000). *Culture and subjective well-being*. Cambridge, MA: MIT Press.
Tov, W., & Diener, E. (2007). Culture and subjective well-being. In S. Kitayama & D. Cohen (Eds.), *Handbook of cultural psychology* (pp. 691–713). New York: Guilford.

Chapter 9
Mental Well-Being in Iran: The Importance of Comprehensive Well-Being in Understanding the Linkages of Personality and Values

Mohsen Joshanloo

In line with the theme of this book, the purpose of this chapter is to highlight the major findings in the field of well-being in Iran. Obviously, it is difficult to do a comprehensive review of a field as broad as well-being in such a dynamic culture. Therefore, this chapter focuses on some selected streams of research. Iranian and western findings are compared in order to draw conclusions and to summarize the Iranian experience. This chapter begins with a review of western conceptualizations of well-being and proceeds with proposing an account of the concept of *the good life* in Islam, with reference to Islamic texts. I argue that the distinction made by western scholars between eudaimonic and hedonic aspects of well-being is applicable to Iranian-Islamic culture in its generality. I then review a few areas of well-being research in Iran. Attention is then directed to some contributions of well-being research in Iran and to the ongoing debates in the field. I argue that the initial Iranian experience with western conceptualizations and scales of well-being has been relatively successful and can be considered as a good first step in this area of research.

Western Conceptualization of Mental Well-Being: Hedonic and Eudaimonic Aspects

It is impossible to map out the entire field of well-being research. Here, I will focus on the distinction between two different perspectives in the study of well-being: hedonic and eudaimonic. The distinction between hedonic and eudaimonic aspects of well-being has repeatedly proved informative and has been held by many to be theoretically and empirically warranted (e.g., see Keyes and Annas 2009; Keyes et al. 2002; Ryan and Deci 2001; Ryan et al. 2008; Waterman et al. 2008). The primary

---

M. Joshanloo (✉)
Victoria University of Wellington & Centre for Applied Cross-Cultural Research,
Kelburn Parade, P.O. Box 600, Wellington 6012, New Zealand
e-mail: mohsen.joshanloo@vuw.ac.nz

C.L.M. Keyes (ed.), *Mental Well-Being: International Contributions to the Study of Positive Mental Health*, DOI 10.1007/978-94-007-5195-8_9,

difference between eudaimonic and hedonic definitions of well-being is that the former is premised on positive functioning and the latter on positive feeling (Keyes and Annas 2009).

Under hedonic theory, well-being is equated with hedonic pleasure or happiness. "Indeed, the predominant view among hedonic psychologists is that well-being consists of subjective happiness and concerns the experience of pleasure versus displeasure broadly construed to include all judgments about the good/bad elements of life" (Ryan and Deci 2001, p. 144). Most research within so-called hedonic psychology have used an assessment of subjective well-being. Subjective well-being (SWB) is generally operationalized as both a predominance of positive over negative affect (i.e., affect balance) and a global satisfaction with life (Diener 1984). In other words, a person is said to have high SWB if that person reports that life is satisfying, experiences frequent pleasant affect, and infrequently experiences unpleasant affect (Diener and Lucas 1999).

Eudaimonic theory, alternatively, draws on virtue ethics. Virtue ethics is an ethical theory that takes virtue as a primary aspect of well-being and asserts that the central question of ethics "How should I live?" can be construed as "What kind of person should I be?" (Bunnin and Yu 2004). This approach to ethics can be traced back to ancient Greek philosophers, including Aristotle. "Virtue ethics is a term of art, initially introduced to distinguish an approach in normative ethics which emphasizes the virtues, or moral character, in contrast to an approach which emphasizes duties or rules (deontology) or one which emphasizes the consequences of actions (utilitarianism)" (Hursthouse 1999, p. 1). This approach locates the origin of ethics in our natural desires and inclinations. According to Devettere (2002), virtue ethics posits that an object functions well or poorly depending on whether or not it achieves its appropriate *telos*, or ends. Almost all versions of virtue ethics hold that our desires aim ultimately at an overriding good, or eudaimonia (i.e., *good fate* or *happiness*). The overriding good is the most important good that makes our lives good on the whole. Humans achieve eudaimonia "whenever the physical, psychological, interpersonal, social, and political aspects of their lives are functioning well and harmoniously… Embedded in their nature are numerous unrealized capabilities or capacities, and they function well when they actualize their innate natural capabilities that make their lives go well" (Devettere 2002, p. 22).

The eudemonistic view maintains that happiness cannot be equated with hedonia. The overriding good cannot be pleasure. Indeed, "happiness in ancient ethical thought is not a matter of feeling good or being pleased; it is not a feeling or emotion at all. It is your life as a whole which is said to be happy or not, and so discussions of happiness are discussions of the happy life" (Annas 2000, pp. 40–41). Annas elucidates why pleasure cannot be what ancient ethicists had in mind while formulating eudaimonia:

> [O]ne point is clear right from the start … Happiness is having a happy life—it applies to your life overall. Pleasure, however, is more naturally taken to be something episodic, something you can feel now and not later. It is something you experience as we perform the activities which make up your life. You can be enjoying a meal, a conversation, even life one moment and not the next; but you cannot, in the ancient way of thinking, be happy one moment and not the next, since happiness applies to your life as a whole. (p. 42)

Virtue ethicists, instead, emphasize the role of virtue in living a eudaimonic life. Eudaimonia is the person's activity that is explicated in terms of living virtuously (Keyes and Annas 2009). In other words, as Solomon and Martin (2004) put it, eudaimonia is a life of activity in accordance with virtue. "A virtue is a disposition that makes us good as a human being in that it makes us perform our functions well" (Hooft 2006, p. 58).

In line with the philosophical tradition of eudaimonism, positive psychologists adhering to the eudemonistic view consider well-being to consist of more than just hedonic pleasure, suggesting that people's reports of happiness (or of being positively affective and satisfied), although beneficial in its turn, do not necessarily mean that they are functioning psychologically and socially well. Eudaimonic view is concerned with living well and actualizing one's human potential (Deci and Ryan 2008).

Some psychologists have tried to formulate eudaimonia. Ryff's (1989) model of psychological well-being, for example, falls into the eudaimonic tradition. Her model stems from extensive literature aimed at defining positive psychological functioning (e.g., the humanistic and existential theories). She tried to integrate these scattered formulations into a multidimensional model of positive psychological functioning, which encompasses the points of convergence in the previous formulations. The model resulting from this distillation contains six components: "positive evaluations of oneself and one's past life (Self-Acceptance), a sense of continued growth and development as a person (Personal Growth), the belief that one's life is purposeful and meaningful (Purpose in Life), the possession of quality relations with others (Positive Relations With Others), the capacity to effectively manage one's life and surrounding world (Environmental Mastery), and a sense of self-determination (Autonomy)" (Ryff and Keyes 1995, p. 720). (For other conceptualizations of eudaimonia by western authors, see Ryan et al. 2008; Vitterso et al. 2010; and Waterman et al. 2008).

Social Components of Human Functioning

According to Keyes and Shapiro (2004), what has been missing in the well-being literature is the recognition that individuals may evaluate the quality of their lives and personal functioning against social criteria. Keyes' (1998) brief review shows that the distinction between public and private life has pervaded social psychological theory. He argues that the private and public life are two potential sources of life challenges, with possibly distinct consequences for judging a well-lived life. Despite this distinction, the "leading conceptions of adult functioning portray well-being as a primarily private phenomenon" (Keyes 1998, p.121) and emphasize private features of well-being. That is, according to Keyes (2002), measures of hedonic well-being often identify individuals' satisfaction, or positive affect, with *life overall* but rarely with facets of their social lives. Dimensions of psychological well-being are also intrapersonal reflections of an individual's adjustment to and outlook on their life. Only one of the six scales of psychological well-being (positive relations with others) reflects the ability to build and maintain intimate, trusting, interpersonal relationship (Keyes 2002). But "individuals remain embedded in social structures and communities, and face countless social tasks and challenges" (Keyes 1998, p. 122). Accordingly, Keyes asserts that there is more to functioning than psychological well-being. He believes that to understand optimal functioning and mental health, social scientists should also investigate individuals' social well-being.

Keyes' (1998) multidimensional model of social well-being is an attempt to conceptualize and assess the social aspect of well-being. This model falls into the eudaimonic perspective and addresses social aspects of human functioning. The model consists of five dimensions that indicate whether and to what degree individuals are functioning well in their social world:

> [S]ocial acceptance is a favorable view of human nature and a feeling of comfort with other people; social actualization is the belief in the evolution of society and the sense that society has potential that is being realized through its institutions and citizens; social contribution is the evaluation of one's value to society; social coherence is the perception of the quality, organization, and operation of the social world and includes a concern for knowing about the world; and social integration is the extent to which people feel they have something in common with others who constitute their social reality (e.g., their neighborhood), as well as the degree to which they feel that they belong to their communities and society. (Robitschek and Keyes 2009, p. 323)

Extant findings regarding the correlates of social well-being confirm the validity and usefulness of this multifaceted model of social well-being. The social well-being scale correlates with variables extracted from earlier formulations of successful aging (e.g., generativity in Erikson's model of human development, Keyes and Ryff 1998), a set of variables reflecting positive functioning in the context of community in which community psychologists are interested (e.g., psychological sense of community, Cicognani et al. 2008; Joshanloo et al. 2006a, b), other aspects of well-being (e.g., life satisfaction, Joshanloo and Ghaedi 2009; Joshanloo and Nosratabadi 2009), and some positive personality traits (e.g., self-efficacy, Joshanloo et al. 2006a, b).

Complete Mental Health

It is important to note that although the hedonic and eudaimonic aspects of well-being are theoretically and empirically distinguishable, many believe that both components of well-being should be included in the research designs, in tandem, to gain a full picture of a well-lived life (Keyes and Annas 2009). Theoretically, feeling and functioning are distinct, yet overlapping. Not surprisingly, empirical investigations suggest that there is overlap between the experience of hedonia and eudaimonia (e.g., see Kashdan et al. 2008). Ryan and Deci (2001) assert that "evidence from a number of investigators has indicated that well-being is probably best conceived as a multidimensional phenomenon that includes aspects of both the hedonic and eudaimonic conceptions" (p. 148). As Strumpfer (2006) pointed out, such a conception would clearly fit well into Keyes' (2002, 2005a) *complete mental health* model. According to this model, each dimension of well-being (hedonic, psychological, and social) represents an important domain of study in itself. Thus, all these scales should be collectively employed to measure the presence and absence of mental health.

Keyes (2002) proposes a mental health continuum ranging from flourishing, moderate, to languishing. Flourishing individuals have high levels on both hedonic and eudaimonic well-being. Languishing individuals have low levels on both types of well-being. Finally, individuals who are neither flourishing nor languishing in life are diagnosed as moderately mentally healthy. These individuals either have moderate levels of both hedonic and eudaimonic well-being or have high level of one and low level of the other. In several studies, Keyes and his colleagues have shown that anything less than flourishing (scoring high on both hedonic and eudaimonic well-being) "is associated with greater burden to self and society" (Keyes and Annas 2009). Results of several studies show that missed days of work, cutbacks in the amount of work, limitations of activities of daily living, prevalence of cardiovascular disease, average number of chronic physical health conditions, and the like are lowest among flourishing individuals, increased among moderately mentally healthy individuals, and highest in languishing individuals (Keyes 2002, 2004, 2005a, b). Findings of another study by Keyes et al. (2002) indicate that when both hedonic and eudaimonic well-being are present in an individual, they complement each other. However, when one is absent, they compensate for each other.

The conceptualizations of well-being outlined above are proposed by western psychologists. Considering the differences between non-western countries and the West, it is not wise to take the utility of these conceptualizations and scales for granted in non-western countries before theoretical and empirical investigations are undertaken. In the sections that follow, I will briefly introduce Iranian culture and closely examine what the Iranian concept of the good life might be like. This analysis is aimed at shedding some light on the question: Is it fruitful or destructive to apply western concepts and scales of well-being to a country like Iran?

The Concept of Mental Well-Being in Iran

Iran is a Muslim country in southwestern Asia, with a population of more than 70 millions. Iran is not an Arab country, and the official language of the country is Persian. Relative to North American and northern European societies, collectivistic values are salient in Iranian social life (Safdar et al. 2006).

Ninety-seven percent of Iran is Muslim (Clawson and Rubin 2005), and the country is currently ruled by a theocratic government. Iranian government has tried to Islamize the population during the last few decades. The constitution of Iran states that no laws, rights, or policies should contradict Islam (Tamadonfar 2001). The foreign policy of the Iranian government is generally anti-western, and such a policy has led to the country's isolation from the West.

A substantial majority of Iranians (about 89%) are Muslims of the Shiite sect, a sect different from Sunni, to which a great majority of Muslims (e.g., most of Arabs) belong. Zoroastrianism (the ancient pre-Islamic religion of Persia) has influenced the Islamic practice and faith among Iranians on a noticeable level (e.g., Stepaniants 2002; Romance 2007). However, the Iranian version of Islam (i.e., Shiism) is identical to mainstream Islam in terms of the fundamental tenets (e.g., belief in the oneness of God, belief in the resurrection day, the belief that the prophet Muhammad is the messenger of God, and that Quran is God's words).

These characteristics of Iranian culture indicate that Iran is different in political regime and culture from most of the countries from which scientific psychological studies come. Accordingly, the relevance of the western notion of the good life to Iran cannot be taken for granted without theoretical and empirical studies supporting this claim. Below, I propose an account of the concept of the good life in Islam with reference to Islamic texts. However, it should be borne in mind that Islam is not the only influential ideology in Iran. Other influential schools of thought are Iranian pre-Islamic religions and philosophies (e.g., Zoroastrianism and Manichaeism), Iranian post-Islamic philosophy, and Persian mysticism which have all influenced the Iranian popular religiosity. However, dealing with all these schools of thought is beyond the scope and purpose of this chapter and is left for future work.

Mental Health in Islam

> I saw a holy man on the seashore who had been wounded by a tiger. No medicine could relieve his pain; he suffered much but he nevertheless constantly thanked God the most high, saying: "Praise be to Allah [=God] that I have fallen into a calamity and not into sin."
>
> If that beloved Friend [=God] decrees me to be slain
> I shall not say that moment that I grieve for life
> Or say: What fault has thy slave committed?
> My grief will be for having offended thee.[1]
>
> —Sa'adi, The Gulistan [The Rose Garden] of Sa'adi (1259 CE)

Islamic view of humankind is dualistic, as humans possess both a perishable body and an everlasting soul (Haque 2004a, b). Islam posits that one of the basic spiritual needs of people is to worship a higher power (Sajedi 2008a). Also, according to Islam, we have two lives, one in this world and one in the hereafter. Our life in the present world is far less important than our eternal life in the afterworld (Quran 6:32). The Islamic concept of the good life needs to take these two important points into account. That is to say, this concept should be formulated in such way that it

[1] Story 12 of Chapter 2, "The Gulistan of Sa'adi" written by one of the most famous and popular Iranian poets Sa'adi. English translation obtained from: http://enel.ucalgary.ca/People/far/hobbies/iran/Golestan/gulistan.pdf

guarantees the satisfaction of individuals' spiritual needs and their happiness in both lives. Clearly, such a concept of mental health and the good life needs to go beyond the absence of mental illness. Indeed, in Islam, mental health is not only the absence of mental disorders but also the presence of positive qualities and virtues (Abou el Azayem and Hedayat-Diba 1994; Haque 2004a, b; Smither and Khordandi 2009). The Islamic view of the good life is consistent with positive psychology's viewpoint in this regard.

The Islamic notion of the good life is more consistent with eudaimonism than hedonism. Islamic texts indicate that to live a good life, one should have faith and put that faith into practice. "[i]t is believed that by following Islamic principles, Muslims can achieve and enjoy the four ingredients of a healthy and balanced life, namely, physical, social, mental, and spiritual health" (Abou el Azayem and Hedayat-Diba 1994, p. 49). All Muslims are obliged to have faith in some principal beliefs of Islam (belief in oneness of God, belief in the resurrection, etc.). Furthermore, Islam is a comprehensive way of life. It covers all aspects of life (individual, spiritual, economic, social, political, and family). Muslims believe that religion cannot be separated from any little aspect of life (Hamdan 2007; Pridmore and Pasha 2004). Only having faith in these beliefs and living based on the ordinances of Islam in all aspects of life can lead to the satisfaction of individuals' spiritual needs and the actualization of their potential. About those who believe and keep their duty to Allah, the Quran (10:64) says "[t]heirs are good tidings in the life of the world and in the hereafter...."[2]

According to Islam, humans are the product of the unification of spirit and body. God has breathed spirit into humans' material body. This divine spirit needs to be actualized. One can freely choose to actualize the divine spirit within oneself by following the ordinances of Islam or choose to indulge in material pleasures. Attainment of a virtuous lifestyle requires relentless patience and constant struggle against our lower nature (Akhtar 2008).

According to Islam, when a child is born, it carries within it a natural belief in God. This natural belief is called the *fitrah*. This innate disposition is considered to be a source of guidance, telling humans when they are wrong (Haque 2004a, b). In a sense, we are preprogrammed to worship God and follow his commands. But, due to environmental pressures, we forget our true nature. Humans are obliged to rediscover their fitrah and follow its guidance. The Quran says (30:30–31):

> So set thy purpose (O Muhammad) for religion as a man by nature upright—the nature (framed) of Allah, in which He hath created man. There is no altering (the laws of) Allah's creation. That is the right religion, but most men know not—Turning unto Him (only); and be careful of your duty unto Him and establish worship, and be not of those who ascribe partners (unto Him).

Obviously, such a viewpoint fits well with the eudaimonic view, which emphasizes actualizing human potential and satisfaction of true human needs.

[2] All the English translation of the Quran verses are obtained from http://www.quranexplorer.com

Islam's emphasis on eudaimonia does not mean that positive emotions and pleasures are not legitimate in Islam. Instead, it holds that by adhering to the Islamic lifestyle, Muslims experience many different positive emotions and pleasures (vitality, peacefulness, gladness, contentment, gratitude, joy, etc.), both in this world and in the hereafter. For example, the Quran says (13:28) "[v]erily in the remembrance of Allah do hearts find rest." Islam holds that one should not pursue hedonistic pleasures as the primary goal of life. In fact, positive emotions and pleasure are considered necessary in Islam, but they are regarded secondary and are placed after eudaimonistic strivings. That is, Muslims should not choose for themselves the goods of this lower life (i.e., evil pleasures of this world) as the goal of life (Q 7:169), since "naught is the life of the world save a pastime…" (Q 6:32). Thus, attempts to maximize positive emotions and pleasures and minimize negative emotions and pains, if not accompanied by eudaimonic strivings, are discouraged.

As it is evident in the excerpt that opened this section, one of the Iranian foremost poets, Sa'adi, finds good reasons to praise a pious man who suffered a long-lasting incurable pain but constantly thanked God because God has destined him to suffer from a calamity and not to a life of committing sin. In other words, although this calamity undermines the hedonic balance of the pious man's life, since it does not interfere with living a virtuous life (as understood by the pious man), he is grateful to God for it. Iranian literature is replete with such stories and sagas, which try to persuade people to choose eudaimonic standards for assessing a well-lived life. But we should also note that gratitude is classified as a positive emotion, which has recently received much attention in positive psychology (e.g., Emmons and McCullough 2004). Thus, Sa'adi is covertly suggesting that even in face of misery and calamity, living a virtuous life (e.g., to be satisfied with God's will and be grateful no matter what happens in one's life) can neutralize the anhedonia caused by misery and replace it with relatively positive emotions (in this case, gratitude).

In sum, no mental health model is adequate in Islam unless it takes eudaimonistic aspects into account. In fact, the most perfect model is one that takes both hedonic and eudaimonic aspects into account. It can be concluded that the distinction between hedonic and eudaimonic well-being and the necessity of both of them in conceptualizing and assessing well-being in Islamic cultures seem to be theoretically warranted. However, there appears to be some variation in the dimensions of eudaimonic and hedonic aspects between western and Islamic cultures or the amount of emphasis that each puts on a single dimension of well-being. For example, whereas autonomy is emphasized more as a basic human need in western culture, the need for worship is emphasized more as a basic need by Islam (Sajedi 2008a).

A detailed discussion of individual symptoms of well-being (positive relations with others, purpose in life, social integration, social contribution, life satisfaction, etc.) and their relevance to Islamic faith is beyond the focus of this chapter. The interested reader is referred to the existing articles and books published by scholars and psychologists in many diverse languages. For example, in an article in Persian, Sajedi (2008a, b) argues that Islam provides Muslims with the mechanisms needed to achieve many high standards posited by western notions of mental health. He cites tens of sayings of Islamic religious leaders and of the Quran to show that many common themes in western models of well-being (e.g., spirituality, positive relations with others, social interest, meaning in life, self-knowledge) are highly valued in Islam. As another example, in an interesting study by Dahlsgaard et al. (2005), philosophical and religious traditions in Confucianism, Taoism, Buddhism, Hinduism, Athenian philosophy, Judaism, Christianity, and Islam were investigated to find common core values. The authors found six core strengths that were valued in all these traditions: courage, justice, humanity, temperance, wisdom, and transcendence. They concluded that "there is convergence across time, place, and intellectual tradition about certain core virtues" (p. 210). Given that these universal values predispose individuals to the good life, these findings indicate that living a virtuous life has some common characteristics, no matter which faith it is lived by.

Especially during the last decade, Persian translations of western scales of hedonic and eudaimonic well-being have been widely used in Iran. Therefore, we can draw on existing empirical literature to evaluate the utility of these scales in Iran. Below, I will provide a brief review of the findings of well-being studies in Iran.

Well-Being Research in Iran

Iranian researchers have used many western scales in their work to assess different aspects of well-being. These studies can be divided into two categories. In the first category, the construct validity and reliability of the translations of these scales are examined. In the second category, the predictors of different aspects of well-being are examined. I will return to the second category of research (specifically, two groups of predictors: personality traits and values) later in this chapter. First, I will briefly review the first category of research, which focuses on the investigation of the validity and reliability of western well-being scales in Iranian samples.

Validity and Reliability of Western Well-Being Scales in Iran

Validity and reliability of some western scales of well-being have been examined in Iran. For example, Joshanloo et al. (2006a) examined the factor structure of 13 symptoms of well-being (including six aspects of Ryff's *psychological well-being* model, five aspects of Keyes' *social well-being* model, *life satisfaction*, and *positive affect*) based on Keyes' (2002) comprehensive model of mental health, described above. Using a sample of 205 Iranian university students, they showed that the three-factor model (viewing psychological, social, and emotional well-being as three separate but correlated factors) showed the best fit to the data. Although, the fit indices were not excellent, some minor modification improved the model's fit.

Shokri et al. (2008) examined the factor structure of 3-, 9-, and 14-item Persian versions of Ryff's Scales of Psychological Well-Being in Iranian university students ($N = 374$). Results of the confirmatory factor analysis revealed that the six-dimensional model of psychological well-being (hypothesizing six distinct yet correlated factors) showed an acceptable fit to the data across all three versions. In that study, the content validity of the items of Ryff's scales was confirmed by some of the professors of psychology at one of the Iranian universities. Interestingly, the six-factor structure of different versions of this scale has not been confirmed in some other countries (e.g., Springer et al. 2006), while the results of this factor analysis conducted in Iran supports the factor structure proposed by Ryff (1989). In another study, Bayani et al. (2008) used an Iranian student sample to examine the reliability and convergent validity of an 84-item version of Ryff's psychological well-being scales. They found 2-month test-retest reliability coefficients greater than 0.71 for six subscales of this scale. They also found that Cronbach's alphas of the six subscales ranged from 0.57 to 0.76. Finally, their results demonstrated that this scale was positively correlated with the Satisfaction with Life Scale, the Oxford Happiness Inventory, and Rosenberg's Self-Esteem Scale.

Bakhshi et al. (2009) examined the construct validity of positive and negative affect scale (Mroczek and Kolarz 1998) in Iranian undergraduates. Their results indicated that scales of positive and negative affect had good reliability and convergent validity. In addition, unidimensional factor structure of positive affect scale was supported by both exploratory and confirmatory factor analyses. As for the negative affect scale, while exploratory factor analysis supported the unidimensional factor structure of this scale, confirmatory factor analysis yielded unacceptable fit indices.

Bakhshipur and Dozhkam (2006) applied confirmatory factor analysis to examine the factor structure of the Positive and Negative Affect Schedule (PANAS; Watson et al. 1988) in a clinical sample of 255 young adults. They found that fit indices for the model that viewed positive and negative affect factors as two separate but correlated factors were superior to those of the single factor model, although the two-factor model's fit indices were lower than the rule-of-thumb recommendation provided in the literature.

The validity of the Satisfaction with Life Scale (Diener et al. 1985) has also been examined in two studies in Iran. Bayani et al. (2007) reported a Cronbach's alpha of 0.83 and a 1-month test-retest reliability of 0.70 for this scale. They also found that this scale had a correlation of 0.71 with the Oxford Happiness Inventory. Joshanloo and Daemi (in press) investigated the construct validity of this scale. Their results indicated that the Satisfaction with Life Scale had a one-factor structure (as proposed by Diener et al. 1985) and acceptable reliability and convergent validity with Iranian student samples.

Hatami et al. (2010) examined the construct validity and reliability of the Multidimensional Students' Life Satisfaction Scale (MSLSS; Huebner 1994) using a sample of 430 students in grades 6–12 in Iran. They applied exploratory and confirmatory factor analyses in their study. They found that the pattern matrix of this Persian adaptation was, by and large, consistent with previous investigations of the MSLSS in other countries. They concluded that this Persian adaptation of the MSLSS offers a reliable and valid means of assessing Iranian middle and high school students' life satisfaction.

The validity and reliability of the Oxford Happiness Inventory (Argyle et al. 1989) have been investigated in a few studies in Iran (e.g., Alipour and Agah Heris 2007; Alipour, and Noorbala 1999; Liaghatdar et al. 2008). Findings of these studies indicate that this scale has satisfactory reliability and convergent validity in Iranian samples, but its factor structure appears to be different from that obtained in other countries. In one of these studies, in order to examine the content validity, a panel of 10 psychologists and psychiatrists were asked to review the items of this scale. All experts confirmed the ability of this scale to assess happiness in Iran (Alipour and Noorbala 1999).

Joshanloo and Ghaedi (2009) examined the psychometric properties of personal growth initiative scale (Robitschek 1998, 1999) in an Iranian university student sample. They found that the internal consistency of the scale was 0.87. Results of the confirmatory factor analyses showed that this scale had a unidimensional factor structure in the sample used. Correlations between this scale and convergent validity scales (positive affect, negative affect, life satisfaction, psychological well-being, and social well-being) were significant and in the expected direction. These results indicate acceptable reliability and validity for the Persian translation of this scale for Iranian university students.

Altogether, the findings of the validation studies done on translations of western well-being scales in Iran indicate that most of these scales are reliable and valid. Most of the Iranian researchers who have conducted these studies assert that these scales can be used in Iranian samples with confidence. The factor structure of these scales, however, has been found in some cases to be different from western versions. Although some might say this is unacceptable, we should bear in mind that this is not specific to Iran. It is sometimes possible that two-factor analytical studies in a single country, on a single scale, yield different results.

Nevertheless, this stream of research can be improved in some ways. Almost all of these studies have used student samples. Future research should examine the validity and reliability of these scales in adult samples. Furthermore, in some cases, it is better to develop some short forms for western scales to be used in Iranian samples by eliminating some items. Some individual items might need further refinement or replacement. Past research indicates that some items of these scales function worse than the rest in Iran. Some statistical techniques, such as factor analysis and Item Response Theory analysis, should be applied to examine how well each individual item functions with Iranian samples and examine the differences in the way each item functions in Iran and other cultures.

In some cases, it seems to be fruitful to add items to the scales to capture some aspects of the construct which are relevant in Iranian culture but are not captured by the original scale. This needs to be done based on some qualitative research and deep theoretical analyses. Finally, some dimensions of well-being, which are relevant to Iranian culture but are not captured by the western scales, should be identified, and new scales should be developed to tap into them. For instance, one likely candidate is spiritual well-being. The Islamic version of spiritual well-being (the satisfaction of the need for worship and surrender to God, having a constructive and positive relationship with God, etc.) should be theoretically and empirically examined to see if it qualifies as an emic aspect of well-being to be applied along with the existing western scales. All these steps may require lots of effort and time, but certainly they will be fruitful for Iranian well-being studies.

In the section that follows, I will turn to the second category of well-being studies in Iran, which focuses on the investigation of various predictors of different aspects of well-being. Due to space constraints, I will focus on two sets of predictors: personality traits and values. First presented is a brief review of the findings from different countries for each set of predictors, followed by a short review of Iranian studies.

Big Five Personality Domains and Self-Esteem as Predictors of Well-Being in Iran

In their recent review of SWB literature, Lucas and Diener (2008) asserted the following:

> [A]fter decades of research on SWB researchers have often arrived at what to some seems like a startling conclusion: The most important factor in determining a person's SWB appears to be the personality with which he or she is born. (p. 801)

Empirical research has shown that external factors (health, income, etc.) have only a modest impact on SWB reports (Diener et al. 1999). Research instead shows that SWB is often strongly correlated with stable personality traits (Diener et al. 2003). In terms of the Big Five personality domains, extraversion (E) and neuroticism (N) have been found to be the strongest predictors of SWB in many countries (for a very brief review, see Schimmack et al. 2002). However, the meta-analyses by DeNeve and Cooper (1998) and Steel et al. (2008) indicated that two other personality traits, namely, agreeableness (A) and conscientiousness (C), predispose individuals toward SWB as well. Openness to experience (O) does not appear to be a strong and consistent predictor of SWB. It has been suggested to be linked positively to both positive affect and negative affect (McCrae and Costa 1991).

Psychological dimensions of eudaimonic well-being have also been linked with personality domains. Schmutte and Ryff's (1997) findings revealed consistent linkages between the domains of personality and psychological well-being. Environmental mastery demonstrated strong negative links with N, as did purpose in life and autonomy, to a lesser degree. Self-acceptance, environmental mastery, and purpose in life were linked with E and C. Personal growth was related to O. Positive relations with others was linked with A and, to a lesser degree, with E. Finally, autonomy was linked with E, C, and O but most strongly with N. Schmutte and Ryff concluded that the "dimensions of psychological well-being are distinct from, yet meaningfully influenced by, personality" (p. 557). One important finding is that O tends to correlate only with eudaimonic aspects of well-being. This is in line with Keyes et al. (2002) results, indicating that those with high levels of eudaimonic well-being (as assessed by psychological well-being scales), but low levels of SWB, were distinguished from their opposite counterpart (high SWB/low psychological well-being) by their high levels of O.

Eudaimonic well-being researchers tend to adopt a more moderate stance on the issue of the relation between personality, environment, and well-being. For example, in her review of the related literature, Ryff (2008) finds good reasons to view both personality traits and environmental factors (e.g., socioeconomic status, gender, marital status, and ethnicity) as operative in understanding variation in well-being. She further asserts that "the comparative advantage ascribed to traits appears premature…" (p. 409).

In sum, the brief review of western findings presented above points to the fact that all the Big Five domains have important implications for well-being. Another remarkable point is that O tends to correlate only with eudaimonic aspects of well-being. From the hedonic point of view, thus, a happy person is most likely to be a person who has high scores on E, C, and A and a low score on N. From a eudaimonic point of view, however, all personality domains, including O, are considered components of a mentally healthy personality.

A number of narrower personality variables are correlated with the components of SWB (see DeNeve and Cooper 1998 for a review). Self-esteem, for example, has been found to be a strong correlate of SWB in many past studies. Campbell (1981) found a correlation of 0.55 between self-esteem and life satisfaction in a US sample. Diener and Diener (1995) found a correlation of 0.47 between self-esteem and life satisfaction in college student samples from 31 countries (see also Kwan et al. 1997; Lucas et al. 1996; Zhang and Leung 2002, for more evidence). Self-esteem has also been suggested by researchers to be the mediator of the relation between personality traits and well-being. Kwan et al. (1997) study shows that for both Chinese and American individuals, self-esteem mediates the relations between four personality traits (E, N, C, and O) and life satisfaction. In a British sample, Furnham and Cheng (2000) found that the influence of E and N on happiness was mediated by self-esteem. In addition to the mediatory role this variable plays in the relationship between personality and SWB, self-esteem also has been found to mediate the influence of a social belief domain (i.e., social cynicism) on life satisfaction (Lai et al. 2007).

Altogether, previous research in different countries indicates that self-esteem is a consistent and relatively strong predictor of aspects of well-being, albeit more so in individualistic cultures. An important issue that needs to be addressed is whether or not we should expect these findings to be replicated in Iran. Below, I provide a brief review which should shed some light on this issue.

Along with validation studies, Iranian researchers have used western well-being scales in many studies in order to find predictors of well-being in Iran. Some studies have investigated the personality predictors of well-being. For example, Joshanloo and Nosratabadi's (2009) study using an Iranian student sample showed that E, N, C, and A could significantly discriminate among the three levels of mental health continuum (i.e., flourishing, moderately mentally healthy, and languishing) based on Keyes' (2002) model of mental health. In another study on Iranian university students (Joshanloo and Rastegar 2007), it was found that eudaimonic well-being (as measured by scales of meaning in life and personal growth) was significantly predicted by C in females and by C, A, and E in males. Results of the hierarchical regression analysis revealed that self-esteem significantly predicted eudaimonic well-being scores over and above the Big Five traits in both sexes.

To the present knowledge, the only examination of the relation between the Big Five personality traits and social well-being is that of Joshanloo et al. (2012). Participants of this study included 236 undergraduates at the University of Tehran. Findings revealed that, among the Big Five personality domains, N was inversely related to social acceptance, social contribution, and social coherence. Interestingly, C was positively related to social contribution, and O was positively related to social contribution and social coherence. Also, A was related to social acceptance and social contribution. Finally, no significant correlation was observed between E and facets of social well-being. Joshanloo et al. (2007), using a sample of Iranian university students, found that high and low levels of social well-being can be significantly discriminated by N and A in females and by E and A in males. The results of hierarchical regression showed that self-esteem significantly predicted social well-being scores over and above the Big Five traits. In another study on social well-being in an Iranian student sample (Joshanloo et al. 2006b), it was found that self-esteem predicted social well-being better than a number of community-related variables (i.e., perceived social support, psychological sense of community, identification with the community, and social participation) and self-efficacy.

The relation between hedonic aspects of well-being and personality domains has been examined in a few studies in Iranian samples. Joshanloo and Afshari's (2011) study with Iranian university students showed that the Big Five personality traits explained about 25% of the variance in life satisfaction scores. Among the Big Five traits, E and N were found to be the strongest correlates of life satisfaction. As well, O was not significantly correlated with life satisfaction. In addition, it was found that self-esteem significantly predicted life satisfaction over and above the Big Five personality traits. Findings also showed that self-esteem completely mediated the influence of conscientiousness and agreeableness on life satisfaction, while the influence of extraversion and neuroticism on life satisfaction was partially mediated by self-esteem. Haghighi et al. (2006) obtained similar results in Iran, with the exception that they found a significant moderate correlation between O and happiness (as assessed by the Oxford Happiness Inventory).

Moghanloo and Aguilar-Vafaie (2009) found that happiness (assessed by a single item) was significantly correlated with E, N, and C. Khanzade et al. (2007) found significant correlations between the Oxford Happiness Inventory and three scales of the Eysenck Personality Inventory. Extraversion was positively, and neuroticism and psychoticism were negatively, correlated with happiness. In another study, it was found that among the Big Five personality traits, N, E, and C significantly predicted hedonic balance in Iranian university students (Joshanloo et al. 2010). In addition, self-esteem predicted hedonic balance over and above the Big Five traits, while perceived social support failed to do so. Finally, in a study by Zaki (2008), self-esteem was found to be a significant correlate ($r=0.48$), of quality of life in Iran (as assessed by Missoula-Vitas Quality of Life Index, Byock and Merriman 1998).

In sum, the findings of studies conducted in Iran indicate that E and N are the strongest correlates of hedonic well-being and C and A are predictors of secondary importance. Furthermore, all five personality traits are significant predictors of eudaimonic (social and psychological) aspects of well-being. Moreover, self-esteem has been repeatedly found to be a strong predictor of both hedonic and eudaimonic well-being. The patterns that have emerged in Iran in this particular line of research (the relation between personality traits and well-being) are mostly in line with the findings that have emerged in other countries, especially western ones.

Values and Well-Being in Iran

As Sagiv and Schwartz (2000) and Vansteenkiste et al. (2006), among others, have pointed out, two lines of research have been followed when examining the relation between values and well-being (see Sagiv et al. 2004, for a review). The main assumption of the first one is that pursuing *healthy* values contributes to well-being and pursuing *unhealthy* ones harms it. In other words, this line of research attempts to find direct effects of value priorities on well-being. Bilsky and Schwartz (1994), for example, suggest that conformity, security, and power values represent deficiency needs, and therefore, priority given to these values is expected to correlate negatively with well-being. Self-direction, universalism, benevolence, achievement, and stimulation, conversely, are classified as representing primarily growth needs, and therefore, pursuing them is expected to boost well-being (Bilsky and Schwartz 1994). These predictions receive partial support in Roccas et al. (2002) study showing that self-direction, stimulation, and universalism were positively, and power and conformity were inversely, related to positive affect. In five large and multicultural samples (two samples from the 2006 European Social Survey, two Basque samples, and a sample of immigrants in the Basque Country), Bobowik et al. (2011) found some support for these predictions. Their results indicate that hedonism, stimulation, and self-direction were weakly related to better well-being, while tradition, power, and conformity were weakly associated with lower well-being.

Findings, however, are sometimes at odds with these predictions. Sagiv and Schwartz (2000), for example, tried to investigate the direct relations between 10 basic values (based on the value theory developed by Schwartz 1992) and SWB. They concluded that "values have some direct influence on SWB. This influence is rather weak and it refers only to the affective aspect of well-being" (p. 186). Haslam et al. (2009) found that, in Australia, negative affect was significantly correlated with none of the values, and life satisfaction was only significantly correlated with stimulation. They also found a positive correlation between security and positive affect, which is inconsistent with the Sagiv and Schwartz's prediction.

Given its assumption that pursuing extrinsic values is detrimental to well-being, research investigating the relation between intrinsic and extrinsic values and well-being also falls into this line of research. Some researchers, self-determination theorists included, have shown that pursuing *intrinsic* values (e.g., self-acceptance and affiliation) benefits one's well-being. In contrast, pursuing *extrinsic* values (e.g., material success and fame) harms it (e.g., Kasser and Ahuvia 2002; Vansteenkiste et al. 2006).

The second line of research followed when examining the relation between values and well-being is focused on the fit between a person's value priorities and the values prevailing in that person's environment. This approach holds that such a fit between a person's values and those emphasized within his or her environment is crucial to a person's well-being. This model has been called congruency model (Sagiv et al. 2004), person-environment fit model (Triandis 2000), or cultural fit model (Lu 2006).

This model is premised on the fact that culture exists at multiple levels. It has been proposed that a distinction should be made between the cultural (or societal) and individual levels of analysis, and both levels should be taken into account (Lu 2006; Ratzlaff et al. 2000; Triandis 2000). In some cases, the results obtained at the two levels of analysis are at odds with each other. For example, it appears that while at the individual level, allocentrism (Triandis et al. 1985) is positively related to SWB, at the societal level, collectivism is negatively related to it (Triandis 2000). "Culture at the ecological level therefore describes mainstream average tendencies; it cannot describe all behaviors of all people in any culture" (Ratzlaff et al. 2000, p. 39). In other words, the individual cultural values of the people in a specific culture might be either congruent or discrepant with the larger societal culture (Lu 2006). Research shows that people differ in the extent to which they internalize existing orientations in a particular culture, as a part of self (e.g., Chirkov et al. 2005; see also Wan, and Chiu 2009). The cultural fit model assumes that to the extent that a person's personal values match the values emphasized in that person's culture, there is a good cultural fit which should boost well-being.

In line with the cultural fit model, and based on a model called *value-as-a-moderator model of SWB*, Oishi et al. (1999b) hypothesized that the relation between domain satisfaction and global life satisfaction would vary, depending on individuals' value orientation. The fundamental postulate of value-as-a-moderator model is that when making life satisfaction judgments, individuals weigh value-congruent domain satisfactions more heavily than value-incongruent domain satisfactions. Consistent with this prediction, Oishi and his colleagues found that value-congruent domain satisfaction was more strongly related to global life satisfaction than was value-incongruent domain satisfaction. For example, they found that satisfaction with social life was a strong predictor of global life satisfaction for those high in benevolence value and satisfaction with family life was a strong predictor for individuals high in conformity values. Their findings also revealed that within-individual variation of day-to-day satisfaction was strongly influenced by daily satisfaction with the most valued domain. For instance, achievement-oriented individuals tended to evaluate a day as good when they excelled in achievement domains. In another study (including data from 39 nations), Oishi et al. (1999a) found support for the value-as-a-moderator model at the cultural level. They showed that, consistent with this model, satisfaction with esteem needs (e.g., the self and freedom) predicted global life satisfaction more strongly among people in individualistic nations than people in collectivistic nations.

In Sagiv and Schwartz's (2000) study, the cultural fit model was tested by comparing a small sample of psychology students with a small sample of business students on the assumption that within these two groups, opposing sets of values would be emphasized. Based on the findings, Sagiv and Schwartz concluded that "personal value priorities contribute significantly to subjective well-being above and beyond their modest direct effects. Congruity between people's values and their environment promotes well-being regardless of the particular values to which people ascribe importance" (p. 194).

Lu (2006) looked closely at the cultural fit model within three diverse samples from Taiwan and mainland China ($N=581$). It was hypothesized that Chinese individual's degree of fit (or lack of discrepancy) between individual culture and societal culture (regarding beliefs in the independent self, the interdependent self, active control, and relationship harmony) would be positively related to SWB. Furthermore, it was hypothesized that Chinese individual's direction of cultural fit would have differential effects on SWB (i.e., being a modernist would promote SWB, whereas being a traditionalist would hinder SWB). Results indicated that the support for the first hypothesis (regarding the magnitude of cultural fit) in the samples used was quite limited. Some isolated effects of magnitude of discrepancy only within certain subgroups of the larger Chinese population were found. Furthermore, after using a Bonferroni correction, no significant correlation remained.

The second hypothesis (the direction of cultural fit), however, was partially supported. Cultural fit regarding the interdependent self and harmony beliefs apparently had no effect on SWB, whereas that regarding the independent self and active control beliefs did. Although findings indicated that people who were in accord with their societal culture generally had higher levels of well-being than those in discord, being a modernist was more advantageous than being a traditionalist. These findings suggest that the direction of cultural fit regarding independent self and active control beliefs is meaningful for SWB in these samples.

Some findings are at odds with the predictions of the cultural fit model. For instance, Kasser and Ahuvia (2002) investigated the relation between extrinsic, materialistic values and well-being in a sample of 92 business students in Singapore, where it is believed that extrinsic, materialistic values are highly supported. Their findings suggest that some types of values may be healthy or unhealthy no matter how congruent they are with the values supported by the environment. Likewise, Vansteenkiste et al. (2006), using a larger sample of business students, found that despite the match between their personal value orientation and the values emphasized within their environments, extrinsically oriented business students displayed lower psychological and physical well-being.

Research on cultural estrangement and its consequences for the individuals' well-being also falls into this line of research. Cultural estrangement is conceptualized as discrepancies between personal value priorities and perceived societal values (Cozzarelli and Karafa 1998). According to the cultural fit model, cultural estrangement is expected to be inversely associated with indicators of mental health. The empirical findings supporting this expectation, however, are scant and inconsistent. Cozzarelli and Karafa (1998), using US samples, found cultural estrangement to be negatively correlated with meaning in life, self-esteem, and life satisfaction. In a British sample, nevertheless, Bernard et al. (2006) found that there was no significant relationship between cultural estrangement and a set of well-being scales (i.e., self-esteem, life satisfaction, and self-actualization).

A rather wide variety of well-being scales have been used in the past studies reviewed above, but generally, researchers have not taken into consideration the distinction between hedonic and eudaimonic aspects of well-being when choosing well-being scales. In addition, the distinction between the two aspects of eudaimonic well-being (social and psychological) also has been totally neglected. In none of the past studies has a social well-being scale been used. Furthermore, no study has been done on the relationship between values and well-being in southern Asia or the Middle East. Therefore, two recent studies were conducted to address limitations of previous research using two Iranian university student samples.

The first one examined the relations between values and aspects of well-being using a sample of 200 Iranian university students (Joshanloo and Ghaedi 2009). Schwartz value survey (Schwartz 1992) was used to assess 10 basic human values (i.e., self-direction, stimulation, hedonism, achievement, power, security, conformity, tradition, benevolence, and universalism). Psychological and social well-being scales were used to assess the eudaimonic aspect of well-being, and the Satisfaction with Life Scale and the affect balance scale were used to assess the hedonic aspect of well-being.

Results revealed that regardless of the value types emphasized within the context, in this Iranian sample, achievement and tradition were significantly correlated with both eudaimonic and hedonic aspects of well-being. Power, self-direction, universalism, benevolence, and conformity also were related only to eudaimonic aspects of well-being. Results of bivariate correlation analysis showed that a larger number of values were correlated with eudaimonic aspects of well-being (seven values) than its hedonic aspects (two values), and the correlations were stronger for eudaimonic aspects. Therefore, it can be concluded that values are more useful variables in predicting eudaimonic well-being than hedonic well-being in this sample. Considering the difference in value correlates of hedonic and eudaimonic aspects of well-being observed in this study, it seems fruitful, and even necessary, to take the distinction between hedonic and eudaimonic aspects of well-being into account in future studies.

One important implication of this study for future well-being studies was the findings regarding the value correlates of social well-being. Self-direction was positively correlated with psychological well-being but negatively related to social well-being. In addition, power, conformity, and benevolence were not significantly correlated with other aspects of well-being but were significantly correlated with social well-being. It can be concluded that two aspects of eudaimonic well-being (psychological and social) differentially relate to various values. Therefore, based on the results of this study, the distinction between psychological and social aspects of eudaimonic well-being is better to be taken into account in future studies.

One other noticeable finding was that in this Iranian sample, conformity was positively correlated with social well-being. This is inconsistent with Bilsky and Schwartz's (1994) hypothesis that conformity, security, and power values represent deficiency needs, and therefore, priority given to these values is expected to correlate negatively with well-being. That security value was unrelated to well-being in this Iranian sample is also inconsistent with this hypothesis. Yet, power was negatively correlated with social well-being and should be considered socially unhealthy. Thus, Bilsky and Schwartz's assumptions pertaining to healthy and unhealthy values, regardless of the values emphasized in the environment, do not appear to be fully applicable to this Iranian sample.

Some findings were inconsistent (while some others were consistent) with self-determination theory's prediction (e.g., Kasser and Ryan 1996) that pursing extrinsic, materialistic values relates to poorer well-being and pursuing intrinsic values leads to higher well-being. Sagiv and Schwartz (2000) suggest that self-direction, benevolence, and universalism values are intrinsic, and the power value is extrinsic. That power had a significant and negative relation to social well-being and benevolence correlated positively with social well-being in this sample was consistent with this hypothesis. However, universalism was inversely related to psychological well-being, and self-direction showed a rather mixed pattern of associations with different aspects of well-being. All in all, these findings cast doubt on the distinction between intrinsic and extrinsic values, as proposed by self-determination theorists, as a basis for relating values to well-being in this Iranian sample. However, it is noteworthy to mention that this study (using Schwartz value survey to measure values) was not an accurate test of Kasser and Ryan's (1996) hypothesis, since as Kasser and Ahuvia (2002) have pointed out, Schwartz value survey does not specifically measure extrinsic, materialistic values as Kasser and Ryans define them.

Altogether, these findings draw our attention to four important points. First, the distinction between hedonic and eudaimonic well-being should be taken into account in studies examining the relation between values and well-being. Second, the distinction between social and psychological well-being should be taken into account in such studies. Indeed, these findings suggest that there are some risks associated with overlooking the social aspects in well-being research. Third, these findings suggest that if we test the existing assumptions regarding the relation between values and well-being, applying more comprehensive scales of well-being (assessing hedonic, psychological, and social well-being), many of the prior assumptions regarding the relation between values and well-being will turn out to be inadequate. Finally, these findings suggest that there are both similarities and differences between Iran and other countries in terms of healthy and unhealthy values. Therefore, based on these findings and those reviewed earlier, any claim of universality in the relation between values and well-being should be made with caution.

In another study (Joshanloo 2010), the cultural fit model was tested in an Iranian student sample ($N=208$). Building on the studies done within this model, this study sought to examine the relation between cultural estrangement and aspects of well-being. As mentioned earlier, cultural estrangement has been found to correlate negatively with some indicators of mental health in a few US samples (Cozzarelli and Karafa 1998), while it has been found to be unrelated to well-being measures in two British samples (Bernard et al. 2006).

In this study, cultural estrangement life satisfaction, hedonic balance, and psychological and social well-being scales were used. Findings revealed that, in this Iranian sample, cultural estrangement was negatively associated with three aspects of well-being, namely, life satisfaction, affect balance, and social well-being. The patterns of relationships indicated that to feel estranged from one's culture undermines emotional well-being and social functioning, while it has no significant effect on individuals' personal functioning (i.e., psychological well-being). The correlations, nevertheless, were rather low. Furthermore, results of regression analysis revealed that aspects of cultural estrangement significantly predicted life satisfaction, affect balance, and social well-being over and above gender. Relative to those of the Big Five personality domains and self-esteem (Joshanloo and Afshari 2011), however, the contribution of cultural estrangement was smaller.

But inconsistent with expectations, psychological well-being was not significantly correlated with cultural estrangement. This might be explained in light of the findings of Joshanloo and Ghaedi's (2009) study reported above. They found a positive association between psychological well-being and self-direction (an individualistic value) in Iranian undergraduates. They also reported a negative correlation between this aspect of well-being and tradition, a collectivistic value. These patterns suggest that, in Iranian culture, psychological well-being (as conceptualized by Ryff 1989) is associated with higher levels of idiocentrism (Triandis et al. 1985). Considering such a dimension as autonomy in Ryff's model, this relation between psychological well-being and idiocentrism is not surprising. It can be suggested that for those who place more emphasis on individualistic values, failure at measuring up to the standards of society does not lead to failure at functioning well in one's personal life. On this basis, the absence of association between psychological well-being and cultural estrangement is perhaps understandable in light of the fact that the psychological well-being scale appears to capture individualistic aspects of human functioning in Iranian culture (relative to the social well-being scale, which is positively associated with such collectivistic values as conformity in Iran).

Alternatively, Cozzarelli and Karafa (1998) suggest that it is possible that cultural estrangement satisfies a person's *need for uniqueness* (Snyder and Fromkin 1980) or produces a sense of *optimal distinctiveness* (Brewer 1991). These models posit that there is a need for individuation and uniqueness in individuals. On this basis, it can be suggested that the negative effects of experiencing cultural estrangement on personal functioning might be neutralized by the sense of uniqueness it triggers in the individual. Bernard et al. (2006) provided empirical evidence supporting this idea. They found that participants who perceived a larger gap between personal and societal values expressed a higher need for uniqueness.

Altogether, the findings of this study suggest that the cultural fit model, in its generality, is applicable to Iranian culture (at least for this student sample), as cultural estrangement correlated inversely with three aspects of well-being. Results of this study also suggest that cultural estrangement has more negative consequences for hedonic aspects of well-being than for eudaimonic well-being. An important point to note is that, in Iranian samples, the significance of personality traits in predicting well-being tends to outweigh that of basic values and cultural estrangement.

Conclusion

In this chapter, I first reviewed the most widely accepted conceptualizations of well-being proposed by western psychologists (i.e., hedonic and eudaimonic well-being). Next, I argued that, consistent with the western conceptualization of well-being, in the implicit view of Islam on mental health, a distinction is made between eudaimonic and hedonic well-being. However, it is important to mention that some aspects of eudaimonic and hedonic well-being endorsed by Islam might be different from that endorsed by western theories. For example, the former emphasizes the satisfaction of the need for worship, but the latter puts more emphasis on the satisfaction of the need for autonomy. One also should bear in mind that although spiritual needs are more emphasized in Islamic contexts, it does not mean that in such cultures a need for autonomy is not recognized. Prior research shows that autonomy is valued in all cultures, but ways in which to satisfy it are different from culture to culture. Ryan and Deci (2008) assert that autonomy, relatedness, and competence are basic psychological needs and therefore "are natural in the sense that they are an invariant, indeed foundational, aspect of the psychological architecture of the human organism, and they are universal in that they apply to all persons regardless of gender, upbringing, or culture" (p. 659) (see also Aik Kwang et al. 2003; Ryan and Deci 2000). They further add that "basic psychological needs may be expressed differently, and the vehicles through which they are satisfied may differ in different societies or stages of life, but their necessity is unchanging" (p. 659). (For empirical support pertaining to the universality of the need for autonomy, see Sheldon et al. 2001). It is also noteworthy that recently, western researchers have started paying more attention to spiritual needs of humankind in their theorizing (e.g., Nelson 2009).

In this chapter, some studies done by Iranian psychologists were reviewed. Although Iranian researchers have conducted survey studies in many areas of psychology, due to space constraints, I chose only three domains to briefly review. The first group of studies I reviewed was those focusing on the validation of western well-being scales in Iranian samples. Although there are some drawbacks in this domain of research, overall, it can be concluded that western scales have evidenced acceptable psychometric characteristics in Iranian samples. Iranian researchers who have validated these scales, or have used them, tend to express their satisfaction with these scales, and their statistical characteristics.

Interestingly enough, although in some other domains (e.g., religiousness) Iranian researchers prefer to develop Iranian scales and have less confidence in western scales, in the well-being domain, it appears that they have no interest in developing new scales. Western scales are widely used in Iranian studies and tend to produce interpretable and replicable results, which are either in line with western findings or are understandably different from them. Generally, Iranian researchers can come up with some relevant and meaningful ideas (such as pointing to different social and cultural characteristics of Iranian society) to explain the cross-cultural differences they find in their studies compared with western findings.

One important question that rises at this point is whether we can think of the Iranian experience with these western scales as a successful one. Considering the anti-western policy of the Iranian government and appreciable differences between Iranian society and the West in terms of culture, religion, political system, language, economical indicators, etc., some prefer to side with the view that emphasizes making indigenous concepts and scales to be used in other such countries. For instance, Haque (2004a, b) argues that given that western psychology has been secularized and has neglected moral and spiritual phenomena within human beings, its concepts are contrary to Islamic theory of human nature in some critical realms. He concludes the following:

> [C]ontemporary psychology presents a serious challenge to Muslim psychologists. Because of its grounding in the secular worldview, present-day psychology cannot be accepted in its entirety by Muslim psychologists. An effort to understand human behavior will lead Muslim psychologists to adhere to the Islamic perspectives of human nature and this will mean taking them back into the history of their ancestors whose works were based on Islamic framework. Psychologists interested in the Islamic perspective need to work both at the theoretical and practical levels to bring back their own indigenous psychology. (pp. 373–374)

Haque's perspective contains some assumptions that are in contrast with my perspective introduced in this chapter. I argued that, at least in the realm of well-being, the distinction made by western psychologists between eudaimonic and hedonic well-being can be applied to Islamic cultures.

It appears that, generally speaking, Iranian well-being researchers tend to side with the perspective that holds that Iranian and western conceptualizations of well-being are rather similar in terms of central assumptions. They see many anecdotal and theoretical similarities between what western scales assess and the Iranian's lay concept of happiness and positive functioning. As reviewed, empirical findings also tend to lend support to the applicability of these scales in Iranian samples. Moreover, the results of Iranians' studies with these scales are interpretable, whether they are in line with western findings or at discord with them. It does not mean that Iranian researchers have accomplished all they need to. As I noted before, these scales can be improved in many different ways. Also, indigenous scales should be developed, and their functionality should be compared against the functionality of western scales. Future research along these lines may help us more thoroughly address this issue.

Another set of findings that I reviewed concerns the relation between personality traits (the Big Five and self-esteem) and different aspects of well-being. It turns out that these studies' results mostly converge with western ones. Among the Big

Five, E and N are the strongest predictors of hedonic well-being. Additionally, O contributes significantly to eudaimonic well-being and not to hedonic well-being. Self-esteem is a strong predictor of different aspects of well-being in Iran.

That self-esteem is one of the most powerful predictors of well-being in Iran might seem counterintuitive. In fact, some researchers have argued that self-esteem is largely a western phenomenon or concept (e.g., Hewitt 2002). Given that Iran is an Asian country where the emphasis on self-esteem is thought to be lower than that in western countries (Myers and Diener 1995), this relatively strong association calls for explanation. Some aspects of Iranian culture help us better understand the pathways from self-esteem to well-being in this culture. Islam highly esteems humankind. According to Islam, God's spirit has been breathed into human form. Humankind has been created of the best stature (Q 95:4) and is God's vicegerent on earth (Q 2: 30). Elsewhere the Quran says "[v]erily we have honored the children of Adam. We carry them on the land and the sea, and have made provision of good things for them, and have preferred them above many of those whom we created with a marked preferment" (17:70).

The Quran consistently reminds Muslims of their worthy nature in order to prevent them from forgetting or losing it: "[T]he losers will be those who lose themselves …" (Q 39:15). Thus, the intrinsic worth of a Muslim, as a unique human being, is respected by God who is the highest authority. Islam's emphasis on the basic and innate human worth is likely to contribute to the idea that one should always treat oneself as a worthy creature. And those who fail to do so are likely to suffer some disadvantages. On this basis, self-esteem is likely to contribute to Iranians' sense of well-being. Self-esteem plays a central role in Islamic ethics, especially as understood by Iranians. Motahhari (1993) (a Shiite writer) argues that self-esteem is at the very root of Islamic ethics. In other words, reminding individuals of their high value is the main strategy of Islamic ethics in order to persuade them to act righteously. Likewise, drawing on the Quran and Shiite texts, Lashgari (2003) concludes that a lack of self-respect is considered to be the source of all sins and vices in Islam.

If this is the case, one might expect self-esteem to be a strong predictor of well-being in all Muslim cultures. Nevertheless, it appears that non-Islamic elements of a Muslim culture can modify the relation between self-esteem and well-being in that culture. For instance, Suhail and Chaudhry (2004) found no significant relation between self-esteem and well-being in Pakistan, Iran's Muslim neighbor (which is of a Buddhist background emphasizing humility and selflessness). In another Lebanese Muslim sample, however, self-esteem was found to correlate positively with SWB (Ayyash-Abdo and Alamuddin 2007). That this aspect of Islam (i.e., self-worth) is highly emphasized in Iran might be because it is consistent with the pre-Islamic Persian tradition of self-respect and honor and, therefore, is emphasized in mainstream Iranian culture today. For example, in Shahnameh,[3] self-worth, honor, objection to any derogatory treatment by others or any self-derogation are introduced among the basic human values. In sum, in line with

[3] "The Book of Kings," written around 1000 AD by the Iranian Poet Ferdowsi, which is the national epic of the Persian-speaking world and is held in high esteem by Iranians.

empirical findings, esteeming oneself has been emphasized in Iranian culture as a way to achieve moral and functional well-being.

The third domain of empirical research that I reviewed in this chapter concerns the relation between values and well-being. Although the research in this area is still nascent in Iran, and although more work is needed to examine this relation more thoroughly, preliminary findings of studies conducted in Iran give us the opportunity to compare the findings with those obtained in other countries. One of the main findings in this domain is that there seem to be similar and different sets of healthy and unhealthy values in diverse countries, including Iran. Furthermore, findings suggest that the cultural fit model is applicable, in its generality, to Iranian student samples.

Although psychological research in Iran is in its infancy and Iranian researchers' share of the contribution to the field has been limited so far, in some cases, Iranian studies have provided interesting input into the ongoing debates in well-being studies. I have touched on some of these contributions earlier throughout the chapter, but it is fruitful to highlight three of them here that are related to my area of work.

First, one of the current debates among well-being researchers is whether hedonic and eudaimonic aspects of well-being are conceptually distinct from each other. Kashdan et al. (2008), for example, maintain that this distinction, which is rooted in philosophy, does not translate well to science. Results of Iranian studies, however, suggest that the two aspects seem to be conceptually distinct, as they differentially relate to the Big Five domains, gender, values, etc. For instance, while women are more satisfied with their life than men in Iran (Joshanloo and Afshari 2011), men score higher than women on social well-being Joshanloo et al. (2012). While O has failed to predict life satisfaction, it has significantly predicted some aspects of social well-being Joshanloo et al. (2012) as well as psychological well-being (Joshanloo and Rastegar 2007). (For more arguments in support of the idea that the distinction between hedonic and eudaimonic well-being is scientifically and philosophically warranted, see Fave and Bassi 2009; Keyes and Annas 2009; Ryan and Huta 2009).

Next, some Iranian studies highlight the necessity for paying due attention to social aspects of eudaimonic well-being in mental health research. In some studies with Iranian university students, psychological and social well-being scales have shown different patterns of relationship with predictors. For instance, in Joshanloo and Ghaedi's (2009) study, as mentioned earlier, self-direction value was positively correlated with psychological well-being and negatively correlated with social well-being. In addition, power, conformity, and benevolence were not significantly correlated with psychological well-being but were significantly correlated with social well-being. While a significant gender difference was found for social well-being Joshanloo et al. (2012), no significant gender difference was found for two aspects of psychological well-being, namely, purpose in life and personal growth (Joshanloo and Rastegar 2007). These findings attest to the significance of a distinction between social and psychological aspects of eudaimonic well-being and demonstrate the need for more attention to be devoted to the social aspect of well-being, which is generally overlooked in well-being studies.

Finally, as I argued elsewhere (Joshanloo 2010), findings emerged in Iran and some other countries regarding the relation between values and aspects of well-being, calling for more attention to be directed to the important point that the relation between values and well-being varies, depending on the way in which well-being is conceptualized and measured. Therefore, it is important to take into account the distinction between aspects of well-being in formulating the relation between well-being and values, a point which has been generally neglected by researchers heretofore.

In sum, although the work done on well-being in Iran is preliminary, sufficient findings have accumulated to conclude that western scales have helped Iranian psychology to produce a sizeable body of literature on well-being in Iran (compared to other research fields in Iran and in other countries of the region). And in some cases, Iranian studies' results have also contributed to the current debates among well-being psychologists. Thus, I believe that Iranian researchers' attempts with western scales have paid off. Even if Iranian researchers decide to modify western scales or develop indigenous ones, their attempt should be partly based on the existing literature produced by using western scales. I briefly reviewed the existing empirical evidence which supports this assertion in this chapter. Fortunately, appreciably more attention has been given to positive human functioning and well-being constructs in Iran over the past few years, and the size of literature is growing on this topic. We are approaching the point of having enough data to allow us to make firmer conclusions. I am hopeful that this line of research in Iran will be able to make more notable and useful contributions and to provide more insight into mainstream psychology in the years to come.

References

Abou el Azayem, G., & Hedayat-Diba, Z. (1994). The psychological aspects of Islam: Basic principles of Islam and their psychological corollary. *The International Journal for the Psychology of Religion, 4*(1), 41–50.

Aik Kwang, N., Ho, D. Y. F., Shyh Shin, W., & Smith, I. (2003). In search of the good life: A cultural odyssey in the east and west. *Genetic, Social, and General Psychology Monographs, 129*(4), 317–363.

Akhtar, S. (2008). *The Quran and the secular mind: A philosophy of Islam*. New York: Routledge.

Alipour, A., & Agah Heris, M. (2007). Reliability and validity of the Oxford Happiness Inventory among Iranians. *Journal of Iranian Psychologists, 3*(12), 287–298 [in Persian].

Alipour, A., & Noorbala, A. (1999). Introductory survey on validity and reliability of Oxford Happiness Inventory in Tehran universities. *Journal of Thought and Behavior, 5*, 55–63 [in Persian].

Annas, J. (2000). *Ancient philosophy: A very short introduction*. Oxford: Oxford University Press.

Argyle, M., Martin, M., & Crossland, J. (1989). Happiness as a function of personality and social encounters. In J. P. Forgas & J. M. Innes (Eds.), *Recent advances in social psychology: An international perspective* (pp. 189–203). Amsterdam: North Holland/Elsevier Science.

Ayyash-Abdo, H., & Alamuddin, R. (2007). Predictors of subjective well-being among college youth in Lebanon. *Journal of Social Psychology, 147*(3), 265–284.

Bakhshi, A., Daemi, F., & Ajilchi, B. (2009). Psychometric properties of the positive and negative affect scales in an Iranian sample. *Journal of Iranian Psychologists, 20*, 343–350 [in Persian].

Bakhshipur, A., & Dozhkam, M. (2006). Confirmatory factor analysis of PANAS. *Journal of Psychology, 9*(4), 351–365 [in Persian].
Bayani, A. A., Kuchaki, A. M., & Gudarzi, H. (2007). The reliability and validity of the satisfaction with life scale. *Journal of Iranian Psychologist, 11*, 259–265 [in Persian].
Bayani, A. A., Koocheky, A. M., & Bayani, A. (2008). Reliability and validity of Ryff's psychological well-being scales. *Iranian Journal of Psychiatry and Clinical Psychology, 14*, 146–151 [in Persian].
Bernard, M. M., Gebauer, J. E., & Maio, G. R. (2006). Cultural estrangement: The role of personal and societal value discrepancies. *Personality and Social Psychology Bulletin, 32*, 78–92.
Bilsky, W., & Schwartz, S. H. (1994). Values and personality. *European Journal of Personality, 8*, 163–181.
Bobowik, M., Basabe, N., Páez, D., Jiménez, A., & Bilbao, M. (2011). Personal values and well-being among Europeans, Spanish natives and immigrants to Spain: Does the culture matter? *Journal of Happiness Studies, 12*(3), 401–419.
Brewer, M. B. (1991). The social self: On being the same and different at the same time. *Personality and Social Psychology Bulletin, 17*, 475–482.
Bunnin, N., & Yu, J. (2004). *The Blackwell dictionary of western philosophy*. Malden: Blackwell Publishing.
Byock, I., & Merriman, M. (1998). Measuring quality of life for patients with terminal illness: The Missoula Quality of Life Index (MVQOLI). *Palliative Medicine, 12*, 231–244.
Campbell, A. (1981). *The sense of well-being in America: Recent patterns and trends*. New York: McGraw Hill.
Chirkov, V. I., Ryan, R. M., & Willness, C. (2005). Cultural context and psychological needs in Canada and brazil: Testing a self-determination approach to the internalization of cultural practices, identity, and well-being. *Journal of Cross-Cultural Psychology, 36*, 423–443.
Cicognani, E., Pirini, C., Keyes, C., Joshanloo, M., Rostami, R., & Nosratabadi, M. (2008). Social participation, sense of community and social well-being: A study on American, Italian and Iranian University students. *Social Indicators Research, 89*(1), 97–112.
Clawson, P. L., & Rubin, M. (2005). *Eternal Iran: Continuity and chaos*. New York: Palgrave Macmillan.
Cozzarelli, C., & Karafa, J. A. (1998). Cultural estrangement and terror management theory. *Personality and Social Psychology Bulletin, 24*(3), 253–267.
Dahlsgaard, K., Peterson, C., & Seligman, M. (2005). Shared virtue: The convergence of valued human strengths across culture and history. *Review of General Psychology, 9*(3), 203–213.
Deci, E. L., & Ryan, R. M. (2008). Hedonia, eudaimonia, and well-being: An introduction. *Journal of Happiness Studies, 9*(1), 1–11.
DeNeve, K. M., & Cooper, H. (1998). The happy personality: A meta-analysis of 137 personality traits and subjective well-being. *Psychological Bulletin, 124*, 197–229.
Devettere, R. J. (2002). *Introduction to virtue ethics: Insights of the ancient Greeks*. Washington, DC: Georgetown University Press.
Diener, E. (1984). Subjective well-being. *Psychological Bulletin, 95*, 542–575.
Diener, E., & Diener, M. (1995). Cross-cultural correlates of life satisfaction and self-esteem. *Journal of Personality and Social Psychology, 68*, 653–663.
Diener, E., & Lucas, R. (1999). Personality, and subjective well-being. In D. Kahneman, E. Diener, & N. Schwarz (Eds.), *Well-being: The foundations of hedonic psychology* (pp. 213–229). New York: Russell Sage.
Diener, E., Emmons, R. A., Larsen, R. J., & Griffin, S. (1985). The satisfaction with life scale. *Journal of Personality Assessment, 49*, 71–75.
Diener, E., Suh, E. M., Lucas, R. E., & Smith, H. E. (1999). Subjective well-being: Three decades of progress. *Psychological Bulletin, 125*, 276–302.
Diener, E., Oishi, S., & Lucas, R. E. (2003). Personality, culture, and subjective well-being: Emotional and cognitive evaluations of life. *Annual Review of Psychology, 54*, 403–425.
Emmons, R. A., & McCullough, M. E. (Eds.). (2004). *The psychology of gratitude*. New York: Oxford University Press.

Fave, A. D., & Bassi, M. (2009). The contribution of diversity to happiness research. *The Journal of Positive Psychology, 4*(3), 205–207.

Furnham, A., & Cheng, H. (2000). Perceived parental behavior, self-esteem and happiness. *Social Psychiatry and Psychiatric Epidemiology, 35*(10), 463–470.

Haghighi, J., Khoshkonesh, A., Shorkrkon, H., Shahani Yeylagh, M., & Neysi, A. (2006). The relation between the Big Five personality traits and happiness in undergraduates at the University of Shahid Chamran. *Journal of Educational and Psychological Sciences, 13*(3), 163–188 [in Persian].

Hamdan, A. (2007). A case study of a Muslim client: Incorporating religious beliefs and practices. *Journal of Multicultural Counseling & Development, 35*(2), 92–100.

Haque, A. (2004a). Psychology from Islamic perspective: Contributions of early Muslim scholars and challenges to contemporary Muslim psychologists. *Journal of Religion and Health, 43*(4), 357–377.

Haque, A. (2004b). Religion and mental health: The case of American Muslims. *Journal of Religion and Health, 43*(1), 45–58.

Haslam, N., Whelan, J., & Bastian, B. (2009). Big five traits mediate associations between values and subjective well-being. *Personality and Individual Differences, 46*, 40–42.

Hatami, G., Motamed, N., & Ashrafzadeh, M. (2010). Confirmatory factor analysis of Persian adaptation of Multidimensional Students' Life Satisfaction Scale (MSLSS). *Social Indicators Research, 98*(2), 265–271.

Hewitt, J. P. (2002). The social construction of self-esteem. In C. R. Snyder & S. J. Lopez (Eds.), *Handbook of positive psychology* (pp. 135–158). Oxford: Oxford University Press.

Hooft, S. V. (2006). *Understanding virtue ethics*. Malta: Gutenberg Press.

Huebner, E. S. (1994). Preliminary development and validation of a multidimensional life satisfaction scale for children. *Psychological Assessment, 6*(2), 149–158.

Hursthouse, R. (1999). *On virtue ethics*. Oxford: Oxford University Press.

Joshanloo, M. (2010). Investigation of the relation between cultural estrangement and hedonic and eudaimonic aspects of well-being in Iranian young adults. *Personality and Individual Differences, 49*(7), 733–737.

Joshanloo, M., & Afshari, S. (2011). Big five personality traits and self-esteem as predictors of life satisfaction in Iranian Muslim university students. *Journal of Happiness Studies, 12*(1), 105–113.

Joshanloo, M., & Daemi, F. (in press). Investigation of statistical characteristics of the satisfaction with life scale in Iranian students. *Journal of behavioral science* [in Persian].

Joshanloo, M., & Ghaedi, G. (2009). The investigation statistical properties of personal growth initiative scale in Iranian students. *Journal of Behavioral Science, 3*(2), 121–125.

Joshanloo, M., & Nosratabadi, M. (2009). Levels of mental health continuum and personality traits. *Social Indicators Research, 90*, 211–224.

Joshanloo, M., & Rastegar, P. (2007). Investigation of the personality Predictors of eudaimonic well-being in male and female university students. *Journal of Iranian Psychologists, 13*, 13–24 [in Persian].

Joshanloo, M., Rostami, R., & Nosratabadi, M. (2006a). Gender differences in social well-being predictors. *Journal of Psychological Sciences, 18*, 166–184 [in Persian].

Joshanloo, M., Rostami, R., & Nosratabadi, M. (2006b). Examining the factor structure of the Keyes' comprehensive scale of well-being. *Journal of Iranian Psychologists, 9*, 35–51 [in Persian].

Joshanloo, M., Nosratabadi, M., & Jafari Kandovan, G. (2007). Social well-being, big five and self-esteem. *Journal of Psychological Sciences, 21*, 66–88 [in Persian].

Joshanloo, M., Daemi, F., & Bakhshi, A. (2010). Examination of the predictors of hedonic balance in Iranian university students. *Advances in Cognitive Science, 12*(2), 40–48.

Joshanloo, M., Rastegar, P., & Bakhshi, A. (2012). Big five personality domains as predictors of social well-being in Iranian university students. *Journal of Social and Personal Relationships, 29*(5), 639–660.

Kashdan, T., Biswas-Diener, R., & King, L. (2008). Reconsidering happiness: The costs of distinguishing between hedonics and eudaimonia. *The Journal of Positive Psychology, 3*(4), 219–233.
Kasser, T., & Ahuvia, A. C. (2002). Materialistic values and well-being in business students. *European Journal of Social Psychology, 32*, 137–146.
Kasser, T., & Ryan, R. M. (1996). Further examining the American dream: Differential correlates of intrinsic and extrinsic goals. *Personality and Social Psychology Bulletin, 22*, 280–287.
Keyes, C. L. M. (1998). Social well-being. *Social Psychology Quarterly, 61*, 121–140.
Keyes, C. L. M. (2002). The mental health continuum: From languishing to flourishing in life. *Journal of Health and Social Behavior, 43*, 207–222.
Keyes, C. L. M. (2004). The nexus of cardiovascular disease and depression revisited: The complete mental health perspective and the moderating role of age and gender. *Aging & Mental Health, 8*, 267–275.
Keyes, C. L. M. (2005a). Mental illness and/or mental health? Investigating axioms of the complete state model of health. *Journal of Consulting and Clinical Psychology, 73*, 539–548.
Keyes, C. L. M. (2005b). Chronic physical disease and aging: Is mental health a potential protective factor? *Ageing International, 30*, 88–104.
Keyes, C. L. M., & Annas, J. (2009). Feeling good and functioning well: Distinctive concepts in ancient philosophy and contemporary science. *The Journal of Positive Psychology, 4*(3), 197–201.
Keyes, C. L. M., & Ryff, C. D. (1998). Generativity in adult lives: Social structural contours and quality of life consequences. In D. P. McAdams & E. de St. Aubin (Eds.), *Generativity and adult development: How and why we care for the next generation* (pp. 227–263). Washington, DC: American Psychological Association.
Keyes, C. L. M., & Shapiro, A. (2004). Social well-being in the United States: A descriptive epidemiology. In O. G. Brim, C. Ryff, & R. Kessler (Eds.), *How healthy are we? A national study of well-being at midlife* (pp. 350–372). Chicago: University of Chicago Press.
Keyes, C. L. M., Shmotkin, D., & Ryff, C. D. (2002). Optimizing well-being: The empirical encounter of two traditions. *Journal of Personality and Social Psychology, 82*, 1007–1022.
Khanzade, A., Moltafet, G., Safikhani, I., & Sadati, S. (2007). Investigation of the relation between personality domains and happiness in university students. *Journal of Psychological Science, 5*(10), 337–351 [in Persian].
Kwan, V. S. Y., Bond, M. H., & Singelis, T. M. (1997). Pancultural explanations for life-satisfaction: Adding relationship harmony to self-esteem. *Journal of Personality and Social Psychology, 73*, 1038–1051.
Lai, J. H., Bond, M. H., & Hui, N. H. (2007). The role of social axioms in predicting life satisfaction: A longitudinal study in Hong Kong. *Journal of Happiness Studies, 8*, 517–535.
Lashgari, M. (2003). Mental health in Islam. *The Journal of Gazvin University of Medical Sciences, 24*, 72–76 [in Persian].
Liaghatdar, M. J., Jafari, E., Abedi, M. R., & Samiee, F. (2008). Reliability and validity of the Oxford Happiness Inventory among university students in Iran. *The Spanish Journal of Psychology, 11*(1), 310–313.
Lu, L. (2006). "Cultural Fit": Individual and societal discrepancies in values, beliefs, and subjective well-being. *The Journal of Social Psychology, 146*(2), 203–221.
Lucas, R. E., & Diener, E. (2008). Personality and subjective well-being. In O. P. John, R. Robins, & L. A. Pervin (Eds.), *Handbook of personality* (3rd ed., pp. 795–814). New York: Guilford.
Lucas, R. E., Diener, E., & Suh, E. M. (1996). Discriminant validity of subjective well-being measures. *Journal of Personality and Social Psychology, 71*, 616–628.
McCrae, R., & Costa, P. T. (1991). Adding Liebe und Arbeit: The full five-factor model and well-being. *Personality and Social Psychology Bulletin, 17*(2), 227–232.
Moghanloo, M., & Aguilar-Vafaie, M. (2009). Domain and facets of the five factor model of personality correlates of happiness, mental health and physical health. *Iranian Journal of Psychiatry and Clinical Psychology, 15*(3), 290–299 [in Persian].
Motahhari, M. (1993). *The philosophy of ethics*. Tehran: Sadra.

Mroczek, D. K., & Kolarz, C. M. (1998). The effect of age on positive and negative affect: A developmental perspective on happiness. *Journal of Personality and Social Psychology, 75*, 1333–1349.

Myers, D. G., & Diener, E. (1995). Who is happy? *Psychological Science, 6*, 10–19.

Nelson, J. M. (2009). *Psychology, religion, and spirituality*. New York: Springer Science+Business Media.

Oishi, S., Diener, E., Lucas, R. E., & Suh, E. M. (1999a). Cross-cultural variations in predictors of life satisfaction: Perspectives from needs and values. *Personality and Social Psychology Bulletin, 25*, 980–990.

Oishi, S., Diener, E., Suh, E., & Lucas, R. E. (1999b). Value as a moderator in subjective well-being. *Journal of Personality, 24*, 1319–1331.

Pridmore, S., & Pasha, M. I. (2004). Psychiatry and Islam. *Australasian Psychiatry, 12*(4), 380–385.

Ratzlaff, C., Matsumoto, D., Kouznetsova, N., Raroque, J., & Ray, R. (2000). Individual psychological culture and subjective well-being. In E. Diener & E. M. Suh (Eds.), *Culture and subjective well-being* (pp. 37–59). Cambridge, MA: MIT Press.

Robitschek, C. (1998). Personal growth initiative: The construct and its measure. *Measurement and Evaluation in Counseling and Development, 30*, 183–198.

Robitschek, C. (1999). Further validation of the personal growth initiative scale. *Measurement and Evaluation in Counseling and Development, 31*, 197–210.

Robitschek, c, & Keyes, C. L. M. (2009). The structure of Keyes' model of mental health and the role of personal growth initiative as a parsimonious predictor. *Journal of Counseling Psychology, 56*(2), 321–329.

Roccas, S., Sagiv, L., Schwartz, S. H., & Knafo, A. (2002). The Big Five personality factors and personal values. *Personality and Social Psychology Bulletin, 28*, 789–801.

Romance, P. (2007). The influence of classical Iranian thought. *Classical Bulletin, 83*(2), 175–181.

Ryan, R. M., & Deci, E. L. (2000). Self-determination theory and the facilitation of intrinsic motivation, social development, and well-being. *American Psychologist, 55*(1), 68–78.

Ryan, R. M., & Deci, E. L. (2001). On happiness and human potentials: A review of research on hedonic and eudaimonic well-being. *Annual Review of Psychology, 52*, 141–166.

Ryan, R. M., & Deci, E. L. (2008). Self-determination theory and the role of basic psychological needs in personality and the organization of behavior. In O. P. John, R. W. Robbins, & L. A. Pervin (Eds.), *Handbook of personality: Theory and research* (pp. 654–678). New York: The Guilford Press.

Ryan, R. M., & Huta, V. (2009). Wellness as healthy functioning or wellness as happiness: The importance of eudaimonic thinking (Response to the Kashdan et al. and Waterman discussion). *The Journal of Positive Psychology, 4*(3), 202–204.

Ryan, R. M., Huta, V., & Deci, E. L. (2008). Living well: A self-determination theory perspective on eudaimonia. *Journal of Happiness Studies, 9*, 139–170.

Ryff, C. D. (1989). Happiness is everything, or is it? Explorations on the meaning of psychological well-being. *Journal of Personality and Social Psychology, 57*, 1069–1081.

Ryff, C. D. (2008). Challenges and opportunities at the interface of aging, personality, and well-being. In O. P. John, R. Robins, & L. A. Pervin (Eds.), *Handbook of personality* (3rd ed., pp. 399–418). New York: Guilford.

Ryff, C. D., & Keyes, C. L. M. (1995). The structure of psychological well-being revisited. *Journal of Personality and Social Psychology, 69*, 719–727.

Safdar, S., Lewis, J. R., & Daneshpour, M. (2006). Social axioms in Iran and Canada: Intercultural contact, coping and adjustment. *Asian Journal of Social Psychology, 9*, 123–131.

Sagiv, L., & Schwartz, S. H. (2000). Value priorities and subjective well-being: Direct relations and congruity effects. *European Journal of Social Psychology, 30*, 177–198.

Sagiv, L., Roccas, S., & Hazan, O. (2004). Value pathways to well-being: Healthy values, valued goal attainment, and environmental congruence. In A. Linley & J. Stephen (Eds.), *Positive psychology in practice*. New York: Wiley.

Sajedi, A. (2008a). Religion and mental health (1). *Journal of Psychology and Religion, 1*, 55–87 [in Persian].
Sajedi, A. (2008b). Religion and mental health (2). *Journal of Psychology and Religion, 2*, 7–35 [in Persian].
Schimmack, U., Radhakrishan, P., Oishi, S., Dzokoto, V., & Ahadi, S. (2002). Culture, personality, and subjective well-being. Integrating process model of life satisfaction. *Journal of Personality and Social Psychology, 82*, 582–593.
Schmutte, P. S., & Ryff, C. D. (1997). Personality and well-being: What is the connection? *Journal of Personality and Social Psychology, 73*, 549–559.
Schwartz, S. H. (1992). Universals in the content and structure of values: Theory and empirical tests in 20 countries. In M. Zanna (Ed.), *Advances in experimental social psychology* (Vol. 25, pp. 1–65). New York: Academic.
Sheldon, K. M., Elliot, A. J., Kim, Y., & Kasser, T. (2001). What is satisfying about satisfying events? Testing 10 candidate psychological needs. *Journal of Personality and Social Psychology, 80*(2), 325–339.
Shokri, O., Kadivar, P., Farzad, V., Daneshvarpour, Z., Dastjerdi, R., & Paeezi, M. (2008). A study of factor structure of 3, 9 and 14-item Persian versions of Ryff's scales psychological well-being in university students. *Iranian Journal of Psychiatry and Clinical Psychology, 14*, 152–161 [in Persian].
Smither, R., & Khordandi, A. (2009). The implicit personality theory of Islam. *Psychology of Religion and Spirituality, 1*, 81–96.
Snyder, C. R., & Fromkin, H. L. (1980). *Uniqueness: The human pursuit of difference*. New York: Plenum.
Solomon, R. C., & Martin, C. W. (2004). *Morality and the good life: Introduction to ethics through classical sources* (4th ed.). New York: McGraw-Hill.
Springer, K. W., Hauser, R. M., & Freese, J. (2006). Bad news indeed for Ryff's six-factor model of well-being. *Social Science Research, 35*(4), 1120–1131.
Steel, P., Schmidt, J., & Shultz, J. (2008). Refining the relationship between personality and subjective well-being. *Psychological Bulletin, 134*, 138–161.
Stepaniants, M. (2002). The encounter of Zoroastrianism with Islam. *Philosophy East & West, 52*(2), 159–173.
Strümpfer, D. J. W. (2006). The strengths perspective: Fortigenesis in adult life. *Social Indicators Research, 77*(1), 11–36.
Suhail, K., & Chaudhry, H. R. (2004). Predictors of subjective well-being in an Eastern Muslim Culture. *Journal of Social and Clinical Psychology, 23*(3), 359–376.
Tamadonfar, M. (2001). Islam, law, and political control in contemporary Iran. *Journal for Scientific Study of Religion, 40*(2), 205–219.
Triandis, H. C. (2000). Cultural syndromes and subjective well-being. In E. Diener & E. M. Suh (Eds.), *Culture and subjective well-being* (pp. 13–36). Cambridge, MA: MIT Press.
Triandis, H. C., Leung, K., Villareal, M., & Clack, F. L. (1985). Allocentric vs. Idiocentric tendencies: Convergent and discriminant validation. *Journal of Research in Personality, 13*, 395–415.
Vansteenkiste, M., Duriez, B., Simons, J., & Soenens, B. (2006). Materialistic values and well-being among business students: Further evidence for their detrimental effect. *Journal of Applied Social Psychology, 36*, 2892–2908.
Vitterso, J., Soholt, Y., Hetland, A., Thoresen, I. A., & Roysamb, E. (2010). Was Hercules happy? Some answers from a functional model of human well-being. *Social Indicators Research, 95*(1), 1–18.
Wan, C., & Chiu, C. (2009). An intersubjective consensus approach to culture: The role of intersubjective norms versus cultural self in cultural processes. In R. Wyer, Y.- Hong, & C.- Chiu (Eds.), *Understanding culture: Theory, research and application* (pp. 79–91). New York: Psychology Press.
Waterman, A. S., Schwartz, S. J., & Conti, R. (2008). The implications of two conceptions of happiness (hedonic enjoyment and eudaimonia) for the understanding of intrinsic motivation. *Journal of Happiness Studies, 9*, 41–79.

Watson, D., Clark, L. A., & Tellegen, A. (1988). Development and validation of brief measures of positive and negative affect: The PANAS scales. *Journal of Personality and Social Psychology, 54*(6), 1063–1070.
Zaki, M. (2008). Quality of life and its relation with self-esteem in female and male students of Esfahan University. *Iranian Journal of Psychiatry and Clinical Psychology, 13*(4), 416–419 [in Persian].
Zhang, L. W., & Leung, J. P. (2002). Moderating effects of gender and age on the relationship between self-esteem and life satisfaction in mainland Chinese. *International Journal of Psychology, 37*(2), 83–91.

Chapter 10
Emotional Well-Being and Self-Control Skills of Children and Adolescents: The Israeli Perspective

Michael Rosenbaum and Tammie Ronen

"People who learn to control inner experience will be able to determine the quality of their lives, which is as close as any of us can come to being happy" (Csikszentmihalyi 2002, p. 2). In almost every human society around the globe, parents want their children to be happy and satisfied with their lives. Yet, it is quite surprising that there is relatively little research on the factors that enhance children's happiness and emotional well-being (Diamond and Aspinwall 2003; Roberts et al. 2005). The dearth of research in this area is probably due to two main reasons. First, young children (in contrast to adolescents) are expected to be happy and satisfied because little demands are put on them, and second, because, in general, researchers in psychiatry and psychology are mostly interested in studying problems and disorders rather than studying the factors that enhance children's well-being.

From a developmental point of view, it appears quite justifiable to focus on the psychological factors that seem to produce ill well-being in children who were happy and relatively problem free in their first years of life. Indeed, extensive research has shown that both acute and chronic negative emotions in children and adults impede the development of effective social and psychological functioning (Fox and Calkins 2003). But, on the other hand, research suggests the many benefits of positive affect may be crucial for healthy psychological and social development (Diamond and Aspinwall 2003; Frederickson 2009). As children grow up, societal demands and pressures increase, and consequently, there is a continuous reduction in emotional well-being from early childhood until adulthood (Chang et al. 2003; Greene 1990). Whereas nearly half of the children ages 12–14 have been defined as

M. Rosenbaum, Ph.D. (✉)
Schwartz Research Center for Health Behavior, Department of Psychology, Tel-Aviv University, Tel Aviv, Israel
e-mail: Miker@post.tau.ac.il

T. Ronen, Ph.D.
Renata Adler Memorial Research Center for Child Welfare and Protection, The Bob Shapell School of Social Work, Tel-Aviv University, Tel Aviv, Israel

C.L.M. Keyes (ed.), *Mental Well-Being: International Contributions to the Study of Positive Mental Health*, DOI 10.1007/978-94-007-5195-8_10,

flourishing (the highest level of mental health, Keyes 2006), at the ages 15–18, only about 40% adolescents have been described as flourishing (Keyes 2006). Among the adult population, less than 20 % of the people were found to be flourishing (Keyes 2002). Klingman (2001), who studied Israeli youth, also found that seventh and eighth graders have more positive feelings (relief, joy, and optimism) than ninth through eleventh graders. Although different self-report measures were used for the different age groups, the current data suggest that there is a decline in positive emotions among young adults compared to adolescents but that there are increases in positive affect with age in samples ranging from 25 to 74 years (Mroczek and Kolarz 1998). As Charles (2010) has noted in a recent article: "Even when age-related upturns in negative affect or downwards in positive affect have been observed, the oldest adults still report better subjective well-being than the youngest adults…" (p. 1071). Although we could not find a longitudinal or a cross-sectional study that assessed well-being from early childhood to old age, it appears that there is a U-shape relationship between age and well-being: The highest points are at early childhood and older adults (however, not for very old people). Nevertheless, there is no evidence for parallel changes in mental illness from early childhood to old age. Twenty one percent of American children and adolescents meet the diagnostic criteria for mental disorder (Novotney 2010), and about 20 % of the adult population has some kind of mental illness and is in need for professional help (Regier et al. 1993). Thus, previous studies suggest (a) that changes in well-being are, at least in part, a function of the person's developmental stage and (b) that it is important to study well-being apart from mental illness.

As a number of authors (e.g., Keyes 2009) have indicated, most research studies focus on mental *illness* and not on mental *health*. Mental health is often equated with the absence of mental disorders. Hence, to increase children's and adolescents' emotional well-being, parents, teachers, and mental health professional aim at diagnosing and treating psychological problems. It is often wrongly assumed that once the child is free of psychological problems, he or she is expected to feel good and to be happy. The heightened awareness of that which is negative and of the flaws of these children leads to greater emphasis on "curing" mental disorders rather than on promoting emotional well-being.

With the emergence of positive psychology in recent decades, it has become clear that mental health is not the obverse of mental illness.

> Mental health is not merely the absence of mental illness, nor is it merely the presence of high well-being. Rather, we defined mental health as a complete state consisting of (a) the absence of mental illness and (b) the presence of high level well-being (Keyes and Lopez 2005, p. 48).

Whereas most individuals are more influenced by negative events than by positive events, there is accumulative evidence that people are also motivated to protect and enhance their self-concept by focusing on the positive (Hepper et al. 2010) and, consequently, on their well-being. Our basic assumption is that children and adults alike are highly motivated to increase their emotional well-being, at least as much as they are motivated to avoid negative feelings. What changes along the lifespan are the specific goals that individuals are trying to achieve at various stages of their lives and the social and psychological resources that are available for them to attain these goals.

In this chapter, we emphasize the role of self-control skills and social factors in enhancing children's and adolescents' emotional well-being. After we define emotional well-being, we will discuss the importance of emotional well-being for the healthy development of children and adolescents. This is followed by a discussion of the role of self-control skills and, in particular, learned resourcefulness in the ability to attain emotional well-being. Then we discuss developmental pattern of EWB as a function of socialization practices. Before we conclude, we will describe the dynamic triad that links self-control, EWB, and social relationship. Each of these processes is assumed to be reciprocally influenced and shaped by each other.

Emotional Well-Being (EWB) or Psychological Well-Being?

Ryff and Singer (2005) noted that the "...discipline of psychology has long been interested in what constitutes positive psychology functioning" (p. 542). Although positive psychology may not be a relatively recent development as is often stated (e.g., Carr 2004), nonetheless, clinical psychology and psychiatry still focus much more on psychological disorders than on psychological well-being. Whereas elaborated and highly complex diagnostic manuals were developed to assess mental illness, there is no widely acceptable diagnostic system to assess mental health. There are some exceptions. For example, Peterson and Seligman (2004) published a *Manual of the Sanities* in a volume titled "Character Strength and Virtues: A Handbook of Classification." It consists of 24 positive strengths and virtues. It is not clear from this scheme how these virtues are related to one's emotional well-being, if at all. For example, do you feel good because you have strengths and virtues?

Ryff and Singer (2005), Peterson and Seligman (2004), and Keyes and Lopez (2005) have adopted the *eudemonic approach* and relate positive human functions to the emergence of mental health and psychological well-being. Keyes and Lopez (2005) clearly stated that "complete mental health is the syndrome that combines high levels of symptoms of emotional well-being, psychological well-being, and social well-being" (Keyes and Lopez 2005, p. 49). These authors distinguish between *emotional well-being* and *positive functioning*. Whereas emotional well-being (EWB) is simply a measure of emotional vitality and good feelings, positive functioning consists of psychological and social well-being. Psychological well-being consists of six dimensions: self-acceptance, personal growth, purpose in life, environmental mastery, autonomy, and positive relations with others. Social well-being consists of social acceptance, social actualization, social contribution, social coherence, and social integration.

In our studies of well-being, and in this chapter, we have adopted the *hedonic approach* (e.g., Diener et al. 2010). Although the term well-being has also been used to indicate psychological and social well-being, we reserve the term EWB to feeling good and energetic (i.e., high levels of positive affect). For example, individuals who have a purpose in life (a part of psychological well-being) and feel that they have something valuable to contribute to society (a part of social well-being, Keyes and Lopez 2005) are not necessarily happy and satisfied with their lives (EWB). As we will discuss later, in order to increase one's EWB, one must have the necessary self-control and social skills as well as the active desire to achieve well-defined targets. Furthermore, in studying children and adolescents, it is not reasonable to expect that they have already reached the developmental stage subsumed under the terms of psychological and social well-being (Erikson 1959).

Another term that has been widely used is *subjective well-being.* It consists of a broad evaluation of one's life (life satisfaction) and self-assessment of positive and negative affect (either momentary feelings or over a period of time). There were found to be two distinct factors that might be the result of different causes, for example, wealthy people might be satisfied with their lives but not feel good. However, people who feel socially acceptable and believe that they have skills to control their lives are likely to report high levels of emotional well-being (Lucas et al. 1996). Furthermore, Updegraff et al. (2004) report that positive affect is positively related to life satisfaction evaluations only among people who have high levels of approach-related motivation and not among people with avoidance-related motivation. These findings suggests an EWB self-maintaining cycle in which positive emotions influence positive evaluations of one's life experiences and where these evaluations, in turn, reinforce good feelings (see also Fredrickson and Joiner 2002). The existence of this reciprocal feeding system is highly dependent on people's disposition to actively pursue positive goals in life, in contrast to people who are predisposed to a defensive approach to life.

EWB Is Not a Luxury But a Necessity for Healthy Development

EWB is assessed by measuring positive and negative affect (PA and NA, respectively). In some cases, EWB is determined only by the level of PA and, in other cases, by the level PA in comparison to the person's reported NA (either by subtraction of NA from PA or by the ratio between the two). Like any psychological construct, PA and NA are defined by the kind of instrument that is used to assess them. By far the most widely used instrument for assessing PA and NA is the positive and negative affect schedule (PANAS, Watson et al. 1988). The child (grades 4–8) version of the PANAS (PANAS-C, Laurent et al. 1999) is highly similar to the adult version, with the exception that it consists of 30 items instead of 20 items. Fifteen items assess PA, and 15 items assess NA. Watson et al. (1999), in a later article, preferred to refer to PA as *pleasant activation* and to NA as *negative activation*. However, they already emphasized the active aspects of PA and NA in their original publication of the PANAS, as can be seen in the following citation:

> High PA is a state of high energy, full concentration, and pleasurable engagement, whereas low PA is characterized by sadness and lethargy. In contrast, Negative Affect (NA) is a general dimension of subjective distress and unpleasurable engagement that subsumes a variety of aversive mood states, including anger, contempt, disgust, guilt, fear, and nervousness (Watson, et al. 1988, p. 1063).

Happiness is an additional indicator of EWB and is also referred to as an active goal-oriented process: "[H]appiness is a characteristic of activities well performed" (Averill and More 1993, p. 620). NA and PA have distinctive functions that are closely associated with dispositional approach and avoidance motivations (cf. Carver and White 1994; Gable et al. 2003). NA has been associated with avoidance motivation. Avoidance motivation primarily serves to keep individuals away from danger. It is reactive in character and is activated when a person is threatened by aversive stimuli of different kinds (e.g., physical or social insult). On the other hand, PA is associated with approach motivation, which mobilizes the individual to obtain physical and social resources. Similarly, Watson et al. (1999) emphasized the motivating force behind PA and NA. For example, PA is both the *cause* and the *effect* of children and adults' EWB. This cycle is maintained by the individual's ability to set and pursue potentially rewarding life goals.

Since Watson's et al.'s (1988) original publication, numerous articles have been published on the benefits of PA. Lyubomirsky et al. (2005), in an extensive review of the literature, concluded that happiness leads to success and not vice versa.

> First, because happy people experience frequent positive moods, they have a greater likelihood of working actively toward new goals while experiencing those moods. Second, happy people are in the possession of past skills and resources, which they have built over time during previous pleasant moods (p. 804).

The review of the numerous published studies indicates that PA and happiness precede success in all major domains of life (i.e., work, love, and health). There is strong evidence that PA fosters the immune system, social skills, and psychological health. PA, in contrast to NA, fosters cognitive and creative functions according to Fredrickson's broaden-and-build theory (Frederickson 1998; Fredrickson and Losada 2005). According to this theory, PA (in contrast to NA) broadens the array of thoughts and actions and encourages behavioral explorations. Also, it is the basis for positive psychological and social actions. PA encourages better knowledge of the environment and the various behavioral alternatives available. That is in sharp contrast to NA, which narrows individuals' attention scope. Fredrickson's research findings clearly suggest that effective child rearing and education should be based on PA and not on NA. Children and adolescents who are happy and high on PA are also likely to be good students in school and well liked by other children.

Although there is compelling evidence for the importance of PA as an active force for social and academic success among college students, there are hardly any published studies that test this hypothesis among school-aged children and adolescents. Reschly et al. (2008) tested aspects of Frederickson's (1998, 2001) broaden-and-build theory of PA in the context of adolescents' engagement at school with learning. As predicted, they found that PA is related to greater student engagement in school activities and more supportive relations with teachers. These factors probably contribute to greater academic success, yet the role of PA in predicting academic success is still not clear. Similarly, Gilman and Huebner (2003) found that life satisfaction evaluations of children and adolescents are highly related to increased social activities and to extraversion, but no evidence is reported on the relationship between life satisfaction and academic success. It should be noted, however, that evaluating one's life as satisfying in general (i.e., global life satisfaction) is not synonymous to a self-report of PA (Diener et al. 2010). For example, Griffin and Huebner (2000) reported no differences in global life satisfaction between adolescent students with *serious emotional disturbance* and *normally achieving* adolescents. Individuals might report that they are satisfied with their life in general but still feel unhappy. However, the only area in which they reported being less satisfied was with peer relations.

After an extensive review of the literature, Diamond and Aspinwall (2003) concluded that PA is a crucial factor in human development. Helping children and adolescents to increase their PA is not a luxury but a necessity, often ignored by teachers and parents. According to these authors, children, from a very early age, have to learn how to control the intricate interplay between negative and positive emotional states. This is a never-ending life task from infancy to adulthood.

> The optimal developmental outcome, therefore, is not maintenance of a stable set point, but rather an enduring capacity for flexibility and change –in one's goals, one's affective states, one's use of different cognitive, behavioral, and social strategies, and one's reliance on intrapsychic versus interpersonal process (Diamond and Aspinwall 2003, p. 149).

Thus, emotional control is a cardinal factor in enhancing PA and EWB.

Self-Control Skills in the Pursuit of EWB

The term *emotional control* comes under the general term of self-control or *self-regulation*. By *self-control*, we mean the process by which human beings control their emotions, thoughts, and behavior. In this chapter, we prefer to use this term because it more clearly carries the notion that individuals exercise control over themselves in order to reach specific targets or goals. Although the practical and theoretical study of self-control process began in the second half of the last century (e.g., Bandura 1978; Kanfer 1971; Thoreson and Mahoney 1974), it has only become a central topic in general psychology during the past two decades.

In the 1970s, self-control was primarily studied by behavior therapists as a self-guided behavior modification of behavior. The general principles of operant conditioning were applied to the process of self-control. Thus, Kanfer (1971) postulated that self-control proceeds through three stages: self-monitoring, self-evaluation, and self-reinforcement. Later, Kanfer and Hagerman (1981) proposed that the self-control process is initiated only if individuals believe that a situation can change based on their own behavior (i.e., *self-efficacy expectancy*, Bandura 1977). Kanfer and Gaelick-Buys (1991), in the best tradition of behavior therapy, clearly emphasized that self-control describes "a person's actions in a specific situation, rather than a personality trait…" (p. 314). In fact, the proponents of behavior therapy strongly objected to conceiving of self-control as a stale personal disposition or as a set of skills and strategies. Rosenbaum (1980a) was among the first behavior therapists to propose that individuals acquire a repertoire of self-control skills and capabilities throughout their lives, which has labeled as *learned resourcefulness* (Rosenbaum and Ben-Ari 1985). This repertoire of self-control skills is considered by Rosenbaum

(1980a) to be a basic repertoire of capabilities from which other skills develop, such as social and academic skills.

Rosenbaum (1983) borrowed the term learned resourcefulness from Donald Meichenbaum. Meichenbaum (1977), a pioneer of cognitive behavior modification, used this term to describe attitudes developed by clients following a stress inoculation training procedure. The major components of the stress inoculation program are (a) self-monitoring maladaptive thoughts, images, feelings, and behaviors; (b) problem-solving skills; and (c) emotion regulation and other self-control skills (Meichenbaum 1985). Meichenbaum (1977) found that persons who have acquired these skills will develop a sense of learned resourcefulness (i.e., the belief that they can effectively deal with *manageable levels of stress*).

The main instrument for the assessment of learned resourcefulness is the self-control schedule (SCS, Rosenbaum 1980a, b). The SCS was later adapted for children (the children self-control scale: CSC) and for adolescents (the adolescents self-control scale; A-SCS; Rosenbaum and Ronen 1991). The three scales tap the same psychological skills but use different wordings in an attempt to adapt it to children's milieu and linguistic abilities. These are self-report questionnaires directed at assessing individual tendencies to apply self-control methods to the solution of behavioral problems (i.e., learned resourcefulness). It has been considered by some researchers as an intraindividual coping resource (White et al. 1996). It covers (a) the use of cognitive restructuring and self-instructions, (b) the use of problem-solving strategies, (c) the ability to delay immediate gratification, and (d) a general belief in one's ability to self-regulate emotions, cognitions, and emotions (i.e., self-efficacy; Rosenbaum 1980a, b). In recent years, a number of researchers have attempted to shorten these scales (e.g., Zauszniewski et al. 2010). Such attempts have in the past proven to adversely affect the validity of these scales. Numerous studies have validated the SCS as measuring self-control skills in various areas of life, such as health behavior (Rosenbaum 1990; Zauszniewski and Chung 2001), behavior therapy for depression (Burns et al. 1994), addictions (Carey et al. 1990), academic performance under stress (Akgun and Ciarrochi 2003), and maintenance of exercise behavior (Kennett et al. 2009). Since learned resourcefulness was predictive of so many diverse areas of behavior that all share the characteristic of performing under stress and coping successfully with temptations and distractions, it became clear that self-control skills are the very basic skills needed for effective functioning in life. Baumeister and Vohs (2004) also echoed our view that "self-regulation holds a pivotal place in self theory and thus is the key to understanding many different aspects of psychological functioning" (p. 3). Furthermore, they expressed the belief that "...the evolution of self-regulation will prove to be one of the defining features of human evolution, contributing to some of the *central abilities* that have made human beings distinctively human" (p. 3, italics were added).

In spite of the extreme importance attached to the development of self-control skills, relatively few research findings have been reported in the social-developmental literature. Early studies of children's self-control were dominated by the concept of *delay of gratification* and *resistance to temptation* (e.g., Mischel 1974). In our theory of learned resourcefulness, delay of gratification is only one of the five major self-control strategies (cognitive restructuring, problem solving, attention control, and self-efficacy). Children and adolescents who reported high levels of resourcefulness were able to more quickly learn how to control their aggression (Ronen and Rosenbaum 2010), to suffer less from depressive symptoms (Chang et al. 2007), and to better deal with the feeling of loneliness, as a result of having a sibling suffer from a serious illness (Hamama et al. 2000, 2008). Adolescents who scored high on the A-SCS were able to cope better with academic stress than those low on this scale (Akgun and Ciarrochi 2003) and were more successful in quitting smoking (Kennett et al. 2006) and in weight loss programs (Kennett and Ackerman 1995).

The theory of learned resourcefulness and the idea of self-control skills was developed 30 years ago (Rosenbaum 1983), when the *psychopathological model* prevailed. The basic assumption was that most people do not succumb to the various interpersonal and intrapersonal factors that lead to mental disorders. People acquire basic self-control skills that help them to effectively cope with various stressors during their lifetime. In more recent years, the focus has shifted, in part, to the study of *positive* aspects of human behavior (positive affect, happiness, etc.). The question now arises: What is the relationship between the use of self-control skills (or learned resourcefulness) and happiness and emotional well-being? Are self-control skills effective mostly because they minimize the adverse effects of negative emotions or because they increase positive affect and EWB? Or both? Although currently there is ample evidence that suggests that people who score high on the self-control scale (Rosenbaum 1980a, b) cope better with various life adversaries compared to people who score low on this scale, the psychological mechanisms behind these findings are not completely clear.

Learned Resourcefulness and Emotional Well-Being

In the last two decades, there has been an upsurge of research on positive and negative emotions and how they are related to self-control. In a recent review of the literature, Charles (2010) strongly asserted that EWB is tied to how well people regulate their emotions (a subset of self-control skills). It should be noted that people usually control their emotions via controlling their thoughts and their behavior (Baumeister et al. 2007). Diamond and Aspinwall (2003) have cogently argued that because positive and negative emotions are governed by different neuropsychological mechanisms, "it makes sense to model their regulatory development separately" (p. 139). PA and NA are different from each other in the way they can be self-controlled.

Unhappiness comes about on its own, but we have to work for happiness. While fear, anger, and sadness are responses to dangers from the external world, our feeling of pleasure has been developed by nature to lure us into desirable situations (Klein 2002, p. 28). Whereas NA is an automatic self-reaction against real or perceived threats to one's physical and psychological well-being (such as receiving a personal insult), PA is a proactive emotion that energizes the organism to pursue happiness and satisfaction in life.

In a number of studies, we investigated the effects of learned resourcefulness as a repertoire of self-control skills on children's and adolescents' PA and NA. For example, Aran (2006) compared the emotional well-being of adolescents who suffer from type 1 diabetes with a healthy group of adolescents. She found that there were no differences in PA between the two groups, but unexpectedly, the healthy adolescents reported higher levels of NA than the diabetics. Whereas among the healthy adolescents, the higher the level of learned resourcefulness, the higher the levels of PA and the lower the levels of NA; among the diabetics, learned resourcefulness was only associated with lower levels of NA but *not* with higher levels of PA. It is interesting to note that among the diabetics was perceived parental support related to higher levels of learned resourcefulness, but not among the healthy group. Ronen and Seeman (2007) also found that the higher one's learned resourcefulness, the higher one's PA. The participants in this study were adolescents who resided in boarding schools in Israel during the waiting period before the American invasion into Iraq in 2003. During this period, the population in Israel was getting prepared for a missile attack from Iraq, a repeat of the 1991 Gulf War.

In a recent study by Shachar (work in progress, 2010), evidence has surfaced that learned resourcefulness skills minimize NA and enhance PA at the same time. The participants in Shachar's study were elementary school students (third to sixth graders) who were trained in self-control skills using sport activities as a medium for such training. The children were assessed at the beginning of the school year (and the beginning of the training) and at the end of the school year that coincided with the end of program. The major goal of this study was to reduce aggressive behavior among the children through the use of sport activities as a tool for training in self-control skills. Compared to the control group, the experimental group significantly exhibited less aggressive behavior by the end of the program than the no treatment control group. NA and PA were also measured. Increases in PA and decreases in NA by the end of the program were associated with decreases in aggressive behavior, but only among children who reported increases in learned resourcefulness. The findings of this study do not suggest that emotions such as NA and PA *cause* behavior but that PA and NA are affected by individual differences in self-control skills (i.e., learned resourcefulness). Those children who were able to control their aggression by self-control methods were likely to feel more efficacious. Perceived self-efficacy of self-control over one's behavior is likely to increase children's EWB (Caprara et al. 2006; MacDonald 2008). Children who are happy and satisfied are less likely to aggress toward other people.

Seeman (2010) found similar results in a study with adolescents living in boarding schools in Israel. In her study, PA mediated the relationship between learned resourcefulness and hostile thoughts and between learned resourcefulness and aggressive behavior (but PA did not mediate the learned resourcefulness–anger relationship). Learned resourcefulness had a direct effect on anger reduction. Seeman added a new variable, *sense of belonging,* which was assessed by a subscale of the social support scale developed by Cohen et al. (1985). She found that PA also mediated the sense of belonging–hostile thoughts relationship. Adolescents who felt that they were welcomed and accepted by their peer group experienced more positive feelings, and these feelings, in turn, lead them to view the world as less hostile. Learned resourcefulness was found to be directly related to increases in sense of belonging and to lower levels of anger and aggressive behavior. These findings suggest that both self-control skills and the belief that one is socially accepted have an impact on hostile thoughts, but only through the mediation of PA. EWB shapes adolescents' views of their social environment. Adolescents who perceive society as less hostile are also likely to be less angry and less aggressive toward their peers (Dodge and Pettit 2003). PA shapes—and is being shaped by—social contacts and by learned resourcefulness, while the latter two are also mutually determined by each other. These processes characterize the development of EWB from birth to adulthood.

As the above studies indicate, children's and adolescents' EWB is related to their ability to be masters of their own behavior. But what about children and adolescents who were born and raised in large families that live under very poor economical conditions and are continuously under the threats of political violence? Intuitively one would expect these children and adolescents to have low levels of EWB and higher levels of trait aggression in comparison to children and adolescents who live in more prosperous and peaceful societies.

To test these hypotheses, we (Rosenbaum et al. 2010) selected three samples of adolescents (13–17 years of age) from three different milieus: First, adolescence who were residing in the Gaza Strip and who were born and raised in Gaza or in the Palestinians refugee camps in the Gaza Strip were selected. These adolescences' families were poor, and they continuously lived under the shadows of war and of political violence either from outside or from inside the Gaza Strip. Second, we selected adolescence who were born and raised in Israeli–Palestinian communities in Israel. The Israeli Palestinians share the same religious and cultural background as the Palestinians who escaped to Gaza in 1948 from their communities in Israel. The economic conditions of the Israeli Palestinians are much better than their counterparts in Gaza, and they live in relatively peaceful atmosphere. The third sample consisted of Jewish Israeli adolescents of the same age as the adolescents of the other two groups. This group was born and raised in Jewish towns in the center of Israel. Relative to the Israeli Palestinians, their families are more prosperous, and they live under the same political conditions as the Israeli Palestinians. All the participants completed a series of questionnaires: (1) the PANAS scale (Watson et al. 1988) that measured their PA and NA—these measures were used to compute the ratio between PA and NA (*the positivity ratio*, Frederickson 2009); (2) the Buss and Perry (1992) aggression questionnaire that assesses trait aggression, trait hostility, and their anger; and (3) the adolescents self-control scale (A-SCS—Rosenbaum and Ronen 1991) that measures their level of learned resourcefulness.

As predicted, the Gaza adolescents received the lowest positivity ratio and the Jewish Israelis received the highest scores of all the groups, with the Israeli Palestinians scoring in between the other two groups. However, in sharp contrast to our expectations, the Jewish Israeli adolescents scored the *highest* on the three subscales of the aggression questionnaire (hostility, anger, and aggressive behavior) and the adolescents from Gaza received the *lowest* scores on these scales. The Israeli Palestinians scored in between those two groups. This pattern of results was not obtained when we assessed learned resourcefulness (A-SCS, Rosenbaum and Ronen 1991). The Israeli Palestinians received, by far, the highest scores on the A-SCS (mean = 25.99) compared to the Jewish Israelis and the Gaza adolescents (means 11.85 and 12.46, respectively). The fact that the Gaza adolescents were the least aggressive compared to the other two groups can be attributed to their assigned role in society in Gaza. In contrast to the Jewish Israeli and the Israeli Palestinian adolescents, the adolescents in Gaza play a major role in promoting the Palestinians goals in their battle against Israel (Barber 2001). In contrast to many adolescents in Western societies (including Israel) who feel alienated from the adult world (Larson 2000), adolescences from Gaza share a collective identity with the adults in their battle for independence. They do not need to resort to aggressive acts against their contemporaries because they experience strong social bonds with their peers who are united in the battle for freedom. Social rejection and social exclusion are the major causes for aggression among adolescents (Twenge et al. 2001). Consequently, they do not have to use self-control skills (learned resourcefulness) in order to control their aggression nor is their EWB a factor in expressing their aggressive tendencies. These speculative ideas received support from the results of our study. Whereas higher levels of learned resourcefulness were associated with lower levels of trait aggression among the Israeli Jewish and Palestinian adolescents, no such relationship was found among the Gaza adolescents, namely, individual differences in learned resourcefulness were not related to trait aggression among the Gaza adolescents. Also, only among the two groups who reside in Israel (Jews and Palestinians), but not among the Gaza group, did the positivity ratio predict reduced levels of aggression. However, in all three groups of adolescents, we found that learned resourcefulness was positively correlated with the positivity ratio of the participants. The more adolescents have self-control skills, the higher is their EWB. This is a rather robust finding in the various studies that measure these two variables. Nevertheless, the three groups of adolescents differed from each in the strength of this relationship. Among the Israeli Palestinians, the learned resourcefulness–positivity ratio relationship was the strongest ($r = 0.42$) compared to the Jewish Israelis ($r = 0.31$) and the Gaza adolescents ($r = 0.20$).

We are not aware of any study that has investigated the relationship between EWB of youth and their involvement in advancing the social and political causes of the adults in their society. Larson (2000) has suggested that when adolescents become more involved in pursuing societal goals, the happier they will be. In fact, the behavior of the adolescents in Gaza exemplifies the success of long-term socialization processes in this society. Gaza adolescents pursue the same goals as Gaza adults. That is obviously not the state of affairs in most Western societies, including Israel. Next, we discuss the role of socialization practices in enhancing EWB among children and adolescents and how self-control skills shape this relationship. A particular emphasis is placed on the goals that these socialization processes attempt to accomplish.

Developmental Patterns of EWB from Birth to Late Adolescence

One can identify differences in socialization practices at different developmental stages of child development, as a function of the temporal hedonic orientation[1] of the socializing agents. As children mature, the socialization practices change their emphases from the present state of EWB to training children with the skills that are required for the maintenance of future EWB (such as preparing for a profession that will be satisfying). "Hedonism of the present" emphasizes current EWB, whereas hedonism of the future "... is concerned with maximizing the expected value of positive *future* events and minimizing the expected value of negative events" (Karniol 2010, p. 95, italics added).

During infancy, mothers and other caregivers are completely oriented toward assuring maximum emotional and physical well-being of infants. The caregivers' efforts are directed at understanding what babies want in order to feel good, and the role of babies is to transmit their preferences. Karniol (2010) named these mother–baby interactions as the *preference game*. Since linguistic tools are unavailable, the infants learn to modulate their emotional responses in such a way as to express their needs through facial expressions, crying, or smiling. These expressions provide the foundations for the development of self-control skills. The caregiver, on the other hand, tries to interpret and understand what their infants prefer for their present well-being. Feldman et al. (1999) noted that positive affect and mutual mother–child regulation are two important features of synchrony that contribute to the development of emotion regulation.

From infancy, self-control, social relationship, and emotional well-being (specifically PA and NA) reciprocally affect each other. The gaze-orienting capacities of infants are related to developmental changes in early social interactions and in self-regulation (Johnson et al. 1991). Rothbart et al. (2011) studied the development of self-regulation from infancy to early childhood. Positive and negative affect can be easily differentiated from infancy. Rothbart et al. (2011) have called PA at this stage of development *extraversion*, defined by "...positive emotionality and approach, including positive anticipation, high intensity pleasure... with a negative loading for shyness" (p. 444). Negative affectivity has been defined as "...discomfort, fear, anger/frustration, and sadness..." (p. 444). Infants' ability to control their orienting responses is the precursor of the development of self-control skills. During the first 4 months, the control of orienting responses is largely in the hands of caregiver presentations (i.e., making sounds and moving objects in front of the infant). By the age of 4 months, infants gain control over their gazes and are able to move these gazes from one location to another (Rothbart et al. 2011). Infants' ability to control their gazes has been associated with lower negative affect and greater ability to be soothed (Johnson et al. 1991). PA, even at this early stage, is associated with

[1] Insko and Schopler (1972), (as cited by Karniol 2010) identified three cultural patterns of temporal hedonic orientations: past, present, and future.

infants' ability to control their attention. It should be noted that attention control has been considered as the primary skill for self-control processes until cognitive processes develop (Sethi et al. 2000).

During infancy, it is apparent that NA and PA have two different functions and that they serve to satisfy two different basic needs. Whereas NA functions mainly to avoid physical distress, PA is, in part, directed at approaching other people. For example, babies' smiles (an expression of PA) attract other people. Eventually, a baby learns to associate smile with social contact. Furthermore, a baby's smile attracts the attention of the caregiver, who in return may try to draw the attention of the baby by making sounds and smiling back. Infants learn to control their gazes initially through their interaction with their caregivers and later with other people. Rothbart et al. (2011) report that "...smiling and laughter in infancy positively predicted both infants' and 7-year-olds approach tendencies" (p. 446). On the other hand, by expressing negative affectivity, they are able to mobilize the caregivers to provide them with their basic needs.

The triad links among self-control skills, EWB, and social relationship become even more noticeable when *effortful control* develops. Effortful control of attention is defined as the "ability to inhibit a dominant response in order to perform a subdominant response" (Rothbart et al. 2011, p. 447). It emerges after infancy during early childhood. Effortful control is an important aspect of self-control, and it has been suggested that effortful control of negative emotions may later be transferred to the control of cognition and behavior (Posner and Rothbart 1998). Effortful control has also been associated with the control of approach behavior, which is, in part, also associated with reward seeking and PA (MacDonald 2008). These are the early foundations of the development of self-control skills.

Socialization goals slowly shift from pursuing present EWB to preparing the child toward the future. The older the child becomes, the less the emphasis on current EWB. Consequently, adolescents' education is directed at preparing them for the future with the implicit assumption that a good education will make them happy adults. Scarifying the current EWB of adolescents for a better and happier future has serious ramifications for adolescents and the society they live in. For example, Larson (2000) reported that, among American adolescents, there were many youth who reported being unhappy, bored, unmotivated, and unexcited about their life. We have no data about Israeli youth, but we believe that it has to be about the same as in the United States. Classes in Israeli schools are overcrowded, and most students are bored and unmotivated in class. The educational authorities are often too busy preparing the adolescents for governmental matriculation examinations while ignoring their well-being in the present. Hence, there is a decrease in EWB from early childhood until early adulthood. Larson (2000) advocates a *positive youth development* program that would emphasize current EWB by providing various activities that are challenging and meaningful for the *present* life of the students. Caprara et al. (2006) also proposed a program that promotes self-efficacy beliefs for adolescents and provides for the successful adaptation from childhood to adulthood. These researchers reported that "...perceived self-efficacy for affect regulation and for management of interpersonal relationships influence adolescents' subjective well-being" (p. 38). It is our view that the regular teaching programs in high schools should be geared toward increasing adolescents' intrinsic motivation and sense of self-determination and thereby blocking the decreases in EWB from childhood to adolescents. As we have already noted, children who are happy and report high levels of EWB are more open and receptive to new learning than children who are low on EWB. Therefore, EWB is a basic requirement for effective learning.

It is interesting to note that while there is a decrease in EWB from early childhood to late adolescents, there is an increase in EWB from early adulthood to old age. Mroczek and Kolarz (1998) found that older people see their future as more bounded compared to younger people, who see their future as open. "This causes older people to gear their lives, especially their social lives, toward maximizing positive and minimizing negative affect" (p. 1333). Through the human lifespan, when people are challenged to self-control their behavior toward meaningful and clear personal goals, their EWB increases.

Final Thoughts

Most studies on well-being treat it as the end result of exposure to factors such as social networking, economic prosperity, and social and political climate. This approach makes sense when we define well-being in terms of how people cognitively evaluate their *satisfaction with life*. However, in this chapter, we discussed well-being in terms of positive (PA) and negative emotions (NA). PA and NA are by no means just the *consequence* of the factors that make us happy (and perhaps also satisfied with life) but the effects of these emotions on the factors that presumably make us happy. Positive and negative emotions provide feedback to the way we have acted and also guide our future actions by creating expectation that if we continue to behave in a certain way, then we will be happy and feel good (Baumeister et al. 2007). As the studies that we have reviewed indicate, self-control behaviors are likely to accentuate PA and decrease NA. When people feel that they can control many aspects of their life, they feel self-efficacious and happy with themselves. It can also be said that PA, in and of itself, enhances the use of self-control methods. When people feel energetic and happy, they are more likely to use their self-control skills.

It should be noted that self-control skills always develop within a social context (Seeley and Gardner 2006). Good social relationships accentuate PA that, in return, reinforces the use of self-control behaviors in a social context and/or enhances one's expectations to feel good when in the company of other people. This *PA feedback loop* is the basis for EWB. However, Csikszentmihalyi (2002) warned against the dependency individuals develop on other people and on society in general. In fact, in order to feel well, a person must self-emancipate from social controls, which "... is the ability to find rewards in the events of each moment. If a person learns to enjoy and find meaning in the ongoing stream of experience,...the burden of social controls automatically falls from ones shoulders" (p. 19). The extent to which social relationship contributes to the EWB of children and adolescents needs to be investigated further. It is likely that during adolescence, more than any other period, peer acceptance is highly associated with one's EWB.

In reading the Israeli newspapers, one is impressed by the fact that among Israeli youth, there is a continuous increase in crime rates, violent acts, bullying, and drug and alcohol use over the past decade. Furthermore, mental health professionals report that more and more youth suffer from depression and suicidal tendencies. However, there are hardly any reports in the public media or in scientific publications on the level of happiness and EWB of Israeli adolescents. Nevertheless, some research findings indicate that adolescents are less happy than young children.

In this chapter, we attributed the reduction of EWB among adolescents to the shifts in emphasis of the socialization agents from focusing on the hedonic present (i.e., assuring current EWB) to hedonism of the future (i.e., assuring future hedonism). During infancy and early childhood, parental efforts in Western society are solely devoted to the enhancement of the well-being of their children. Once children reach an age in which they can go to school, the EWB of children becomes weaker with the advancement of the years in school when schoolwork becomes more and more demanding. Parents in our society are faced with the following dilemma almost on a daily basis: "Should we force our children to devote more time and energy to school work or should we let them do what really makes them happy (playing soccer with their friends, playing games on the computer, etc.)"? When parents feel responsible for the future of their children, they tend to value more academic achievements than present well-being. Adolescents are often expected to delay current pleasurable activities, such as sports and music, in favor of success in school. However, as has been reviewed here, with the advent of positive psychology in the last two decades, there is now scientific evidence that positive emotions are not only good for accentuating well-being but also for the enhancement of new learning and creativity (Csikszentmihalyi 1993, 2002; Frederickson 2009). Nevertheless, there appears to be a consensus among parents and teachers that school achievements and grades are more important than current happiness and emotional well-being. Is this really an unresolved dilemma? Do children and adolescents have to delay current happiness for a happier and more gratifying future?

To resolve the happiness dilemma, schools should adopt the dual role of transmitting knowledge and increasing the level of EWB of their students. The concept of *flow* that has been proposed by Csikszentmihalyi (2002) appears to be most suited to what schools should provide their adolescent students. Flow describes feelings that arise when there is "...concentration, absorption, deep involvement, joy, a sense of accomplishment..." (Csikszentmihalyi 1993, p. 176). In another place, the author describes the situations in which flow feelings are likely to arise as "...situations in which attention can be freely invested... (with) no threat for the self to defend against" (Csikszentmihalyi 2002, p. 40). Flow experiences are likely to arise when students are taught and challenged to explore and gain new knowledge of the world through intrinsic motivation. According to Csikszentmihalyi (1993, pp. 208–213), in order to experience flow (and happiness), one has to set clear personal goals, develop skills to achieve these goals, become fully immersed in the activities leading toward these goals, be open and attentive to the immediate experience, and learn the joys of new discoveries. Learning in school should be built on principles of self-determination and intrinsic motivation and not on teachers' or parental determination only (Larson 2006; Ryan and Deci 2000). If these principles are applied to school settings, both teachers and students will be more satisfied and happy in their joint adventure of gaining new knowledge. By empowering teachers to explore new teaching methods and students to be the investigators of the world around them and of past knowledge, they will enrich their self-control skills and their EWB.

We have applied the *empowerment approach* in helping adolescents to reduce their aggressive behavior through the acquisition of self-control skills (learned resourcefulness; Ronen and Rosenbaum 2010). In line with the present discussion, we hypothesized that most children who aggress in school do so because they want to be accepted by their peers and because they fear social rejection. They simply do not know how to materialize their desire to be part of the group. Hence, we developed a program by which they are taught to become part of their group of peers by empowering them with self-control and social skills. The empowerment training takes place in small groups under the teachers' guidance. These teachers were trained on how to empower children and adolescents to become their own agents of change. Adolescents and children who graduated from 12 group sessions in our program of empowerment became much less aggressive and were accepted by their peer group. Although, at the time, we did not assess their EWB, the general impression of the group leaders was that these adolescents became happier individuals with stronger feelings of self-determination. We are currently investigating the role of EWB in reducing aggressive behavior in schools.

In the last 100 years, children and adolescents in the Western world were freed from participating in the work force of the adult world but were required to attend schools for many years in order to acquire knowledge as an introduction to learning a profession. In these schools, they are not trained to become autonomous, agentic adults, as it is done in most non-Western societies (Larson 2000). In these schools, the emphasis is on achievement and on tests that compare the scholastic achievements of students across the nation (and even in comparison to other nations). Hardly any attention is given to children's EWB, in contrast to the teachings in kindergartens. As one could easily expect, various surveys have shown that during schoolwork, adolescents report low intrinsic motivation, high rates of boredom, and little challenges (Larson 2000).

It is high time for educators and teachers to change the school system into a place where adolescents are challenged and become deeply involved in the subjects they choose to study. Children and adolescents will come alive in activities in which they can control and be guided with minimal adult supervision. Children and adolescents feel good when they are challenged to use their skills to complete a difficult task, and once they succeed, they feel efficacious. Positive feelings are not only related to a general sense of well-being but also contribute to increases of intrinsic motivation and to greater creativity. In addition, happy children and adolescents are most likely to have more friends and social support. As we have suggested, the mutual triad of emotional well-being, self-control skills, and social relations enhances flourishing among children and adolescents, at least in Western societies. So far, we have little information on what leads to flourishing in non-Western societies in which children and adolescents are assigned adult roles from very early adolescence.

References

Akgun, S., & Ciarrochi, J. (2003). Learned resourcefulness moderates the relationships between academic stress and academic performance. *Educational Psychology, 23*, 287–294.

Aran, O. (2006). *The connection between personal and interpersonal resources and subjective well-being in diabetic and healthy adolescents (in Hebrew).* Unpublished Ph.D. dissertation, Tel Aviv University, Tel Aviv.

Averill, J. R., & More, T. A. (1993). Happiness. In M. Lewis & J. M. Haviland (Eds.), *Handbook of emotions* (pp. 617–629). New York: The Guilford Press.

Bandura, A. (1977). Self-efficacy: Toward a unifying theory of behavioral change. *Psychological Review, 84*, 191–215.

Bandura, A. (1978). The self system in reciprocal determinism. *American Psychologist, 33*, 344–358.

Barber, B. K. (2001). Political violence, social integration, and youth functioning: Palestinian youth from the Intifada. *Journal of Community Psychology, 29*(3), 259–280.

Baumeister, R. F., & Vohs, K. D. (Eds.). (2004). *Handbook of self-regulation: Research, theory, and application.* New York: Guilford Press.

Baumeister, R. F., Vohs, K. D., DeWall, N. C., & Zhang, L. (2007). How emotion shapes behavior: Feedback, anticipation, and reflection, rather than direct causation. *Personality and Social Psychology Review, 11*(2), 167–203.

Burns, D. D., Rude, S., Simons, A. D., Bates, M. A., & Thase, M. E. (1994). Does learned resourcefulness predict the response to cognitive behavioral therapy for depression? *Cognitive Therapy and Research, 18*, 277–291.

Buss, A. H., & Perry, M. (1992). The aggression questionnaire. *Journal of Personality and Social Psychology, 63*, 452–459.

Caprara, G. V., Steca, P., Gerbino, M., Paciello, M., & Vecchio, G. M. (2006). Looking for adolescents' well-being: Self-efficacy beliefs as determinants of positive thinking and happiness. *Epidemiologia E Psichiatria Sociale, 15*(1), 30–43.

Carey, M. P., Carey, K. B., Carnrike, C. L., & Meisler, A. W. (1990). Learned resourcefulness, drinking, and smoking in young adults. *Journal of Psychology, 124*, 391–395.

Carr, A. (2004). *Positive psychology: The science of happiness and human strength.* New York: Brunner-Routledge.

Carver, C. S., & White, T. L. (1994). Behavioral inhibition, behavioral activation, and affective responses to impending reward and punishment: The BIS / BAS scales. *Journal of Personality and Social Psychology, 67*, 319–333.

Chang, L., McBride-Chang, C., Stewart, S. M., & Au, E. (2003). Life satisfaction, self-concept, and family relations in Chinese adolescents and children. *International Journal of Behavioral Development, 27*, 182–189.

Chang, H.-J., Zauszniewski, J. A., Heinzer, M. M., Musil, C. M., & Tsai, W.-C. (2007). Adaptive functioning and depressive symptoms in school-aged children. *Journal of Advanced Nursing, 60*(5), 502–512.

Charles, S. T. (2010). Strength and vulnerability integration: A model of emotional well – being across adulthood. *Psychological Bulletin, 136*(6), 1068.

Cohen, S., Mermelstein, R., Kamarck, T., & Hoberman, H. M. (1985). Measuring the functional components of social support. In I. G. Sarason & B. R. Sarason (Eds.), *Social support: Theory, research, and applications* (pp. 73–94). The Hague: Martinus Nijhoff.

Csikszentmihalyi, M. (1993). *The evolving self: The psychology for the third millennium.* New York: Harper Perennial.
Csikszentmihalyi, M. (2002). *Flow: The classic work on how to achieve happiness* (Rev. and updated revision ed.). London: Rider.
Diamond, L. M., & Aspinwall, L. G. (2003). Emotion regulation across the life span: An integrative perspective emphasizing self-regulation, positive affect, and dyadic processes. *Motivation and Emotion, 27*(2), 125–156.
Diener, E., Ng, W., Harter, J., & Arora, R. (2010). Wealth and happiness across the world: Material prosperity predicts life evaluation, whereas psychosocial prosperity predicts positive feelings. *Journal of Personality and Social Psychology, 99*(1), 52–61.
Dodge, K. A., & Pettit, G. S. (2003). A biopsychosocial model of the development of chronic conduct problems in adolescence. *Developmental Psychology, 39*(2), 349–371.
Erikson, E. (1959). Identity and the life cycle. *Psychological Issues, 1*, 18–164.
Feldman, R., Greenbaum, C. W., & Yirmiya, N. (1999). Mother-infant affect synchrony as an antecedent of the emergence of self-control. *Developmental Psychology, 35*, 223–231.
Fox, N. A., & Calkins, S. D. (2003). The development of self-control of emotion: Intrinsic and extrinsic influences. *Motivation and Emotion, 27*(1), 7–26.
Frederickson, B. L. (1998). What are positive emotions? *Review of General Psychology, 2*, 300–319.
Frederickson, B. L. (2001). The role of positive emotions trigger upward spirals toward emotional well-being. *Psychological Science, 13*, 172–175.
Frederickson, B. L. (2009). *Positivity*. New York: Crown Publishing.
Fredrickson, B. L., & Joiner, T. (2002). Positive emotions trigger upward spirals toward emotional well – being. *Psychological Science, 13*(2), 172–175.
Fredrickson, B. L., & Losada, M. F. (2005). Positive affect and the complex dynamics of human flourishing. *American Psychologist, 60*(7), 678–686.
Gable, S. L., Reis, H. T., & Elliot, A. J. (2003). Evidence for bivariate systems: An empirical test of appetition and aversion across domains. *Journal of Research in Personality, 37*(5), 349–372. doi:10.1016/S0092-6566(02)00580-9.
Gilman, R., & Huebner, S. (2003). A review of life satisfaction research with children and adolescents. *School Psychology Quarterly, 18*(2), 192–205.
Greene, A. L. (1990). Patterns of affectivity in the transition to adolescence. *Journal of Experimental Child Psychology, 50*, 340–356.
Hamama, R., Ronen, T., & Feigin, R. (2000). Self-control, anxiety, and loneliness in siblings of children with cancer. *Social Work in Health Care, 31*, 63–83.
Hamama, L., Ronen, T., & Rahav, G. (2008). Self-control, self-efficacy, role overload and stress responses among siblings of children with cancer. *Health & Social Work, 33*, 121–132.
Hepper, E. G., Gramzow, R. H., & Sedikides, C. (2010). Individual differences in self-enhancement and self-protection strategies: An integrative analysis. *Journal of Personality, 78*(2), 781–814.
Insko, C. A., & Schopler, J. (1972). *Experimental social psychology*. New York: Academic Press.
Johnson, M. H., Posner, M. I., & Rothbart, M. K. (1991). Components of visual orienting in early infancy: Contingency learning, anticipatory looking, and disengaging. *Journal of Cognitive Neuroscience, 3*(4), 335–344.
Kanfer, F. H. (1971). The maintenance of behavior by self-generated stimuli and reinforcement. In A. Jacob & L. B. Sachs (Eds.), *The psychology of private events* (pp. 39–57). San Diego: Academic.
Kanfer, F. H., & Gaelick-Buys, L. (1991). Self-management methods. In F. H. Kanfer & A. P. Goldstein (Eds.), *Helping people change: A text book of methods* (pp. 305–360). New York: Pergamon Press.
Kanfer, F. H., & Hagerman, S. (1981). The role of self-regulation. In L. P. Rehm (Ed.), *Behavior therapy for depression* (pp. 143–179). San Diego: Academic.
Karniol, R. (2010). *Social development as preference management: How infants, children, and parents get what they want from one another*. New York: Cambridge University Press.

Kennett, D. J., & Ackerman, M. (1995). Importance of learned resourcefulness to weight loss and early success during maintenance: Preliminary evidence. *Patient Education and Counseling, 25*, 197–203.

Kennett, D. J., Morris, E., & Bangs, A. M. (2006). Learned resourcefulness and smoking cessation revisited. *Patient Education and Counseling, 60*, 206–211.

Kennett, D. J., Worth, N. C., & Forbes, C. A. (2009). The contributions of Rosenbaum's model of self-control and Trans-theoretical model to the understanding of exercising behavior. *Psychology of Sport and Exercise, 10*, 602–606.

Keyes, C. L. M. (2002). The mental health continuum: From languishing to flourishing in life. *Journal of Health and Social Behavior, 43*, 207–222.

Keyes, C. L. M. (2006). Mental health in adolescence: Is America's youth flourishing? *The American Journal of Orthopsychiatry, 76*(3), 395–402.

Keyes, C. L. M. (2009). The nature and importance of positive mental health in America's adolescents. In R. H. Gilman, E. Scott, & M. J. Furlong (Eds.), *Handbook of positive psychology in schools* (pp. 9–23). New York: Routledge/Taylor & Francis Group.

Keyes, C. L. M., & Lopez, S. J. (2005). Toward a science of mental health: Positive directions in diagnosis and interventions. In C. R. Snyder & S. J. Lopez (Eds.), *Handbook of positive psychology* (p. 45). New York: Oxford University Press.

Klein, S. (2002). *The science of happiness*. New York: Marlow & Company.

Klingman, A. (2001). Stress responses and adaptation of Israeli school-age children evacuated from homes during massive missile attacks. *Anxiety, Stress and Coping, 14*(2), 149–172.

Larson, R. W. (2000). Toward a psychology of positive youth development. *American Psychologist, 55*(1), 170–183.

Larson, R. (2006). Positive youth development, willful adolescents, and mentoring. *Journal of Community Psychology, 34*(6), 677–689.

Laurent, J., Catanzaro, S. J., Joiner, T. E., Rudolph, K. D., Potter, K. I., Lambert, S., Osborne, L., & Gathright, T. (1999). A measure of positive and negative affect for children: Scale development and preliminary validation. *Psychological Assessment, 11*(3), 326–338.

Lucas, R., Diener, E., & Suh, E. (1996). Discriminant validity of well-being measures. *Journal of Personality and Social Psychology, 71*, 616–628.

Lyubomirsky, S., King, L., & Diener, E. (2005). The benefits of frequent positive affect: Does happiness lead to success? *Psychological Bulletin, 131*(6), 803–855.

MacDonald, K. B. (2008). Effortful control, explicit processing, and the regulation of human evolved predispositions. *Psychological Review, 115*(4), 1012–1031.

Meichenbaum, D. (1977). *Cognitive-behavior modification: An integrative approach*. New York: Plenum.

Meichenbaum, D. (1985). *Stress inoculation training*. New York: Pergamon.

Mischel, W. (1974). Process in delay gratification. In L. Berkowitz (Ed.), *Advances in experimental social psychology* (Vol. 7, pp. 247–292). New York: Academic.

Mroczek, D. K., & Kolarz, C. M. (1998). The effects of age on positive and negative affect: A developmental perspective on happiness. *Journal of Personality and Social Psychology, 75*, 1333–1349.

Novotney, A. (2010, September). Pediatrics urged to screen more closely for mental health problems. *Monitor on Psychology, 41*, 10.

Peterson, C., & Seligman, M. E. P. (2004). *Character strengths and virtues*. Washington, DC/New York: American Psychological Association and Oxford University Press.

Posner, M. L., & Rothbart, M. K. (1998). Attention, self-regulation, and consciousness. *Philosophical Transactions of the Royal Society of London B, 353*, 1915–1927.

Regier, D. A., Narrow, W. E., Rae, D. S., Manderscheid, R. W., Locke, B. Z., & Goodwin, F. K. (1993). The de Facto US Mental and Addictive Disorders Service System: Epidemiologic catchment area prospective 1-year prevalence rates of disorders and services. *Archives of General Psychiatry, 50*(2), 85–94.

Reschly, A. L., Huebner, E. S., Appleton, J. J., & Antaramian, S. (2008). Engagement as flourishing: The contribution of positive emotions and coping to adolescents' engagement at school and with learning. *Psychology in the Schools, 45*(5), 419–431.

Roberts, M. C., Brown, K. J., Johnson, R. J., & Reinke, J. (2005). Positive psychology for children: Development, prevention, and promotion. In C. R. Snyder & S. J. Lopez (Eds.), *Handbook of positive psychology* (pp. 663–675). New York: Oxford University Press.

Ronen, T., & Rosenbaum, M. (2010). Developing learned resourcefulness in adolescents to help them reduce their aggressive behavior: Preliminary findings. *Research on Social Work Practice, 20*, 410–426.

Ronen, T., & Seeman, A. (2007). Subjective well-being of adolescents in boarding schools under the threat of war. *Journal of Traumatic Stress, 20*, 1053–1062.

Rosenbaum, M. (1980a). A schedule for assessing self-control behaviors: Preliminary findings. *Behavior Therapy, 11*, 109–121.

Rosenbaum, M. (1980b). Individual differences in self-control behaviors and tolerance of painful stimulation. *Journal of Abnormal Psychology, 89*(4), 581–590.

Rosenbaum, M. (1983). Learned resourcefulness as a behavioral repertoire for the self-regulation of internal events: Issues and speculations. In M. Rosenbaum, C. M. Franks, & Y. Jaffe (Eds.), *Perspectives on behavior therapy in the eighties* (pp. 54–73). New York: Springer.

Rosenbaum, M. (Ed.). (1990). *Learned resourcefulness: On coping skills, self-control, and adaptive behavior*. New York: Springer.

Rosenbaum, M., & Ben-Ari, K. (1985). Learned helplessness and learned resourcefulness: Effects of noncontingent success and failure on individuals differing in self-control skills. *Journal of Personality and Social Psychology, 48*(1), 198–215.

Rosenbaum, M., & Ronen, T. (1991, November). *Development of a rating scale for assessment of children's self-control skills (CSC)*. Paper presented at the Annual Meeting of the Association for the Advancement of Behavior Therapy.

Rosenbaum, M., Ronen, T., Abuelaish, I., & Agbaria, Q. (2010). *Adolescents' trait aggression and political violence: The role of personal dispositions and gender*. Unpublished raw data.

Rothbart, M. K., Ellis, L. K., & Posner, M. I. (2011). Temperament and self-regulation. In K. D. Vohs & R. F. Baumeister (Eds.), *Handbook of self-regulation: Research, theory, and application* (2nd ed., pp. 441–460). New York: The Guilford Press.

Ryan, R. M., & Deci, E. L. (2000). Self-determination theory and the facilitation of intrinsic motivation, social development and well-being. *American Psychologist, 55*, 68–78.

Ryff, C. D., & Singer, B. (2005). From social structure to biology: Integrative science in pursuit of human health and well-being. In C. R. Snyder & S. J. Lopez (Eds.), *Handbook of positive psychology* (pp. 541–555). New York: Oxford University Press.

Seeley, E. A., & Gardner, W. L. (2006). Succeeding at self-control through a focus on others: The roles of social practice and accountability in self-regulation. In K. D. Vohs & E. J. Finkel (Eds.), *Self and relationship: Connecting intrapersonal and interpersonal processes* (pp. 407–425). New York: The Guilford Press.

Seeman, A. (2010). *Are happy adolescents less aggressive? The moderating role of self-control skills and sense of belonging on the happiness – Aggression relationship*. Unpublished raw data Tel Aviv University.

Sethi, A., Mischel, W. W., Aber, J. L., Shoda, Y., & Rodriguez, M. L. (2000). The role of attention deployment in development of self-regulation: Predicting preschoolers' delay of gratification from mother-toddler interactions. *Developmental Psychology, 36*(6), 767–777.

Shachar, K. (2010). *The reduction in aggression among children through the use of training in sport*. Unpublished raw data University of Tel Aviv.

Thoreson, C. E., & Mahoney, M. J. (1974). *Behavioral self-control*. New York: Holt, Rinehart & Winston.

Twenge, J. M., Baumeister, R. F., Tice, D. M., & Stucke, T. S. (2001). If you can't join them, beat them: The effects of social exclusion on aggressive behavior. *Journal of Personality and Social Psychology, 81*, 1058–1069.

Updegraff, J. A., Gable, S. L., & Taylor, S. E. (2004). What makes experiences satisfying ? The interaction of approach – Avoidance motivations and emotions in well – being. *Journal of Personality and Social Psychology, 86*(3), 496–504.

Watson, D., Clark, L. A., & Tellegen, A. (1988). Development and validation of brief measures of positive and negative affect: The PANAS scales. *Journal of Personality and Social Psychology, 54*(6), 1063–1070.

Watson, D., Wiese, D., Vaidya, J., & Tellegen, A. (1999). The two general activation systems of affect: Structural findings, evolutionary considerations and psychobiological evidence. *Journal of Personality and Social Psychology, 76*(5), 820–838.

White, R., Tata, P., & Burns, T. (1996). Mood, learned resourcefulness and perceptions of control in type 1 diabetes mellitus. *Journal of Psychosomatic Research, 40*(2), 205–212. doi:10.1016/0022-3999(95)00515-3.

Zauszniewski, J. A., & Chung, C. (2001). Resourcefulness and health practices of diabetic women. *Research in Nursing and Health, 24*(2), 113–121.

Zauszniewski, J. A., Bekhet, A. K., & Bonham, E. (2010). Psychometric testing of the children's resourcefulness scale. *Journal of Child and Adolescent Psychiatric Nursing, 23*(3), 181–188.

Chapter 11
The Nature of Happiness: Nature Affiliation and Mental Well-Being

Andrew J. Howell and Holli-Anne Passmore

> Appreciating the beauty of a blossom, the loveliness of a lilac, or the grace of a gazelle are all ways in which people can, in some small measure, fill their daily lives with evolutionarily inspired epiphanies of pleasure (Buss 2000, p. 22).

It has been over 25 years since E. O. Wilson (1984) wrote *Biophilia*, in which he argued for an evolved inclination among humans to affiliate with nature. Wilson reasoned that, because our ancestors' survival and reproduction depended upon access to natural resources, selection pressures favored those who had an affinity to orient toward nature. Findings in support of Wilson's biophilia hypothesis have emerged (Kaplan and Kaplan 1989; Ulrich 1993), including evidence for human preference for savannah-like landscapes, beneficial physiological responses to natural environments relative to manufactured environments, and improvements in cognitive functioning and restorative effects on mental well-being as a result of exposure to nature (see review by Joye 2007).

Additional support for Wilson's (1984) idea that we have a deep-rooted connection to nature comes from the fact that only recently in our evolutionary history have we separated ourselves from a hunter-gatherer way of life which was immersed daily in nature (Burns 2005; Frumkin 2001; Gullone 2000; Kahn 1997; Kellert 1997; Nesse and Wiliams 1996). There is dissociation between human biology and modern urban life. As Gelter (2000) writes, "[t]he time-span in our habitat change from the natural world setting into the technological habitat is too short for the evolutionary processes to permit any major biological adaptations" (p. 86). Within this context, affiliating with nature is framed as a basic human need.

Unfortunately, humanity is increasingly neglecting this instinctual preference or need. In 1847, Emerson lamented that "[w]e do not know an edible root in the woods. We cannot tell our course by the stars, nor the hour of the day by the sun" (p. 249). In

A.J. Howell (✉) • H.-A. Passmore
Department of Psychology, Grant MacEwan University,
Edmonton, AB, Canada
e-mail: HowellA@macewan.ca

C.L.M. Keyes (ed.), *Mental Well-Being: International Contributions to the Study of Positive Mental Health*, DOI 10.1007/978-94-007-5195-8_11,

2013, some 160-odd years later, our disengagement from nature is even more pronounced, widespread, and lamentable. The World Health Organization (WHO) announced in 2009 that more than half of the world's population now lives in an urban, rather than rural, environment; WHO projects this will increase to 65% by 2030 (WHO, 2011). In Canada, for example, the 50% urbanization mark was passed in 1941, and today, more than 80% of Canadians live in urban areas (Human Resources and Skills Development Canada 2007). On average, Canadians spend almost 90% of their time indoors (Environment Canada 2005), and a Kaiser Family Foundation study (2010) reported that the average child (aged 8–18) in the United States spends over 7 h a day plugged into some form of entertainment media. Both time-criterion and nature-knowledge-criterion studies show that nature-based recreation is on the decline in many countries (Charles and Louv 2009; Pergams and Zaradic 2008). Terms such as *nature deficit disorder* (Louv 2005) and *nature starvation* (Royal Society for the Protection of Birds 2010) have been coined to reflect our increasing disconnection from nature. In a recent survey of 1,000 United Kingdom citizens, only 55% of those over the age of 35, and 37% of those under the age of 35, reported feeling "connected to the natural world" (Royal Society for the Protection of Birds 2010).

But, does this epoch of industrialization really matter? Are we, both individually and as a species, poorer because of this protracted divorce from nature? Evidence is mounting that answers these questions with a resounding "yes." Nature affiliation and exposure to elements of the natural environment clearly, and significantly, impact our physical health and overall well-being in a positive manner.

> We need the tonic of wildness. (Thoreau 1854/1989, p. 339)

In the last decade alone, several lines of inquiry have explored the relationship between physical health and engagement with, or proximity to, elements of the natural world. For example, Pretty (as cited in Mind 2007) found that *green exercise*—exercising while viewing photographs or pictures of nature—reduced blood pressure to a greater degree than did exercising in the absence of such photos or in the presence of less green rural or urban photos.

Takano et al. (2002) showed that longevity was greater among senior citizens living in areas with walkable green spaces. Five year survival rates for 3,144 Tokyo seniors, born in 1903, 1908, 1913, or 1918, were analyzed. Variables such as age, sex, marital status, socioeconomic status, and baseline physical ability were controlled. Having walkable green streets and spaces near the seniors' residences showed significant predictive value for elderly survival over the 5 years of the study. It appears that character Carrie Watts (played by actress Geraldine Page), in *The Trip to Bountiful,* justly proclaimed, "I bet I can live to a hundred if only I can get outdoors again."

Historical data concerning over 10,000 people in Holland was analyzed by de Vries et al. (2003) to explore the relationship between green space and health. Respondent information was used only if the degree of urbanism in their neighborhood had remained constant over the time period that the data had been originally collected and if respondents had lived in their current location for over 12 months. These two exclusion criteria left 10,197 respondents from 1,155 different neighborhoods. Three global health indicators were used: number of symptoms experienced in the past 2 weeks, perceived general health rated on a 5-point scale, and the Dutch version of Goldberg's 1972 Global Health Questionnaire. Several demographic and socioeconomic variables were controlled, as was level of urbanism. A strong relationship between health and greenness of environment was shown; people living in a greener environment, regardless of level of urbanism, reported fewer physical symptoms and greater perceived general health. Of particular note, de Vries et al. found that "assuming a causal relation between greenspace [*sic*] and health, 10% more greenspace [*sic*] in the living environment leads to a decrease in the number of symptoms that is comparable with a decrease in age by 5 years" (p. 7). A subsequent study conducted by Maas et al. (2006) involved the review of records for 250,782 Dutch citizens being treated by 104 general practitioners; the relationship between health and green space was confirmed. Maas et al. reported that "health differences in residents of urban and rural municipalities are to a large extent explained by the amount of green space" in the individuals' direct living environment (p. 591). Moreover, the relation between green space and health was found to be stronger for lower socioeconomic groups.

Similar findings emerged in a recent study by Mitchell and Popham (2008), which examined socioeconomic factors in relation to health inequalities and access to green space. In this study, mortality records for 366,348 individuals of the population of England at younger than retirement age were classified into groups based on income deprivation and exposure to green space. (Exposure to green space was calculated using England's generalized land use database.) Based on the analyses of these data, Mitchell and Popham reported that "[p]opulations that are exposed to the greenest environments also have lowest levels of health inequality related to income deprivation" (p. 1655).

> There was a great joy—to be out in the air—for I had not been outside in almost a month. [...] Some part of me came alive [...] which had been starved, and died, perhaps without my knowing it (Sacks, as quoted in Frumkin 2001, p. 236).

A sizeable body of accumulated research corroborates neurologist Oliver Sacks' eloquent description of nature's restorative effect on our well-being. Ulrich (1993), whose own work is seminal in this area, provided a summary of the proposed theoretical platform for the restorative capacity of our biophilic responses. Maller et al. (2005) provided a summary of substantiating research findings, including stress reduction after urban park or wilderness excursions; reduction in feelings of anger and aggression after viewing color photographs of nature scenes, as well as subsequent to viewing urban scenes with salient natural elements such as trees and other vegetation; and decreased postoperative anxiety among patients exposed to nature pictures depicting an open water view.

The Kaplans' influential work (Kaplan 1993, 2001, 1995; Kaplan and Kaplan 1989), based on attention restoration theory (ART), has linked exposure to nature with restoration of stress and attentional fatigue, resulting in improved cognitive functioning and well-being. This body of work has provided additional empirical support for nature's restorative effect. For example, office workers with a window view encompassing natural elements reported higher job satisfaction and fewer physical ailments than did office workers with a window view of urban scenes lacking natural elements (Kaplan 1993). Other researchers have also reported a positive effect on individuals' cognitive functioning when tasks are performed in rooms with windows affording views of nature (see Chalquist 2009). Ulrich (as cited in Chalquist 2009) found that the introduction of flowers and plants into a workplace increased cognitive functioning, resulting in a reported "15% rise in innovative ideas and more creative, flexible problem-solving than that of the control group without greenery nearby" (p. 2).

Professionals in a variety of disciplines are beginning to investigate ways of utilizing these research findings by building exposure to nature into components of treatment plans for an array of diagnoses. For example, building on the Kaplan's work with ART and exposure to nature, Taylor et al. (2001) explored the benefits of "greening" play areas as part of a treatment plan for children diagnosed with attention deficit disorder (ADD) or attention deficit/hyperactivity disorder (ADHD). In this study consisting of 96 parents of children aged 7–12 years diagnosed with ADD/ADHD, contact with nature was systematically related to a decrease in the children's attention deficit symptoms—"the 'greener' a child's play area, the less severe his or her attention deficit symptoms" (p. 54). Kuo and Taylor (2004) replicated these findings in a national study of 452 parents/guardians of children aged 5–18 years who had been diagnosed with ADHD. Regardless of age, gender, income, community type, and geographic region, findings were consistent: "green outdoor activities reduced [ADD/ADHD] symptoms significantly more than did activities conducted in other settings, even when activities were matched across settings" (p. 1580).

Therapeutic gardening, formalized as horticulture therapy, is used in a number of treatment settings, including community based programs, geriatric programs, prisons, developmental disabilities programs, and special education (Mattson, as cited in Frumkin 2001). One such setting is the healing garden at the Swedish University of Agricultural Sciences' Alnarp campus (Grahn et al. 2007; Stigsdotter and Grahn 2003), designed specifically for use in a treatment program for individuals who have been unable to work or study for over 2 years due to "burnout" or depression. The treatment program runs 8 weeks, during which time patients interact with the therapeutic team (consisting of a horticultural therapist, a landscape architect, an occupational therapist, a physical therapist, a physician, and a psychotherapist) while working and spending time in the garden 3 h and 30 min a day, 4 days a week.

In his biophilia hypothesis, Wilson (1984) also suggested that we have an innate urge to affiliate with other forms of life; indeed, the subtitle of *Biophilia* is *The Human Bond with Other Species*. This bond between humans and animals is recognized by therapists and counselors in the emerging field of Animal-Assisted Therapy (AAT), wherein animals or pets are an integral part of the therapy program and help to engage the client in the therapeutic process (Fine, as cited in Wesley et al. 2009; Walsh 2009). Several studies have demonstrated that AAT enhances both the therapeutic relationship and positive therapy outcomes when used with diverse populations in a variety of therapy settings, such as psychiatric inpatients, substance abuse populations in residential group therapy, and couples and family therapy (Hooker et al. 2002; Marr et al. 2000; Walsh 2009; Wesley et al. 2009).

A few counseling psychologists, most notably George Burns (1998, 2009) and Ronen Berger (Berger and McLeod 2006), are incorporating elements of nature into their therapy work with clients who are struggling with issues involving relationship difficulties, chronic pain, autism, and depression.

> [As] psychologists we have heard but little about gardens, about foliage, about forests and farmland. ... Perhaps this resource for enhancing health, happiness, and wholeness has been neglected long enough. (Kaplan and Kaplan 1989, p. 189)

Most of the research thus far presented has focused on the reduction of dysfunction—be it stress, anxiety, anger, depression, substance abuse, or inattention. Mental health, however, is more than the absence of mental illness (Keyes 2005); therefore, we now expand our focus to look at not just the restorative, but also the additive, effects of nature. In line with this, nature affiliation has recently emerged as an interest within positive psychology. For example, in their classification of character strengths, Park et al. (2006) describe *appreciating beauty and excellence* as being related to nature involvement; Keltner and Haidt (2003, see also Shiota et al. 2007) include nature among the most common elicitors of the experience of awe; in their introduction to positive psychology, Gable and Haidt (2005) referred to *exposure to green spaces* (p. 104) as a potential means of boosting well-being; and Fredrickson (2009) lists *find nearby nature* as Tool 6 in her tool kit of proven strategies to increase one's level of positivity (p. 177). Nonetheless, the role of nature affiliation in positive functioning is often overlooked (Herzog and Strevey 2008). We next examine evidence for such a role.

Measures of Nature Affiliation

Nature affiliation has been viewed as a *trait*, that is, as a stable disposition capturing important differences between persons. This trait has been defined as "individuals' experiential sense of oneness with the natural world" (Mayer and Frantz 2004, p. 504). Nature affiliation has also been characterized as "dynamic, changing from day to day and moment to moment as a function of experiences with nature" (Weinstein et al. 2009, p. 1316) and can thus be conceptualized as a *state*. The recent development of reliable and valid measures of both trait and state conceptualizations of nature affiliation has significantly aided research on nature affiliation and positive indices of well-being.

The 14-item Connectedness to Nature Scale, developed by Mayer and Frantz (2004), assesses nature affiliation as a relatively stable disposition or trait. Items (e.g., "I often feel a sense of oneness with the natural world around me"; "Like a tree can be part of a forest, I feel embedded within the broader natural world") assess a sense of oneness with the natural world and are rated on 5-point scales with endpoints 1 = *strongly disagree* and 5 = *strongly agree*. Total scores are calculated by summing across items after reverse-scoring oppositely worded items; higher scores denote greater nature affiliation. Mayer and Frantz reported a coefficient α of 0.84 and demonstrated that factor analysis consistently yielded a one-factor solution. Mayer and Frantz validated their measure in a series of five studies with both community members and university students by establishing a nomological web of positive and negative correlates (e.g., time spent outdoors, degree of environmental concern, endorsement of consumerism, and other explicit and implicit measures of nature connectedness). Scores on the scale are not related to social desirability, and no gender difference has emerged. The entire scale is included in the appendix of the article by Mayer and Frantz.

Recently, Mayer et al. (2009) created a 13-item version of the Connectedness to Nature Scale in order to assess the acute state of nature affiliation, which has proven to have good internal stability (coefficient α=0.91). Items (e.g., "Right now I'm feeling a sense of oneness with the natural world around me"; "At the moment, I'm feeling that the natural world is a community to which I belong") are rated on a 7-point scale with endpoints 1 (*strongly disagree*) and 7 (*strongly agree*). The state version was validated among three samples of undergraduate psychology students by evidencing positive associations with environmental self-awareness, private self-awareness, ability to reflect, and attentional capacity; and a negative association with public self-awareness. The state version of the Connectedness to Nature Scale is available in the article by Mayer et al. (2009).

The Nature Relatedness Scale is a 21-item scale developed by Nisbet et al. (2009), in order to assess individual differences in people's "appreciation for and understanding of our interconnectedness with all other living things on the earth" (p. 4). Items (e.g., "I enjoy digging in the earth and getting dirt on my hands"; "I don't often go out in nature") are rated on a scale with endpoints 1=*disagree strongly* and 5=*agree strongly*. While factor analysis has suggested a 3-factor structure (i.e., internalized identification with nature, nature-related worldview, and familiarity with the natural world), an overall score is calculated by summing across all items, with higher scores denoting greater nature relatedness. The scale has good internal stability (coefficient α of 0.87) and good test-retest stability (0.85). The scale was validated by Nisbet et al. with undergraduate psychology students against related measures (e.g., ecology scales) and behaviors (e.g., buying organic food, choosing fair trade products, owning a pet, adopting vegetarianism, belonging to an environmental organization, participating in nature activities). Scores correlate positively with measures of extraversion, agreeableness, conscientiousness, and openness, as well as with measures of humanitarianism, love of animals, and considering future consequences of behavior. Among public and private sector executives, scores were shown to correlate positively with experience-sampling measures of time spent outdoors and in nature. This scale has been made available to researchers through contact with the scale developers.

Leary et al. (2008) devised a 16-item Allo-Inclusive Identity Scale, adopted from Aron et al.'s (1992) Inclusion of Other in the Self Scale (see also Schultz 2001, for a briefer such adoption). Eight items address the extent to which nature is incorporated into one's identity, and eight items address the extent to which other people are incorporated into one's identity (the latter scale is not discussed further here).

Items (e.g., "The connection between you and the Earth"; "The connection between you and a tree") are rated by choosing one of seven diagrams depicting increasing degrees of overlap between a circle labeled *you* and one labeled *other*. Leary et al. reported a coefficient $\alpha > 0.75$ for the Nature subscale and generated preliminary evidence of the subscale's validity (e.g., significant correlations with kindness, spirituality, and ecological concern; independence from socially desirable responding). The Allo-Inclusive Identity Scale is available within Leary et al.'s chapter.

Clayton (2003) described the content and validation of the Environmental Identity Scale, devised to assess the incorporation of the natural environment into one's identity. This scale is composed of 24 items, such as "I really enjoy camping and hiking outdoors" and "Living near wildlife is important to me; I would not want to live in a city all the time." Clayton established the internal reliability of the scale (coefficient $\alpha > 0.90$ across three studies) and showed that scores on the scale correlate positively with proenvironmental behaviors and choices and with measures of ecocentrism and the value of *universalism*. Scale items appear in the appendix of Clayton's chapter.

Finally, Diessner et al. (2008) constructed the Engagement with Beauty Scale, which is composed of a 4-item Natural Beauty subscale in addition to Moral Beauty and Artistic Beauty subscales (the latter two subscales are not discussed further here). Items (e.g., "I notice beauty in one or more aspects of nature"; "When perceiving beauty in nature I feel changes in my body, such as a lump in my throat, an expansion in my chest, faster heart beat, or other bodily responses") are rated on a 5-point scale with endpoints 1 (*very unlike me*) to 7 (*very much like me*). As employed with a sample of undergraduate students, the subscale has adequate internal reliability ($\alpha = 0.80$) and test-retest reliability ($r = 0.79$) and is inversely associated with materialistic values while directly related to both spiritual transcendence and gratitude (Diessner et al.). Items comprising the Natural Beauty subscale are presented in the appendix of Diessner et al.'s article.

Nature Affiliation and Well-Being

> The pursuit of 'the good life' is through our broadest valuational experience of nature. (Kellert 1993, p. 60)

Commensurate with the development of reliable and valid measures of nature affiliation, the last decade has seen an increase in both correlational and experimental research linking nature affiliation with well-being. The correlational approach to examining nature involvement and well-being assesses the association between individual differences in nature affiliation and aspects of well-being (e.g., life satisfaction; positive affect; psychological, emotional, and social well-being.) A significant correlation between trait nature affiliation and life satisfaction was demonstrated in a study by Mayer and Frantz (2004) aimed at validating their dispositional Connectedness to Nature Scale. Diessner et al.'s (2008) Natural Beauty subscale of the Engagement with Beauty Scale was shown to correlate, among undergraduate students, with a measure of life satisfaction. However, Leary et al. (2008) did not find that life satisfaction correlated significantly with scores on the Allo-Inclusive Identity—Nature scale.

State (but not trait) nature affiliation was significantly associated with positive affect in three studies conducted by Mayer et al. (2009); in the second of these studies, state nature affiliation was also significantly inversely associated with negative affect. In one of their two studies, Nisbet et al. (2009) demonstrated a positive correlation between Nature Relatedness scores and scores on an extraversion measure (which includes a tendency toward positive affect).

The majority of correlational studies examining individual differences in nature affiliation and well-being have focused upon positive affect and life satisfaction. These studies, as presented above, have yielded mixed results. This mixed pattern of findings may be understandable in terms of the differences drawn by some theorists concerning hedonic versus eudaimonic aspects of well-being (Kashdan et al. 2008; Keyes and Annas 2009; Waterman 2008). Hedonic well-being refers to attaining pleasure or feeling well and is measured with indices of life satisfaction and positive affect. Eudaimonic well-being refers to functioning well in either the private or public domain (Keyes and Annas 2009). Eudaimonia is concerned with how one lives one's life and thus focuses on concepts such as meaning, growth, and social relatedness; it is measured, in part, with indices of psychological and social well-being (Keyes and Annas 2009). It may be that aspects of well-being beyond hedonic positive affect and life satisfaction are most associated with nature affiliation. It is also possible that nature affiliation relates to some aspects of hedonic functioning (e.g., awe and vitality) more than others.

Howell et al. (2011) conducted two studies examining associations among various measures of nature affiliation and Keyes' (2005) comprehensive measure of well-being, which assesses emotional well-being via ratings of positive affect and ratings of life satisfaction (e.g., Diener et al. 1999); psychological well-being via ratings of self-acceptance, positive relations with others, personal growth, purpose in life, environmental mastery and autonomy (Ryff 1989); and social well-being via ratings of social acceptance, social actualization, social contribution, social coherence, and social integration (Keyes 1998). In a first study with Canadian undergraduate psychology students, correlations between the Connectedness to Nature Scale and both psychological and social well-being were significant (albeit small in magnitude), whereas no relationship emerged with emotional well-being. In a second study with Canadian undergraduate psychology students, all three forms of well-being were significantly associated with three measures of nature affiliation: the Connectedness to Nature Scale, the Nature Relatedness Scale, and the Allo-Inclusive Identity—Nature scale.

Additional findings have emerged for the relationship between nature affiliation and eudaimonic aspects of well-being, such as personal growth, engagement, and meaning. Herzog and Strevey (2008) measured undergraduate students' self-reported degree of contact with nature and correlated it with numerous indices of well-being. They showed that contact with nature was associated with positive affect and with the personal growth subscale of Ryff's (1989) psychological well-being scales. In research expanding on their previous work, Nisbet et al. (2011) had undergraduate students (study 1) and government and business executives (study 2) complete the Nature Relatedness Scale, as well as measures of positive affect, life satisfaction, and psychological well-being. Nature relatedness was not significantly associated with life satisfaction, but was significantly associated with positive affect, autonomy, personal growth, and purpose in life. And in research conducted by Peterson et al. (2007), engagement and meaning aspects of well-being were reliable correlates of the character strength of appreciating beauty.

Famed naturalist John Muir (1901) encouraged us to "[c]limb the mountains and get their good tidings. Nature's peace will flow into you as sunshine flows into trees. The winds will blow their own freshness into you, and the storms their energy…" (p. 56). Recent research provides empirical support for Muir's notion that relating to nature is associated with greater feelings of vitality. Ryan et al. (2010) conducted (in addition to three experiments described below) two correlational studies examining associations between outdoor activity and subjective vitality. In study 4, undergraduate students completed a diary study in which they logged, on a daily basis, their level of vitality; they also recorded whether they spent more than 20 min outside, whether they exercised for more than 20 min, and whether they engaged in social interaction for more than 20 min. Participants were also paged at random times to record whether or not the activity they were engaged in took place outside, took place in a natural or artificial setting, involved social activity, or involved physical activity. Regardless of the influence of exercise and social activity, results showed that for diary measures, greater vitality was associated with spending more than 20 min outdoors. Similarly, paging measures revealed that, controlling for social, physical, and outdoor activity, behaviors involving nature predicted greater vitality. In study 5, undergraduate students completed a 4-day experience-sampling procedure in which they were paged randomly six times per day and recorded the number of people they were interacting with, the extent of their physical activity, whether they were indoors or outdoors, the presence of natural and non-natural environmental elements, and their subjective vitality. As in study 4, results showed that participants experienced greater vitality if they were exposed to nature and that simply being outdoors was not predictive of vitality if this did not involve contact with nature.

It appears that the cognitive aspect of relating to nature also has a vitalizing effect. In study 3 by Nisbet et al. (2011), students enrolled in a university course related to the environment were contrasted with students enrolled in non-environment-related courses. Results revealed that students in classes pertaining to the environment reported higher levels of vitality than did students in other courses. This higher level of vitality was accounted for by students maintaining a stronger sense of connectedness to nature (compared to other students) during a time period of stressful school exams and weather that was less amenable to outdoor activity.

Overall, correlational studies suggest reliable relationships between nature affiliation and eudaimonic aspects of well-being; however, vitality may be a specific aspect of emotional well-being that also correlates with nature affiliation. As we explore further on, another aspect of emotional well-being, awe, also appears to correlate with nature affiliation.

The experimental approach to studying associations between nature affiliation and well-being involves manipulating exposure to nature (e.g., via nature video clips or slides, plant-filled rooms, visualization involving nature settings, virtual experiences of nature, and, of course, actual experiences in real nature settings) and examining the resulting impact on indices of well-being. In addition to examining direct effects on well-being, mediator variables are also often examined and identified. A mediator variable helps to clarify the relationship between a manipulated or predictor variable and an outcome variable. For example, in study 3 by Nisbet et al. (2011) described above, environmental courses (predictor variable) led to an increased sense of nature relatedness (mediator), which resulted in higher levels of vitality (outcome variable). Therefore, increased nature relatedness mediated the relationship between environmental education and higher levels of vitality.

In recent years, several experimental studies have explored nature's effect on people's well-being. Mayer et al. (2009) conducted three experiments in which they manipulated participants' immersion in nature and then had the participants complete scales of positive and negative affect along with the state version of the Connectedness to Nature Scale. In study 1, psychology undergraduate students were randomly assigned to spend 15 min in either a nature preserve or in an urban setting. In study 2, undergraduate psychology students were randomly assigned to spend 10 min in a nature setting or to watch a 10-min video clip of either the same setting experienced by those in the first group or a 10-min video clip of an urban setting. In study 3, undergraduate psychology students were randomly assigned to either a nature walk or to watch a video clip of the same walk. In all three of these studies, the nature condition had no effect on negative affect, but participants' positive affect was boosted compared to those in the control conditions. Moreover, in all three of these studies, state nature affiliation was shown to mediate the effect of nature immersion on well-being: immersion in nature influenced positive affect via its effects on state nature affiliation.

Berman et al. (2008) randomly assigned undergraduate students to spend 50 min walking in either a park or a downtown, urban setting, before and after which they completed (among other measures) a self-report of positive affect. Mood was shown to increase for participants in the nature-walk condition but not for those in the urban-walk condition. This boosting of positive affect following immersion in nature held true in an experiment conducted by Valtchanov et al. (2010), in which undergraduate psychology students were randomly assigned to either a virtual experience of nature or to a virtual experience of abstract paintings immediately after a stress-induction experience. (The virtual experience of nature was an interactive computer-generated forest, of which its 1,600 m^2 could be explored using a head-mounted display and a wireless mouse. The experience was enhanced with somatosensory stimulation via a rumble platform which shook with each "step" a participant took and olfactory stimulation via a forest-scented air freshener.) Positive affect and skin conductance (among other measures) were assessed prior to and following the experience. Results showed that the computer-generated nature immersion significantly reduced participants' skin conductance and elevated their positive affect relative to participants in the control condition. Similar findings emerged in a replication of this research by Valtchanov and Ellard (2010).

Participants' levels of a variety of positive emotions were boosted in Saraglou et al. (2008) experiment that involved exposing psychology undergraduate students to film clips of varying subject matter and emotional content. Students who had viewed nature-oriented clips (e.g., childbirth, panoramic views of natural landscapes) reported higher levels of ecstasy, respect, and wonder compared to students who had viewed clips that were humorous or neutral in content. In a quasi-experiment conducted by Han (2009), Taiwanese children whose classroom was beautified with several plants were compared to a second group of children whose classroom had not been modified with the addition of plants. Although no difference between these two groups of children emerged on a specific measure of well-being, after two and a half months, the children in the "plant" classroom reported greater feelings of preference, comfort, and friendliness in relation to their classroom setting.

It has been shown that exposure to nature can also increase one's endorsement of intrinsic goals such as closeness and community (which are associated with greater well-being), decrease one's endorsement of extrinsic goals such as fame and fortune (the pursuit of which are associated with lower well-being), and cause an increase in generous behavior toward others. Weinstein et al. (2009) evidenced these beneficial effects in a series of four experiments. In studies 1 and 2, adults were randomly assigned to look at a series of four slides (for 2 min each) depicting either nature scenes or manufactured environments while following instructions to encourage immersion in the materials. A measure of intrinsic versus extrinsic aspirations was completed both before viewing the slides and after. In study 3, adult participants randomly assigned to view either nature or non-nature slides completed self-report measures of intrinsic and extrinsic aspirations, then engaged in a behavioral decision task in which their distribution of funds could be coded as reflecting an intrinsic aspiration (valuing another person) or an extrinsic aspiration (valuing money). In study 4, students were exposed to a 5-min period of relaxation in either a plant-laden or plant-free laboratory prior to completing self-report and behavioral measures of intrinsic and extrinsic aspirations. In all four studies, participants in the nature conditions endorsed more intrinsic and less extrinsic values, and these well-being effects on goal aspirations were mediated by state Connectedness to Nature scores. In study 1, results showed that degree of immersion in the materials interacted with the conditions in predicting change in aspirations, such that those who were exposed to nature slides and who experienced high immersion in the materials reported higher intrinsic aspirations and lower extrinsic aspirations than those in the non-nature conditions. In both studies 3 and 4, individuals immersed in nature behaved more generously toward others relative to individuals not immersed in the nature conditions. Indeed, Thomas Fuller's assertion in 1732 that "he that plants trees loves others beside himself" (p. 89) appears to hold true even today and even with less active involvement in nature.

In conjunction with their correlational research (described previously in this chapter), Ryan et al. (2010) conducted a series of three experiments examining the impact of experiences in nature on subjective vitality. In study 1, undergraduate students imagined themselves in situations depicted in a subset of 8 of 64 total vignettes that varied randomly along three independent dimensions: physical activity versus no physical activity, social activity versus solitary activity, and indoor activity versus outdoor activity. For each vignette, participants rated the extent to which vitality was experienced. Results showed that vitality was impacted by all three of the dimensions varied in the vignettes—higher vitality was felt in relation to vignettes involving physical activity, the outdoors, and the presence of others. Importantly, these findings suggest that outdoor activity singly is related to vitality. In study 2, undergraduate students were randomly assigned to walk for 15 min either indoors or outdoors. Measures of vitality taken before and immediately after the walk revealed that vitality increased following the outdoors walk but not following the indoors walk. And in study 3, undergraduate students completed the measure of vitality before and after imagining themselves in either an outdoor natural setting or an outdoor manufactured environment. Results showed that vitality increased for those students exposed to imagined natural scenes but decreased for those exposed to imagined scenes of manufactured settings.

As demonstrated by these experimental research findings, nature affiliation and exposure to elements of the natural world affects our well-being in several ways: by boosting our positive affect; by eliciting feelings of ecstasy, respect, and wonder; by fostering feelings of comfort and friendliness; by heightening our intrinsic aspirations and generosity; and by increasing our vitality. An overall pattern is evident in both the correlational and experimental research: exposure to nature is, quite simply, good for us.

Expanded Relationships

> We may achieve our most fulfilling and enriching humanity by celebrating our secular as well as spiritual bonds with other life and creation. (Kellert 2002, p. 50)

Given that relationships between nature affiliation and well-being have begun to be established, the natural next step for research is to expand the study of mediators and moderators of this relationship.

It is possible that nature affiliation and well-being are mediated by meaning and/or purpose in life. Historical and literary figures have often credited nature with providing a sense of cohesiveness, meaning, and purpose to their lives. Many of Admiral Bird's diary entries from his winter 1934 Antarctic expedition speak to how the power of this natural environment awakened a sense of purpose in his life: "Here were imponderable processes and forces of the cosmos, harmonious and soundless. […] It was enough to catch that rhythm, momentarily to be myself a part of it. […] The conviction came that […] there must be a purpose in the whole and that man was part of that whole and not an accidental off-shoot" (as cited in Storr 1988, p. 36). Thomas Merton reflected that "[o]ne has to be alone, under the sky, before everything falls into place and one finds his own place in the midst of it all.

We have to have the humility to realize ourselves as part of nature" (1968/1989, p. 294). And Kalnin (2008) wrote that "there are times when the beauty and tranquility of places allow us to see the world and our part in it from a completely different perspective" (p. 15).

Scientists, philosophers, therapists, and researchers have echoed, and have provided empirical support for, these sentiments. For example, Vernon (2008) proposed that "there are ways of living in the world that make more sense than others; there are patterns to be discerned in nature that express deep order: that it is not just facts that count but values" (p. 31). Berger and McLeod (2006) advised that the use of nature analogies and embedding clients' experiences "in a larger natural story of life" can help clients bestow and extract meaning to guide them through change (p. 91). Kaplan and Kaplan (1989) discuss how the deepest instances of nature affiliation elicit "reflections on one's life, on one's priorities and possibilities, on one's actions and one's goals" (p. 197). As described previously, Peterson et al. (2007) showed that *appreciating beauty and excellence* was associated with a greater sense of meaning, and Nisbet et al. (2011) showed that purpose in life was a correlate of nature affiliation. It may be that those who are highly nature affiliated derive a sense of meaningful existence and/or purpose in life from their closeness with nature, and that this, in turn, boosts well-being. This parallels recent research in another domain, religiosity, which has shown that purpose in life mediates the association between religious beliefs and well-being (Byron and Miller-Perrin 2009; Steger and Frazier 2005).

> To be directly in touch with cranes, grebes, wolves, cougars, and other fauna and flora within their natural habitats is to be directly in touch with historically evolved reality and nature and human origins—an ultimate spiritual or religious experience, laced with deep emotional and aesthetic valences, including a sense of tragedy and loss (Donnelley 2002, p. 169).

Norenzayan and Shariff (2007) found that individuals primed with concepts of God behaved in a more prosocial way (i.e., allocating more money to strangers in an anonymous economic game) than individuals in the control condition. This parallels Weinstein et al.'s (2009) findings described previously that individuals immersed in nature behaved more generously than did their control counterparts. Tendencies toward, and concepts of, religiosity, spirituality, and nature affiliation are commonly intertwined. Indeed, validated measures of spirituality commonly include items relating to nature. Examples include Gomez and Fisher's (2003) Spiritual Well-Being Questionnaire (e.g., items pertaining to "developing connection with nature" and "developing oneness with nature"), Underwood and Teresi's (2002) Daily Spiritual Experience Scale (e.g., "I am spiritually touched by the beauty of creation"), and Delaney's (2005) Spirituality Scale (e.g., "I believe that nature should be respected").

This intertwining of spirituality and nature appears to be true even for those individuals who eschew a belief system involving a deity, such as architect Frank Lloyd Wright, who once quipped that he believed in God, just that he spelled it "nature," or Vincent Van Gogh who wrote that he turned to painting the stars when he was in need of religion. Caldwell-Harris et al. (2008) found that atheists agreed with statements which measured aspects of spirituality construed as "respect for nature" to the same extent as did Catholics and Buddhists. Furthermore, approximately one-third of the atheists endorsed the term *spirituality* in relation to an appreciation of nature, and nature was the most frequently cited source of wonderment. Douglas Todd (2008), asserting that "spirituality and nature are inextricably linked in the public's mind," noted that "many of those who [...] attend religious institutions [...] take frequent breaks from the pews to venture out into the great outdoors" (p. 19). "Thus biophilia may be difficult to tease apart from what some people call a relationship with 'spirit' or 'God'" (Soulé 1993, p. 444).

In the Saraglou et al. (2008) research described previously, spirituality was also assessed as a function of nature immersion. Specifically, in a second experiment with psychology undergraduate students randomly assigned to watch a video clip of either childbirth, nature, humor, or one of neutral content, those in the childbirth and nature conditions scored higher on a measure of spirituality than did those in the remaining two conditions. In a qualitative study of participants' perceptions of a wilderness experience (Fox, as cited in Heintzman 2003), "nature inspired spiritual experiences that were connected to self and nature, wonderment, awe, and natural beauty" (p. 29). This relationship between nature and spirituality has also emerged in other research areas. In Shiota et al.'s (2007) research on awe, participants were asked to think of either a recent time when they were in a natural setting they felt was beautiful (nature condition) or a recent time when they felt pride (accomplishment condition). Participants in the nature condition, as compared to the accomplishment condition, gave higher ratings to statements such as "I felt the presence of something greater than myself." Additionally, Diessner et al.'s (2008) research on appreciating beauty evidenced significant associations between nature affiliation and spirituality.

Future research could further examine the relationship between hope, spirituality, religiosity, nature affiliation, and well-being. The thread of hope arises from, and is interwoven with, both spirituality and nature. Robert Lifton (as cited in Scioli 2007) includes seeking salvation in spiritual beliefs and bonding with the eternal cycles of nature as ways to increase hope. Kalnin (2008) links nature, hope, and spirituality in that "[n]ature expands to embrace infinite possibilities. Ideas about spirituality do the same" (p. 15). Studies have established connections between spirituality and well-being (see Gomez and Fisher 2005), between hope and well-being (see Snyder 2002), between hope and spirituality (Vailant, as cited in Scioli 2007), and, as described in this chapter, between nature and both well-being and spirituality. However, to date, much of the scientific study on the relationship between nature and spirituality is correlational and refers to nature in the context of wilderness experiences, where solitude and escape from hectic daily life play a significant role (Heintzman 2003). For example, Brayley and Fox (as cited in Heintzman 2003) found that close to 46% of backpackers visiting one Canadian national park reported that "the opportunity to reflect on spiritual values" played an important part in their decision to spend time in the backcountry (p. 27). In the future, experimental research could test the hypothesis that exposure to nature in an everyday context (e.g., indoor plants) will increase self-reports of spirituality, religiosity, and hope, and, in turn, increase well-being.

It is also possible that the relationship between nature affiliation and well-being is mediated by the extent to which important basic psychological needs are met through contact with nature (see also Clayton 2003). Kellert (1997) speculated that involvement with nature may satisfy needs similar to those of competence, autonomy, and relatedness; these are the very needs underscored in self-determination theory (e.g., Deci and Ryan 2000). Regarding competency needs, outdoor educational and therapy programs capitalize on the unlimited opportunities nature provides for individuals to "learn to demonstrate personal competencies" through activities such as wilderness camping adventures (Newes and Bandoroff 2004, p. 9). Urban nature experiences also lend themselves to helping fulfill individuals' competency needs, through activities such as outdoor or container gardening (Hunter 2006). Competency, as a result of learning about the world in general, is readily fostered by nature experiences. For example, educator David Sobel uses local nature excursions to teach children a myriad of skills (Sobel 1998). One class trip to the local nature area involved activities such as a hike along the stream bed—this not only helped the children learn mapmaking skills and reinforced fundamental concepts of topographic maps, it also provided them with "the thrill of posing a question and working directly to find the answer." As Louv (2005) advised, when heading outdoors with children, we need to encourage them to "pay attention," rather than warn them to "be careful." Interacting with nature also contributes indirectly to fulfilling our competency needs, in that the feelings of vitality nature inspires in us spill over into other areas of our lives, prompting us to "roll up our sleeves" and tackle new projects—resulting in expanded opportunities for accomplishment.

Although "the complexity and interdependence of contemporary life often thwarts the realization of personal distinctiveness, [t]he natural world continues to afford opportunities for people to achieve feelings of autonomy and individuality" (Kellert 1997, p. 130). This view is echoed by Ridder (2005), who suggested that while many people struggle with the values imposed on them by society, and come to feel that their lifestyle is "excessively mediated by external influences rather than priorities determined by personal values, beliefs, and experience of life" (p. 7), nature is associated with spontaneity, self-organizing processes, and freedom. This *nature-inspired autonomy* (Ridder 2005, p. 1) is of symbolic significance for people, as illustrated by the portrayal of nature in literature as inspiring "downtrodden citizens to seek personal freedom" from authoritarian societies (Drew, as cited in Ridder 2005, p. 5). Experimental evidence has emerged that links the experience of nature with increased autonomy. In studies conducted by Weinstein et al. (2009) described previously, the more participants were immersed in nature contexts, the more autonomous they felt.

Regarding relatedness needs, nature affiliation and well-being may be mediated by a greater sense of social connectedness. In writings describing his mostly solitary life at Walden Pond, Thoreau (1854/1989) several times refers to this sense of social connectedness that nature provides: "the most sweet and tender, the most important and encouraging society may be found in any natural object, even for the poor misanthrope and most melancholy man"; "I enjoy the friendship of the seasons"; "I was suddenly sensible of such sweet and beneficent society in Nature [...] an infinite and unaccountable friendliness all at once like an atmosphere sustaining me" (p. 202–203). Lending scientific credence to these literary references are findings from Shiota et al.'s (2007) study that participants in the *nature* condition gave higher ratings to such statements as "I felt connected with the world around me." Robert Sommer (2003) presented a variety of evidence from several studies demonstrating how tree planting programs in urban areas can enhance social connectedness by building "local identity, turning a street of strangers into a community. [...] Trees create a canopy over residential streets, putting a 'roof' over a neighborhood, forming natural bridges that unite two sides of a street" (p. 182).

Our bonds with animals, particularly our pets, also help to fulfill our social relatedness needs. In an edited book by Podberscek et al. (2000), numerous authors explored evidence of how animals can be highly significant social companions to people of all ages in a diverse array of cultures and countries. The role that pets play in meeting individual's social relatedness needs was also examined in a study by Epley et al. (2008), in which participants selected three traits that best described their pet (or a pet they knew) subsequent to viewing a short video clip that induced feelings of either social disconnection, fear, or neutrality. Individuals in the social disconnection condition were more likely to attribute humanlike mental states or traits to pets than were individuals in the other conditions. Many people find that the companionship of nonhuman animals enriches their lives. As Epley et al. demonstrated, this natural connection may be heightened for individuals who feel socially disconnected. Heeding the words of Richard Nelson, that our isolation from the natural community has created for us a "profound and imperiling loneliness" (Nelson 1993, p. 221), further research is needed regarding the hypothesis that feeling connected to the natural world may help to fulfill individuals' relatedness needs, in addition to needs of competency and autonomy. Of particular focus could be socially marginalized individuals and those who are socially introverted.

Finally, nature affiliation and well-being may be mediated by improved physical functioning. As described earlier, there is evidence from large-scale cohort studies that exposure to green spaces is associated with many indicators of physical health (de Vries et al. 2003; Maas et al. 2006; Mitchell and Popham 2008; Takano et al. 2002). Perhaps exposure to public parks and tree-lined streets (with concomitant increases in nature affiliation) improves physical health, which, in turn, boosts mental well-being.

> Some people walk in the rain, others just get wet. (Miller n.d.)

There may also be variables (called moderators) that strengthen or weaken the relationship between nature affiliation and well-being. One such variable is the extent to which nature affiliation is shared within one's immediate social group. The relationship between nature affiliation and well-being may be stronger among those surrounded by others who value nature. For example, Sagiv and Schwartz (2000) found that psychology students value *universalism* (which includes unity with nature) to a greater degree than do business students and that well-being was higher among psychology students when their valuing of universalism exceeded their valuing of power. This well-being finding did not hold true for business students, who tended to value power over universalism.

Cultures may also differ on the degree to which they value nature involvement. Despite conceptualizations of nature affiliation being cross-culturally ubiquitous, the tendency to affiliate with nature requires cultivation (Wilson 1984); certain cultures may foster nature affiliation more than others. For example, rooted deeply in the cultures of Norway and Sweden is the concept of *friluftsliv*, a word that translates to *free-air life* meaning "a philosophical lifestyle based on experiences of the freedom in nature and spiritual connectedness with the landscape" (Gelter 2000, p. 78); *friluftsliv* stems from "the self-image of Scandinavians as nature loving people" (Sandell and Sorlin, as cited in Gelter 2000, p. 79). It is possible that it is only among those nations highly valuing nature that robust associations between nature affiliation and well-being would emerge. "Thus," as Kellert (1997) suggests, "the different aspects of biophilia are best viewed as products of 'biocultural' evolution—inborn tendencies shaped by the mediating influence of learning, culture, and experience" (p. 4).

A final potential moderator that we examine concerns mindfulness. It is possible that involvement in nature is conducive toward well-being mostly among those who are highly mindful. Mindfulness is "the tendency to be highly aware of one's internal and external experiences in the context of an accepting, nonjudgmental stance toward those experiences" (Cardaciotto et al. 2008, p. 205). Mindfulness enhances the richness and vitality of moment-to-moment experiences (Brown and Ryan 2003; see also Brown et al. 2007) and thus allows the full experience of nature to be attended to and appreciated. The enhanced sensory impact of experiences in nature fostered by mindfulness may strengthen the impact of nature on well-being. For example, Wilson (1984) wrote, in describing the state of mind of a naturalist, "He goes alone into a field or woodland and closes his mind to everything but that time and place, so that life around him presses in on all the senses and small details grow in significance" (p. 103). Attention toward, and awareness of, such detail may enrich the experience of nature, thereby enhancing well-being.

Nisbet et al. (2009) showed that openness to experience (a correlate of mindfulness; Brown and Ryan 2003) is associated with nature affiliation, Mayer et al. (2009) showed that attentional capacity (a facet of mindfulness) is related to trait nature connectedness, Herzog and Strevey (2008) showed that contact with nature predicted higher attentiveness, and Leary et al. (2008) showed that internal state awareness is related to nature affiliation. As stated by Leary et al., "Perhaps high internal state awareness is associated with greater sensitivity to one's feelings of connection, appreciation, and awe with respect to animals and nature" (p. 142). In the most direct test of the association between mindfulness and nature affiliation, Howell et al. (2011) established mindfulness as a significant correlate of nature affiliation.

Where to From Here?

> "Viewed as an amenity, nature may be readily replaced by some greater technological achievement. Viewed as an essential bond between humans and other living things, the natural environment has no substitutes" (Kaplan and Kaplan 1989, p. 203).

Anthropologist Richard Nelson (as cited in Kahn 1997) described our society as being alienated from nature due to our viewing the natural world from "a great distance of mind" (p. 13). As the rate and spread of industrialization and urbanization increases, this distance is extending from the mental to the physical, with our experiences of nature increasingly mediated by technology such as 3D-IMAX movies, virtual nature walks, and nature shows on high-definition television. Interactive technical-nature experiences are also now possible. For example, an online telegarden, developed at the University of Southern California, was active from 1995 to 2005; in its first year alone, over 9,000 people remotely accessed this live garden, planting and cultivating it (see http://www.telegarden.org/tg/ for archival videos). One can even hunt and kill live animals from one's living room by telehunting, although public outcry has caused some jurisdictions to ban this practice (Associated Press 2007). Consumer-level robotic pets are now readily available (Engber 2008).

Researchers have begun to study how these technologically mediated experiences of nature differ from experiences of direct exposure to the natural world in their effect on our health and well-being (Kahn et al. 2005, 2006; Levi and Kocher 1999; Melson et al. 2005; Valtchanov et al. 2010; Valtchanov and Ellard 2010). One recent study by Kahn et al. (2008) involved 90 participants working on four low-level stress tasks in one of three conditions: a room with a high-definition plasma screen real-time view of nature, a room with the same view of nature but through a glass window, or a windowless room. Participants' physiological reactions (e.g., heart rates) were measured and harmonized with coding of the frequency and duration with which each participant looked at either the plasma window, the glass window, or the blank wall. Results showed that while heart-rate recovery was faster in the glass window condition compared to the blank wall, there was no difference in heart-rate recovery time between the plasma window and the blank wall condition. Although participants glanced at the plasma window and the glass window the same number of times, the glass window held participants' attention for a significantly longer period of time than did the plasma window. Furthermore, no relationship was found between heart-rate recovery time and duration of viewing the plasma window; but for participants viewing the glass window, the more time a participant looked at the glass window, the faster was their heart-rate recovery time.

Findings from these studies are consistent with other similar studies (for a review, see Kahn et al. 2009) in suggesting that while virtual nature can offer us some of the benefits and enjoyments of affiliating with actual nature, there may be inherent negative consequences to increasingly replacing exposure to the live, natural world with technologically mediated experiences. Winston Churchill admonished that "[n]ature will not be admired by proxy," and Kahn et al. (2008) caution that "it is important to address the issue of whether such adaptations are not just different but impoverished from the standpoint of human functioning and flourishing, and whether such technological systems and resulting interactions are shifting the very baseline of what we can recognize as impoverishment" (p. 198).

We cannot stop the progression of urbanization or technological innovation, nor should we necessarily want to impede them. For example, Valtchanov et al. (2010; see also Valtchanov and Ellard 2010) suggest that computer-generated virtual-reality nature may assist researchers in developing methods and environments with possible therapeutic applications in scenarios where access to real nature is limited. And many of the advances in technology and urban living over the last hundred years have increased our lifespan (e.g., advanced medical diagnostics), improved communication (e.g., telephones and email), and improved the quality of life for many individuals (e.g., teleworking from home). However, "quality of life isn't measured only by what we gain, but also by what we trade it for" (Louv 2005, p. 59). We need to recognize the limitations of technology, as Kahn et al.'s (2008) and others' research demonstrates. We need, as Canadian wildlife artist and environmentalist Robert Bateman (2000) wrote, "a new definition of Progress, one that is more elegant and sophisticated, one that values our heritage, both natural and human" (p. ix).

GPI Atlantic, a Canadian research organization, is currently working on defining progress in just such a balanced and expanded way with the development of their Genuine Progress Index (GPI Atlantic 2007). GPI measures sustainability, quality of life, and well-being and is put forth as an alternative to the commonly used measure of Gross Domestic Product (GDP). Six main categories make up the GPI: living standards, population health, time use, community vitality, education quality, and environmental quality. Another similar measure to replace GDP is Gross National Happiness (GNH). GNH has been the national priority of the kingdom of Bhutan since 1972; Bhutan's GNH program includes reserving at least 60% of its lands as natural forest. GPI Atlantic shared its research and measurement tool with the government of Bhutan at an international conference in 2004 on "Operationalizing Gross National Happiness" (Kavanagh 2004). This GNH measure of progress is also receiving interest in France, the United Kingdom, and the United States; a grassroots group in Vermont has established an organization called "Gross National Happiness USA" with a mandate of raising awareness of alternative measures of progress.

What these new measures of progress have in common is the recognition that our physical health and mental well-being are impacted by the environment in which we live. As presented previously in this chapter, population-based research has evidenced a positive relationship between green space and physical health and longevity (de Vries et al. 2003; Maas et al. 2006; Mitchell and Popham 2008; Takano et al. 2002). Evidence continues to mount in this area, with the research scope of focus broadening to include various indicators of mental well-being. For example, Grahn and Stigsdotter (as cited in Mind 2007) found an "inverse relationship between proximity of open green spaces in urban areas and levels of stress" (p. 3), and Wells and Evans (as cited in Chalquist 2009) reported that "the impact of life stress [was] lower among children [living] in the midst of natural features of the landscape than among those with little nature nearby" (p. 6). The MIND Institute

(Mind 2007) has stated that "inequality of access to green space should be addressed as a human rights, social justice and discrimination issue" (p. 31). Bolstering this recommendation are not only findings (presented earlier) that the relation between green space and health is stronger for lower socioeconomic groups (Maas et al. 2006; Mitchell and Popham 2008), but also findings pertaining to the effect that green space in impoverished, inner city neighborhoods has on social interaction, crime, and individuals' mental outlook. In studies utilizing data collected at two large public housing developments in Chicago (located in some of the poorest neighborhoods in the United States), it was found the following: that there was proportionately more social activity in green spaces surrounding individual buildings than in barren spaces that surrounded some of the buildings, regardless of the location of the spaces (Sullivan et al. 2004); that the greener a building's surroundings, the fewer the crimes—both property and violent—recorded by police for that building, even when controlling for varying number of apartments in the buildings (Kuo and Sullivan 2001); and that "residents living in buildings without trees and grass reported more procrastination in facing their major issues, and assessed their issues as more severe, less soluble, and more long-standing than did their counterparts living in greener surroundings" (Kuo 2001, p. 5).

In light of these findings, Sullivan et al. (2004) recommend that "guidelines for developing and maintaining green neighborhood spaces" be included in public housing development designs and that government agencies responsible for public housing "actively promote neighborhood greening efforts" (p. 697). Psychologists Diener et al. (2008) have urged business leaders and government officials to develop national well-being accounts that will "help determine where, what type, and how much nature is necessary for optimal functioning of society" (p. 47). These national well-being accounts could be published as a set of guidelines for *Daily Nature Exposure*, analogous to publications such as *Canada's Food Guide* (a guideline for daily food consumption based on recommended daily allowances of vitamins and minerals.) Evidence continues to mount that "[r]egular contact with nature may be as important to our psychological and social health as the regular consumption of fruit and vegetables is to our physical health" (Kuo 2001, p. 29).

To date, research in the nature–well-being area has focused on visual stimuli comprising the natural world. Research is needed on the effects of exposure to polysensory experiences of nature, of infusing our auditory and tactile senses with the sounds and feels of nature as well as her rich sights. There may be effective mood-enhancing experiences in simple actions such as smelling the fragrance of a lilac bush, walking barefoot in the grass, or listening to the sounds of birds chirping to greet the morning. Musician Murray Schafer said that "[t]he world is as alive with sound as it is with anything, yet most of us automatically tune out much of what we hear. Focusing on sound is another excellent way to connect us with the present. Any step we take to increase our awareness brings us more in tune with the totality of creation" (as cited in Kalnin 2008, p. 134). Taking this as a starting point, future research could include combining mindfulness training with exposure to various modal experiences of nature (via touch, sound, smell, cognition) under experimentally controlled conditions, in order to examine not only the effect of each modal experience of nature on various indicators of well-being but also to assess the moderating influence of mindfulness. Of assistance in this area of research will be utilizing tools and measures such as the Sensual Awareness Inventory (as Burns 2005, suggests), modified versions of instruments developed to measure immersion in present environments (such as those that Weinstein et al. 2009, used), well-being measures, and the various nature affiliation scales presented in this chapter.

Longitudinal experimental studies are needed to assess the long-term effects of exposure to nature, as well as the effects of prolonged immersion in, or contact with, elements of the natural world. Consistent with the review of Lyubomirsky et al. (2005), affiliation with nature, promoted through greater involvement in nature, may complement other *intentional activities*, such as gratitude expression, shown to be conducive to the cultivation of well-being. "The key for long lasting changes to well-being is to engage in activities that provide small and frequent [well-being] boosts" (Mochon et al. 2008, p. 641). Taken alongside experimental evidence of the positive effects for well-being of immersion in nature, the ready availability of experiences in nature suggests that such activity, occurring frequently across large numbers of individuals, may have modest but important consequences for well-being.

To that end, we suggest that connecting with nature in a variety of ways can enrich the journey along each of the three paths to happiness proposed by Seligman (2002): the pleasant life, the engaged life, and the meaningful life. Research is needed to develop, test, and validate a detailed Nature Immersion Therapy aimed at enriching individuals' levels of well-being. The foundation for this work could be existing therapy plans built upon the numerous validated positive psychology interventions for increasing well-being (e.g., *Positive Psychotherapy* developed by Seligman et al. 2006; *Happiness 101: A How-to Guide in Positive Psychology for People who are Depressed, Languishing, or Flourishing* developed by Lambert 2009), as well resources specific to connecting to nature developed by researchers in other fields (e.g., *Nature as a Guide: Using Nature in Counseling, Therapy, and Education* developed by Nebbe 1991; *Coyote's Guide to Connecting with Nature: For Kids of All Ages and Their Mentors* developed by Young et al. 2008).

> In every walk with nature one receives far more than he seeks. (Muir 1918 p.128)

We are not born *tabula rasa*; we are a product of our evolutionary past and carry the seeds of many innate tendencies—including biophilia. We must not, for the benefit of ourselves as individuals and as a species, allow these biophilic seeds to lie fallow within us. Rather, we must nourish and cultivate this tendency in order to become complete and flourishing. There is much research yet to be done in this area of nature affiliation and well-being.

> May the sun bring you new energy by day,
> May the moon softly restore you by night,
> May the rain wash away your worries,
> May the breeze blow new strength into your being,
> May you walk gently through the world and know its beauty all the days of your life.
>
> Apache Blessing

References

Aron, A., Aron, E. N., & Smollen, D. (1992). Inclusion of other in the self scale and the structure of interpersonal closeness. *Journal of Personality and Social Psychology, 63*, 596–612.

Associated Press. (2007). *Should killing be merely a mouse click away?* Retrieved June 27, 2010, from http://www.nytimes.com/2007/03/11/sports/othersports/11hunt.htmlei=5088&en=37373e4c91554cd6&ex=1331269200&partner=rssnyt&emc=rss&pagewanted=print

Bateman, R. (2000). *Thinking like a mountain*. Toronto: Penguin.

Berger, R., & McLeod, J. (2006). Incorporating nature into therapy: A framework for practice. *Journal of Systemic Therapies, 25*, 80–94.

Berman, M. C., Jonides, J., & Kaplan, S. (2008). The cognitive benefits of interacting with nature. *Psychological Science, 19*, 1207–1212.

Brown, K. W., & Ryan, R. M. (2003). The benefits of being present: Mindfulness and its role in psychological well-being. *Journal of Personality and Social Psychology, 84*, 822–848.

Brown, K. W., Ryan, R. M., & Creswell, J. D. (2007). Mindfulness: Theoretical foundations and evidence for its salutary effects. *Psychological Inquiry, 18*, 211–237.

Burns, G. W. (1998). *Nature-guided therapy: Brief integrative strategies for health and well-being*. Philadelphia: Brunner/Mazel.

Burns, G. W. (2005). Naturally happy, naturally healthy: The role of the natural environment in well-being. In F. A. Huppert, N. Baylis, & B. Keverne (Eds.), *The science of well-being* (pp. 405–431). New York: Oxford University Press.

Burns, G. W. (2009). Can you be happy in pain? Applying positive psychology, mindfulness, and hypnosis to chronic pain management. In G. W. Burns (Ed.), *Happiness, healing, enhancement: Your casebook collection for applying positive psychology in therapy* (pp. 202–213). Hoboken: Wiley.

Buss, D. M. (2000). The evolution of happiness. *American Psychologist, 55*, 15–23.

Byron, K., & Miller-Perrin, C. (2009). The value of life purpose: Purpose as a mediator of faith and well-being. *Journal of Positive Psychology, 41*, 64–70.

Caldwell-Harris, C. L., Wilson, A., LoTempio, E., & Beit-Hallahmi, B. (2008) *Exploring the Atheist personality: Well-being, awe, and magical thinking in Atheists, Buddhists, and Christians*. Unpublished manuscript.

Cardaciotto, L., Herbert, J. D., Forman, E. M., Moitra, E., & Farrow, V. (2008). The assessment of present-moment awareness and acceptance: The Philadelphia mindfulness scale. *Assessment, 15*, 204–223.

Chalquist, C. (2009). A look at the ecotherapy research evidence. *Ecopsychology, 1*, 1–11.

Charles, C., & Louv, R. (2009, September). Children's nature deficit: What we know—and don't know. *Children & Nature Network, 2009*, 1–32.

Clayton, S. (2003). Environmental identity: A conceptual and an operational definition. In S. Clayton & S. Opotow (Eds.), *Identity and the natural environment: The psychological significance of nature* (pp. 45–66). Cambridge, MA: MIT Press.

De Vries, S., Verheij, R. A., Groenewegen, P. P., & Spreeuwenberg, P. (2003). Natural environments—healthy environments? An exploratory analysis of the relationship between greenspace and health. *Environment and Planning, 35*, 1717–1731.

Deci, E. L., & Ryan, R. M. (2000). The "what" and "why" of goal pursuits: Human needs and the self-determination of behavior. *Psychological Inquiry, 11*, 227–268.

Delaney, C. (2005). The spirituality scale: Development and psychometric testing of a holistic instrument to assess the human spiritual dimension. *Journal of Holistic Nursing, 23*, 145–167.

Diener, E., Suh, E. M., Lucas, R. E., & Smith, H. L. (1999). Subjective well-being: Three decades of progress. *Psychological Bulletin, 125*, 276–302.

Diener, E., Kesebir, P., & Lucas, R. (2008). Benefits of accounts of well-being—for societies and for psychological science. *Applied Psychology: An International Review, 57*, 37–53.

Diessner, R., Solom, R. C., Frost, N. E., Parsons, L., & Davidson, J. (2008). Engagement with beauty: Appreciating natural, artistic, and moral beauty. *The Journal of Psychology, 142*, 303–329.
Donnelley, S. (2002). Leopold's Darwin: Climbing mountains, developing land. In S. R. Kellert & T. J. Farnham (Eds.), *The good in humanity: Connecting science, religion, and spirituality with the natural world* (pp. 161–174). Washington, DC: Island Press.
Emerson, R. W. (1847). *Essays by R. W. Emerson* (Second Series). Boston: Tickner and Fields.
Engber, D. (2008, December 16). Rrrrrrobots! The search for the ideal animatronic pet. Slate. Retrieved from http://www.slate.com/id/2206604
Environment Canada. (2005). Retrieved May 13, 2010, from http://www.ec.gc.ca/cleanair-airpurIndoor_Air_Pollution-WS1280FDA8-1_En.htm
Environment Canada. (2007). Regulatory framework for air emissions. [Brochure]. Ottawa, ON: Author.
Epley, N., Akalis, S., Waytz, A., & Cacioppo, J. T. (2008). Creating social connection through inferential reproduction. *Psychological Science, 19*, 114–120.
Fredrickson, B. (2009). *Positivity*. New York: Random House.
Frumkin, H. (2001). Beyond toxicity: Human health and natural environment. *American Journal of Preventive Medicine, 20*, 234–240.
Fuller, T. (1732/2003). *Gnomologia, adagies and proverbs, wise sentences and witty sayings, ancient and modern, foreign and British*. Whitefish: Kessinger Publishing.
Gable, S. L., & Haidt, J. (2005). What (and why) is positive psychology? *Review of General Psychology, 9*, 103–110.
Gelter, H. (2000). Friluftsliv: The Scandinavian philosophy of outdoor life. *Canadian Journal of Environmental Education, 5*, 63–76.
Gomez, R., & Fisher, J. W. (2003). Domains of spiritual well-being and development and validation of the spiritual well-being questionnaire. *Personality and Individual Differences, 35*, 1975–1991.
Gomez, R., & Fisher, J. W. (2005). Item response theory analysis of the spiritual well-being questionnaire. *Personality and Individual Differences, 38*, 1107–1121.
GPI Atlantic. (2007, September 14). The Genuine Progess Index: A better set of tools. Retrived from http://gpiatlantic.org/about.htm
Grahn, P., Bengtsson, I. -L., Welen-Andersson, L., Lavesson, L., Lindfors, L., Tauchnitz, F., & Tenngart, C. (2007). Alnarp rehabilitation garden: Possible health effects from the design, from the activities and from the therapeutic team. In *Open space conference summary paper.* Retrieved June 13, 2010, from http://www.openspace.eca.ac.uk/conference2007/PDF/Summary_Paper__P_Grahn._AB_edit.W-out_trackg.pdf
Gullone, E. (2000). The biophilia hypothesis and life in the 21st century: Increasing mental health or increasing pathology. *Journal of Happiness Studies, 1*, 293–321.
Han, K. T. (2009). Influence of limitedly visible leafy indoor plans on the psychology, behavior, and health of students at a junior high school in Taiwan. *Environment and Behavior, 41*, 658–692.
Heintzman, P. (2003). The wilderness experience and spirituality: What recent research tells us. *The Journal of Physical Education, Recreation & Dance, 74*, 27–31.
Herzog, T. R., & Strevey, S. J. (2008). Contact with nature, sense of humor, and psychological well-being. *Environment and Behavior, 40*, 747–776.
Hooker, S. D., Freeman, L. H., & Stewart, P. (2002). Pet therapy research: A historical review. *Holistic Nursing Practice, 17*, 17–23.
Howell, A.J., Dopko, R., Passmore, H.-A. & Buro, K. (2011). Nature connctendess: Associations with well-being and mindfulness. *Personality and Individual Differences*, 51, 166–171
Human Resources and Skills Development Canada. (2006, March 12). Canadians in context-geographic distribution. Retrived from http://www4.hrsdc.gc.ca/.3ndic.1t.4r@-eng.jsp?iid =34
Hunter, D. (2006). *Healing children, adolescents and families nature-ly*. VISTAS 2006, American Counseling Association. Retrieved June 25, 2010, from http://counselingoutfitters.com/vistas/vistas_2006_Title.htm

Joye, Y. (2007). Architectural lessons from environmental psychology: The case of biophilic architecture. *Review of General Psychology, 11*, 305–328.
Kahn, P. H. (1997). Developmental psychology and the biophilia hypothesis: Children's affiliation with nature. *Developmental Review, 17*, 1–61.
Kahn, P.H. Jr., Friedman, B., Alexander, I.S., Freier, N.G., & Collett, S. L. (2005). The distant gardener: What conversations in the Telegarden reveal about human-telerobotic interaction. IEEE *International Workshop on Robot and Human Interactive Communication*. ROMAN 2005. DOI: 10.1109/ROMAN.2005.1513749
Kahn, P. H., Jr., Friedman, B., Perez-Granados, D. R., & Freier, N. G. (2006). Robotic pets in the lives of preschool children. *Interaction Studies, 7*, 405–436.
Kahn, P. H., Jr., Friedman, B., Gill, B., Hagman, J., Severson, R. L., Freier, N. G., Feldman, E. N., Carrere, S., & Stolyar, A. (2008). A plasma display window? The shifting baseline problem in a technologically mediated natural world. *Journal of Environmental Psychology, 28*, 192–199.
Kahn, P. H., Jr., Severson, R. L., & Ruckert, J. H. (2009). The human relation with nature and technological nature. *Current Directions in Psychological Science, 18*, 37–42.
Kaiser Family Foundation. (2010). Generation M2: Media in the lives of 8-18-year olds [Brochure]. Menlo Park, California: Author
Kalnin, J. (2008). *The spirituality of nature*. Kelowna: Northstone Wood Lake Publishing Inc.
Kaplan, R. (1993). The role of nature in the context of the workplace. *Landscape and Urban Planning, 26*, 193–201.
Kaplan, S. (1995). The restorative benefits of nature: Toward an integrative framework. *Journal of Environmental Psychology, 15*, 169–182.
Kaplan, R. (2001). The nature of the view from home: Psychological benefits. *Environment and Behavior, 33*, 507–542.
Kaplan, R., & Kaplan, S. (1989). *The experience of nature: A psychological perspective*. New York: Cambridge University Press.
Kashdan, T. B., Biswas-Diener, R., & King, L. A. (2008). Reconsidering happiness: The costs of distinguishing between hedonics and eudaimonia. *Journal of Positive Psychology, 3*, 410–422.
Kavanagh, P. (2004). *Happiness and progress: Measuring human well-being in Bhutan and Canada*. The International Development Research Centre. Retrieved June 6, 2010, from http://www.idrc.ca/en/ev-61364-201-1-DO_TOPIC.html
Kellert, S. R. (1993). The biological basis for human values of nature. In S. R. Kellert & E. O. Wilson (Eds.), *The biophilia hypothesis* (pp. 42–69). Washington, DC: Island Press.
Kellert, S. R. (1997). *Kinship to mastery: Biophilia in human evolution and development*. Washington, DC: Island Press.
Kellert, S. R. (2002). Values, ethics, and spiritual and scientific relations to nature. In S. R. Kellert & T. J. Farnham (Eds.), *The good in humanity: Connecting science, religion, and spirituality with the natural world* (pp. 49–64). Washington, DC: Island Press.
Keltner, D., & Haidt, J. (2003). Approaching awe, a moral, spiritual, and aesthetic emotion. *Cognition and Emotion, 17*, 297–314.
Keyes, C. L. M. (1998). Social well-being. *Social Psychology Quarterly, 61*, 121–140.
Keyes, C. L. M. (2005). Mental illness and/or mental health? Investigating the axioms of the complete state model of health. *Journal of Consulting and Clinical Psychology, 73*, 539–548.
Keyes, C. L. M., & Annas, J. (2009). Feeling good and functioning well: Distinctive concepts in ancient philosophy and contemporary science. *Journal of Positive Psychology, 4*, 197–201.
Kuo, F. E. (2001). Coping with poverty: Impacts of environment and attention in the inner city. *Environment and Behavior, 33*, 5–34.
Kuo, F. E., & Sullivan, W. C. (2001). Environment and crime in the inner city. Does vegetation reduce crime? *Environment and Behavior, 33*, 343–367.
Kuo, F. E., & Taylor, A. F. (2004). A potential natural treatment for attention-deficit/hyperactivity disorder: Evidence from a national study. *American Journal of Public Health, 94*, 1580–1586.
Lambert, L. (2009). *Happiness 101: A how-to guide in positive psychology for people who are depressed, languishing, or flourishing*. Bloomington: Xlibris Corporation.

Leary, M. R., Tipsord, J. M., & Tate, E. B. (2008). Allo-inclusive identity: Incorporating the social and natural worlds into one's sense of self. In H. A. Wayment & J. J. Bauer (Eds.), *Transcending self-interest: Psychological explorations of the quiet ego* (pp. 137–147). Washington, DC: APA.

Levi, D., & Kocher, S. (1999). Virtual nature: The future effects of information technology on our relationship to nature. *Environment and Behavior, 31*, 203–226.

Louv, R. (2005). *Last child in the woods: Saving our children from nature-deficit disorder*. Chapel Hill: Algonquin Books.

Lyubomirsky, S., Sheldon, K. M., & Schkade, D. (2005). Pursuing happiness: The architecture of sustainable change. *Review of General Psychology, 9*, 111–131.

Maas, J., Verheij, R. A., Groenewegen, P. P., de Vries, S., & Spreeuwenberg, P. (2006). Green space, urbanity, and health: How strong is the relation? *Journal of Epidemiology and Community Health, 60*, 587–592.

Maller, C., Townsend, M., Pryor, A., Brown, P., & St. Leger, L. (2005). Healthy nature, healthy people: 'Contact with nature' as an upstream promotion intervention for populations. *Health Promotion International, 21*, 45–54.

Marr, C. A., French, L., Thompson, D., Drum, L., Greening, G., Mormon, J., Henderson, I., & Hughes, C. W. (2000). Animal-assisted therapy in psychiatric rehabilitation. *Anthrozoos, 13*, 43–47.

Mayer, F. S., & Frantz, C. M. (2004). The connectedness to nature scale: A measure of individuals' feeling in community with nature. *Journal of Environmental Psychology, 24*, 504–515.

Mayer, F. S., Frantz, C. M., Bruehlman-Senecal, E., & Dolliver, K. (2009). Why is nature beneficial? The role of connectedness to nature. *Environment and Behavior, 41*, 607–643.

Melson, G. F., Kahn, P. H. Jr., Beck, A. M., Friedman, B., Roberts, T., & Garrett, E. (2005, 2–7 April). Robots as dogs? Children's interactions with robotic dog Aibo and a live Australian Shepherd. In *CHI, conference, Portland*. http://www.chi2005.org/

Merton, T. (1968/1989). *Conjectures of a guilty bystander*. New York: Doubleday.

Miller, R. Retrieved July 20, 2011, from http://thinkexist.com/quotation/some_people_walk_in_the_rain-others_just_get_wet/224618.html

Miller, R. (n.d). BrainyQuote.com. Retrieved Auguest 25, 2012, from http://www.brainyquote.com/quotes/r/rogermille107155.html

Mind. (2007). *Ecotherapy: The green agenda for mental health*. London: Author

Mitchell, R., & Popham, F. (2008). Effect of exposure to natural environment on health inequalities: An observational population study. *The Lancet, 372*, 1655–1660.

Mochon, D., Norton, M. I., & Ariely, D. (2008). Getting off the hedonic treadmill, one step at a time: The impact of regular religious practice and exercise on well-being. *Journal of Economic Psychology, 29*, 632–642.

Muir, J. (1901/2006). *Our national parks*. New York: Cosimo, Inc.

Muir, J. (1918). Steep trails. Boston, MA: Houghton Mifflin.

Nebbe, L. L. (1991). *Nature as a guide: Using nature in counseling, therapy, and education*. Minneapolis: Educational Media Corporation.

Nelson, R. (1993). Searching for the lost arrow: Physical and spiritual ecology in the hunter's world. In S. R. Kellert & E. O. Wilson (Eds.), *The biophilia hypothesis* (pp. 201–228). Washington, DC: Island Press.

Nesse, R. M., & Wiliams, G. C. (1996). *Evolution and healing: The new science of Darwinian medicine*. London: Phoenix.

Newes, S., & Bandoroff, S. (2004). What is adventure therapy? In S. Bandoroff & S. Newes (Eds.), *Coming of age: The evolving field of adventure therapy* (pp. 1–30). Boulder: Association for Experimental Education.

Nisbet, E. K., Zelenski, J. M., & Murphy, S. A. (2009). The nature relatedness scale: Linking individuals' connection with nature to environmental concern and behavior. *Environment and Behavior, 41*, 715–740.

Nisbet, E. K., Zelenski, J. M., & Murphy, S. A. (2011). Happiness is in our nature: Exploring nature relatedness as a contributor to subjective well-being. *Journal of Happiness Studies, 12*, 303–322.

Norenzayan, A., & Shariff, A. F. (2007). God is watching you: Priming god concepts increases prosocial behavior in an anonymous economic game. *Psychological Science, 18*, 803–809.
Park, N., Peterson, C., & Seligman, M. E. P. (2006). Character strengths in fifty-four nations and the fifty US states. *Journal of Positive Psychology, 1*, 118–129.
Pergams, O. R. W., & Zaradic, P. A. (2008). Evidence for a fundamental and pervasive shift away from nature-based recreation. *Proceedings of the National Academy of Sciences of the United States of America, 105*, 2295–3000.
Peterson, C., Ruch, W., Beermann, U., Park, N., & Seligman, M. E. P. (2007). Strengths of character, orientations to happiness, and life satisfaction. *Journal of Positive Psychology, 2*, 149–156.
Podberscek, A. L., Paul, E. S., & Serpell, J. A. (2000). *Companion animals and us: Exploring the relationships between people and pets*. Cambridge: Cambridge University Press.
Ridder, B. (2005). Reorienting environmentalism to nature-inspired-autonomy. *Griffith Journal of the Environment, 1*, 1–26.
Royal Society for the protection of Birds. (2010, January 7). 'Nature stravation' threatens the well-being of young people. Retrieved from http://www.rspb.org.uk/news/details.aspx?id=tcm:9-238307#credits
Ryan, R. M., Weinstein, N., Bernstein, J., Brown, K. W., Mistretta, L., & Gagne, M. (2010). Vitalizing effects of being outdoors and in nature. *Journal of Environmental Psychology, 30*, 159–168.
Ryff, C. D. (1989). Happiness is everything, or is it? Explorations on the meaning of psychological well-being. *Journal of Personality and Social Psychology, 57*, 1069–1081.
Sagiv, L., & Schwartz, S. H. (2000). Value priorities and subjective well-being: Direct relations and congruity effects. *European Journal of Social Psychology, 30*, 177–198.
Saraglou, V., Buxant, C., & Tilquin, J. (2008). Positive emotions as leading to religion and spirituality. *Journal of Positive Psychology, 3*, 165–173.
Schultz, P. W. (2001). The structure of environmental concern: Concern for self, other people, and the biosphere. *Journal of Environmental Psychology, 21*, 327–339.
Scioli, A. (2007). Hope and spirituality in the age of anxiety. In R. J. Estes (Ed.), *Advancing quality of life in a turbulent world* (pp. 135–152). Dordrecht: Springer.
Seligman, M. E. P. (2002). *Authentic happiness*. New York: Free Press.
Seligman, M. E. P., Rashid, T., & Parks, A. C. (2006). Positive psychotherapy. *American Psychologist, 61*, 774–788.
Shiota, M. N., Keltner, D., & Mossman, A. (2007). The nature of awe: Elicitors, appraisals, and effects on self-concept. *Cognition and Emotion, 21*, 944–963.
Snyder, C. R. (2002). Hope theory: Rainbows in the mind. *Psychological Inquiry, 13*, 249–275.
Sobel, D. (1998). Beyond ecophobia. *Yes!* Retrieved July 1, 2010, from http://www.yesmagazine.org/issues/education-for-life/803
Sommer, R. (2003). Trees and human identity. In S. Clayton & S. Opotow (Eds.), *Identity and the natural environment: The psychological significance of nature* (pp. 179–204). Cambridge, MA: MIT Press.
Soulé, M. E. (1993). Biophilia: Unanswered questions. In S. R. Kellert & E. O. Wilson (Eds.), *The biophilia hypothesis* (pp. 441–455). Washington, DC: Island Press.
Steger, M. F., & Frazier, P. (2005). Meaning in life: One link in the chain from religiousness to well-being. *Journal of Counseling Psychology, 52*, 574–582.
Stigsdotter, U. A., & Grahn, P. (2003). Experiencing a garden: A healing garden for people suffering from burnout diseases. *Journal of Therapeutic Horticulture, 14*, 38–49.
Storr, A. (1988). *Solitude: A return to the self.* New York: Ballantine Books.
Sullivan, W. C., Kuo, F. E., & Depooter, S. F. (2004). The fruit of urban nature: Vital neighborhood spaces. *Environment and Behavior, 36*, 678–700.
Takano, T., Nakamura, K., & Watanabe, W. (2002). Urban residential environments and senior citizen's longevity in megacity areas: The importance of walkable green spaces. *Journal of Epidemiology and Community Health, 56*, 913–918.
Taylor, A. F., Kuo, F., & Sullivan, W. C. (2001). Coping with ADD: The surprising connection to green play settings. *Environment and Behavior, 33*, 54–77.

Thoreau, H. D. (1854/1989). *Walden and other writings by Henry David Thoreau*. New York: Bantam Books.
Todd, D. (2008). *Cascadia-the elusive Utopia: Exploring the spirit of the Pacific Northwest*. Vancouver: Ronsdale Press.
Ulrich, R. (1993). Biophilia, biophobia, and natural landscapes. In S. Kellert & E. O. Wilson (Eds.), *The biophilia hypothesis* (pp. 73–137). Washington, DC: Island Press.
Underwood, L. G., & Teresi, J. A. (2002). The daily spiritual experience scale: Development, theoretical description, reliability, exploratory factor analysis, and preliminary construct validity using health-related data. *Annals of Behavioral Medicine, 24*, 22–33.
Valtchanov, D., & Ellard, C. (2010). Physiological and affective responses to immersion to virtual reality: Effects of nature and urban settings. *Journal of CyberTherapy and Rehabilitation, 3*, 359–373.
Valtchanov, D., Barton, K. R., & Ellard, C. (2010). Restorative effects of virtual nature settings. *Cyberpsychology, Behavior, and Social Networking, 13*, 503–512.
Vernon, M. (2008). *Well-being*. Durham: Acumen Publishing.
Walsh, F. (2009). Human-animal bonds II: The role of pets in family systems and family therapy. *Family Process, 48*, 481–499.
Waterman, A. S. (2008). Reconsidering happiness: A eudaimonist's perspective. *Journal of Positive Psychology, 3*, 234–252.
Weinstein, N., Przybylski, A. K., & Ryan, R. M. (2009). Can nature make us more caring? Effects decline time spent in nature of immersion in nature on intrinsic aspirations and generosity. *Personality and Social Psychology Bulletin, 35*, 1315–1329.
Wesley, M. C., Minatrea, N. B., & Watson, J. C. (2009). Animal-assisted therapy in the treatment of substance dependence. *Anthrozoos, 22*, 137–148.
Wilson, E. O. (1984). *Biophilia*. Cambridge, MA: Harvard University Press.
World Health Organization (2009). Retrieved July 20, 2011, from http://www.who.int/gho/urban_health/situation_trends/urban_population_growth_text/en/index.html
World Health Organization. (2011, July 20). Global Health Observatory (GHO). Retrieved from http://www.who.int/gho/urban_health/situation_trends/urban_population_growth_text/en/index.html
Young, J., McGown, E., Haas, E., & Yu, K. (2008). *Coyote's guide to connecting with nature: For kids of all ages and their mentors*. Duvall: Wilderness Awareness School.

Chapter 12
Physiological Correlates of Mental Well-Being

Petra Lindfors

Despite the rapidly growing interest in positive aspects of human functioning, the research on physiological correlates of mental well-being is still quite scarce. Comparing the extensive number of studies that delineate the physiological correlates of mental disorders with the modest number of studies that focus on physiological correlates of mental well-being, the lack of research that is physiologically oriented becomes particularly clear. This lack of knowledge of the physiological correlates of mental well-being results from research primarily focused on alleviating human suffering by detecting physiological changes linked to mental disorders and to tailoring effective medical treatment that target relevant physiological systems (e.g., Dockray and Steptoe 2010; Ryff and Singer 1998). However, recent research makes it clear that the absence of mental disorder does not necessarily equal mental well-being, as characterized by thriving and flourishing. Instead, mental functioning has turned out to be more complex, with some individuals who exhibit concurrent mental disorder and mental well-being, others who show no mental disorder but who demonstrate low levels of mental well-being, and still others who flourish and live meaningful and happy lives (Keyes 2002). Research on the linkages between bodily processes and mental well-being allows descriptions to be formatted of important similarities and differences between human functioning, in terms of mental disorder and mental well-being. Importantly, studies of the physiological correlates to mental well-being can help to clarify why some individuals maintain health during adversity, while others fall ill (cf. Ryff et al. 2006).

The purpose of this chapter is to offer a review of research that investigates the physiological underpinnings of mental well-being. The chapter starts out by providing a rationale for the study of physiological correlates of mental well-being. It then

P. Lindfors (✉)
Stockholm University, Stockholm, Sweden
e-mail: pls@psychology.su.se

C.L.M. Keyes (ed.), *Mental Well-Being: International Contributions to the Study of Positive Mental Health*, DOI 10.1007/978-94-007-5195-8_12,

proceeds to provide a basic framework for understanding different physiological systems and related physiological indicators that have been included in empirical studies of mental well-being. The chapter then moves on to introducing common physiological indicators that have been included in empirical research on mental well-being. Having introduced basic physiology and having presented the two broad well-being orientations and their related definitions of mental well-being, the subsequent section describes and summarizes research on physiological correlates relating to three different aspects of mental well-being. The chapter ends with an integration of the field and suggestions for future research.

Why a Focus on Physiological Correlates?

Although the research on physiological correlates of mental well-being is scarce, an increasing number of studies show that positive psychological functioning is related to good physical health, reduced mortality, and longevity (Chida and Steptoe 2008; Cohen and Pressman 2006; Dockray and Steptoe 2010; Ryff and Singer 1998, 2008; Steptoe et al. 2009). In addition to research on factors pertaining to resilience, such as optimism (Seligman 1998) and sense of coherence (Antonovsky 1985, 1987), positive affective states have been more consistently linked to various physical health outcomes (for reviews, see Pressman and Cohen 2005; Cohen and Pressman 2006; Steptoe et al. 2009). A now classic example is the longitudinal study of catholic nuns by Danner et al. (2001), which showed that positive emotional content expressed in writing by nuns in their early twenties was inversely associated with risk of mortality 60 years later. These relationships between various types of positive psychological functioning and physical health outcomes are likely to be coupled with physiological processes (e.g., Ryff and Singer 1998; Steptoe et al. 2005). This assumption also draws on the fact that mental disorders, apart from deteriorating psychological functioning, most often involve physiological changes reflected in deviations at the neurophysiological, hormonal, or other bodily levels (Ganzel et al. 2010; McEwen 2007). With this in mind, delineating how mental well-being relates to physiology will advance the knowledge of health-promoting and protective bodily processes.

When it comes to explaining the nature of the relationships between positive psychological functioning and physical health, different mechanisms have been suggested (Pressman and Cohen 2005; Ryff and Singer 1998; Steptoe et al. 2005). Among these are mechanisms including behavioral and psychobiological processes, respectively. A mechanism focusing on behavioral factors suggests that mental well-being may be coupled with health-promoting behaviors, including a healthy lifestyle, which, in turn, promote better physical health. According to mechanisms including psychophysiological processes, the interaction between mental well-being and physical health involve psychobiological processes, including various bodily systems and their functioning, which, in turn, influence physical health.

Physiological Indicators

Physiological indicators can be used to investigate bodily functioning and health-related outcomes. Considering that the brain plays a central role in interpreting, evaluating, and responding to daily life challenges and demands, central physiological processes relating to an individual's interpretation, evaluation, and response to situations in daily life reverberate through the body, which, in turn, signal back to the brain. This means that there is a constant ongoing interaction between central and peripheral processes that is reflected in central and peripheral physiological activity (e.g., Ganzel et al. 2010; McEwen 2007). From this, physiological indicators can be measured at different levels (McEwen and Seeman 1999). In describing the different levels of physiological correlates, it is useful to distinguish between peripheral and central indicators. While central indicators reflect central functioning in terms of brain activity, peripheral indicators reflect physiological functioning in the rest of the body (Ganzel et al. 2010). Since valid assessment of central indicators typically requires careful measurements using technically advanced and sophisticated equipment, the assessment of central indicators is commonly restricted to the laboratory setting. In contrast, the development of portable devices has facilitated the assessment of peripheral indicators reflecting, for instance, cardiovascular functioning in different settings, including situations in daily life and controlled experimental settings (Andreassi 2006). Other peripheral indicators, for instance, that assess functioning within the endocrine system are commonly measured in blood, saliva, or urine. These indicators can thus be measured in different settings, including both laboratory and daily life settings. Also the use of saliva and urine for the assessment of physiological indicators is noninvasive, which allows for intensive repeated sampling over time without causing any harm to study participants (Lundberg 2005). Among the commonly studied peripheral physiological indicators are physiological indicators that reflect activity within the cardiovascular, endocrine, metabolic, and immune systems. Physiological indicators from these different systems have independently and together been linked to various health outcomes (Ganzel et al. 2010; McEwen and Seeman 1999).

The cardiovascular system consists of the heart, systemic circulation, and pulmonary circulation with the primary function of supplying blood and transporting oxygen, nutrients, and other substances to different bodily organs and tissues (e.g., Andreassi 2006). The cardiovascular system is influenced by activity within the sympathoadrenomedullary (SAM) system, which involves brain mechanisms and plays a central role in physiological arousal. Commonly assessed indicators of the functioning of the cardiovascular system include systolic and diastolic blood pressure and heart rate. Increased levels of blood pressure and heart rate have repeatedly been associated with adaptive responses to acute challenges and demands. However, chronically high levels of cardiovascular activity, such as high blood pressure, have been identified as a risk factor for physical ill health and disease.

Apart from influencing activity within the cardiovascular system, the SAM system influences the endocrine system and the release of the catecholamines adrenaline and noradrenaline. Both adrenaline and noradrenaline are secreted peripherally into the blood by the adrenal medulla and then circulated around the body. Besides catecholamines, there is another set of endocrine markers: glucocorticoids. Glucocorticoids are released peripherally into the blood from the adrenal cortex upon activation of the hypothalamic-pituitary-adrenal (HPA) axis. Cortisol is one of the most important and well-researched glucocorticoids, and cortisol receptors are found in all major organs and bodily tissues. This means that cortisol can have a major impact on bodily functioning. By stimulating the peripheral release of endocrine markers, the central mechanisms of the SAM system and the HPA axis trigger a set of coordinated physiological changes that have an adaptive function and increase an individual's readiness to respond to and act on challenges or demands in the environment. Such acute physiological changes are adaptive. In contrast, long-term physiological activity, characterized by chronic changes in endocrine activity, has been associated with bodily wear and tear. Cortisol, in particular, has diversified short-term and long-term effects on bodily functioning with chronic changes being linked to various diseases, including type 2 diabetes, hypertension, cardiovascular diseases, depression, and autoimmune conditions (Ganzel et al. 2010; McEwen and Seeman 1999).

The metabolic system is involved in distributing energy resources throughout the body. These energy resources include glucose and blood lipids such as cholesterol and triglycerides. Generally, different types of cholesterol are distinguished, the main types being low-density (LDL) lipoproteins and high-density (HDL) lipoproteins, with total cholesterol as a measure reflecting the total amount of lipids circulating in the blood stream. While HDL is considered to promote health and to protect against atherosclerosis, high levels of triglycerides might be a risk factor for disease. Additionally, LDL and total cholesterol are associated with cardiovascular ill health. Triglycerides are another commonly investigated blood lipid, reflecting fat deposits, with higher values associated with diabetes and obesity. In addition to blood lipids, measures of glucose are also included among metabolic indicators. Glycosylated hemoglobin (HbA1c) is an integrated measure reflecting an individual's glucose metabolism during the previous 30–90 days and that has been linked to diabetes.

Recent research underscores the importance of immune system functioning and inflammatory mechanisms underlying various diseases, including cardiovascular disease (Kiecolt-Glaser 2009; Glaser and Kiecolt-Glaser 2005). The immune system plays a central role as a barrier, active in defending and protecting the body from infections and other threats. There are a number of immune system markers, including several different cytokines, which have their specific functions in the complex process of protecting the body. These processes are further complicated by the fact that acute and long-term responses of the immune system involve diverse parts of the immune system.

In addition to investigating separate physiological systems and focusing on physiological indicators reflecting activity within a specific system, the concept of allostatic load has been proposed as a complementary approach that underscores the mutual interactions between different bodily systems by describing how physiological functioning within theses bodily systems relates to health and disease (e.g., McEwen

2007; McEwen and Seeman 1999). The allostatic load model also takes into account the ability of bodily systems to reach stability through change and distinguishes between the effects of acute and chronic responses. While acute responses that are necessary to adapt to current challenges and demands have a protective effect when they are followed by periods of rest and recovery, prolonged activation of different bodily systems increases the wear and tear of bodily resources. Partly, such wear and tear is related to natural life course changes and the reduced flexibility of aging bodily systems. Young and healthy functioning bodily systems respond with activity within a given and optimal range. However, daily wear and tear may, over time, result in physiological dysregulation. Dysregulation in multiple bodily systems, characterized by activity deviating from the optimal range or by increased difficulties in returning to baseline levels (or resting levels) after various bodily challenges, may result in allostatic load. Such cumulative dysregulation may result in an allostatic load that, in turn, increases the risk for future ill health and disease and reduces the chances for long-term physical health. To reflect the multisystems approach, allostatic load has been operationalized as a summary indicator of physiological challenge across multiple bodily systems (McEwen and Seeman 1999). Typically, a measure of allostatic load includes one or several physiological indicators of cardiovascular, endocrine, immune, and metabolic system functioning. To date, research has shown that high allostatic load is associated with different health-related outcomes, including cardiovascular disease, cognitive decline, and mortality (Ganzel et al. 2010).

Different Aspects of Mental Well-Being

Based on how mental well-being is defined, the research within the field can be divided into two broad orientations (Deci and Ryan 2008; Ryan and Deci 2001). Each of these orientations focuses on different, yet overlapping, aspects of well-being, namely, hedonic aspects of well-being and eudaimonic aspects of well-being (Kashdan et al. 2009; Keyes et al. 2002). While the hedonic orientation focuses on subjective well-being, the eudaimonic orientation underscores the pursuit of growth, human fulfillment, and psychological well-being. The differences between the two orientations become clear when looking at how these different aspects of mental well-being are defined and assessed (e.g., Ryan and Deci 2001). Subjective well-being is commonly associated with happiness. The assessment of subjective well-being includes measures of positive affect, affect balance, happiness, and life satisfaction (Diener 1984; Ryan and Deci 2001). In contrast, psychological well-being refers to a broader conceptualization, including characteristics of the optimally functioning individual. Over the past several decades, psychological well-being has mainly been measured using the six well-being dimensions included in the Ryff scales (Ryff 1989; Ryff and Keyes 1995). However, other ways of measuring psychological well-being cover individual strengths relating to meaningfulness, such as sense of coherence (Antonovsky 1985, 1987). Theoretical reviews (Deci and Ryan 2008; Kashdan et al. 2009; Ryan and Deci 2001) comparing the philosophical underpinnings, measures, and empirical findings of the two orientations conclude that in investigating different aspects of mental well-being using different yet slightly overlapping self-report measures, the two lines of research complement each other. This complementary perspective is supported by empirical studies of mental well-being profiles, including measures of both subjective and psychological well-being (Keyes et al. 2002).

Hedonic Well-Being and Its Physiological Correlates

Most of the existing research on physiological correlates of mental well-being has focused on the hedonic aspects of well-being in terms of positive affect and positive emotions (for detailed reviews, see Pressman and Cohen 2005; Steptoe et al. 2009). In contrast, the research investigating physiological correlates of more complex aspects of hedonic well-being, such as life satisfaction and subjective well-being which go beyond pure ratings of emotions or affect, is scarce. In part, this results from psychology's primary concern with emotion and affect. However, with regard to the linkages to various health-related outcomes, emotion and affect have been suggested to explain how psychosocial stress can influence physical health (Pressman and Cohen 2005).

Research on central physiological correlates (i.e., brain functioning) of positive affect draws on findings showing that there is a differentiation between positive and negative emotional processes in the brain. The prefrontal cortex has been identified as a part of the brain that is involved in emotional processes, and so this part of the brain appears to be particularly important for mental well-being (Davidson 2004). Studies on mental well-being have also focused on such measures as those used in earlier findings relating to asymmetric activity between the left and right hemispheres. As regards levels of activity in the brain, a study focusing on mental well-being has shown that greater left than right activation of the prefrontal cortex is associated with higher levels of positive affect. However, activation of the left and right frontal hemispheres was shown to not be associated with positive affect (Urry et al. 2004).

As regards cardiovascular indicators, systematic reviews show that positive affect and positive emotions are related to increases in cardiovascular responses (Pressman and Cohen 2005). These relationships have been found both in experimental and correlational studies. However, increases in blood pressure have been established in both experimental and correlational research, while increases in heart rate have been found in experimental studies only. When it comes to the size of the increase, the magnitude is typically relatively small. A related line of research investigating the form and function of positive emotions has shown that the experience of positive emotions, by restoring autonomic activity to midrange levels, decreases the duration of cardiovascular arousal and thus facilitates physiological recovery, which, in turn, may hinder detrimental processes and promote health (Fredrickson 1998, 2004; Fredrickson et al. 2000). However, other experimental studies have failed to replicate these findings (Steptoe et al. 2005).

For endocrine measures, including cortisol and catecholamines (adrenaline and noradrenaline), experimental research inducing positive affect by active techniques, including study participants' experiences, results in increased cortisol levels (Pressman and Cohen 2005). Yet, laboratory studies inducing positive affect by passive techniques (showing film clips, listening to music, or similar) show no consistent cortisol increases but rather a decrease or no change at all. In contrast, research in real-life settings typically shows that positive affect is associated with lower cortisol levels. However, these results tend to be stronger for trait positive affect than for state positive affect. As regards catecholamines, positive affect (trait and state) has been coupled with lower levels of both adrenaline and noradrenaline in studies conducted in real-life settings; however, some studies have shown null findings. For laboratory studies, the findings on catecholamines are mixed, with some studies showing positive affect as being associated with higher noradrenaline levels or both higher levels of adrenaline and noradrenaline, while other studies show null findings. As for cortisol, the mixed laboratory findings can be explained by differences in inducing positive affect, with active techniques being associated with a clear increase, while results for passive techniques are less clear (Pressman and Cohen 2005; Steptoe et al. 2009). It is important to bear the differences in mind for individuals who are reacting emotionally to active and passive experimental techniques, as well as the potential differences between state and trait positive affect, when transferring the research findings between settings and when evaluating the associations between positive affect and health outcomes.

There are several potential indicators of immune system functioning (Kiecolt-Glaser 2009). Cytokines constitute a larger group of immune system markers that have been found to be helpful in measuring physical health. The existing laboratory studies suggest that induced positive affect is linked to changes in immune system response. So far, only a few field studies have included immune system indicators, but these studies suggest that both trait and state positive affect are related to higher secretory immunoglobulin A (SIgA) levels (Pressman and Cohen 2005; Steptoe et al. 2009).

To conclude, an increasing number of studies that have investigated the physiological correlates of positive affect and positive emotions have shown that positive affect is linked to physiology. Importantly, the relationships between positive affect and emotions recur across different physiological systems, including both central and peripheral physiological indicators, such as brain activity and cardiovascular, endocrine, and immune system markers. Although additional research is needed to clarify patterns of physiological correlates and to delineate how these patterns relate to health over time, the findings clearly show that there are physiological correlates of mental well-being in terms of positive affect and positive emotions that are central to physical health.

Eudaimonic Well-Being and Its Physiological Correlates

Eudaimonic well-being includes meaning, purpose, and actualization of individual potential. In contrast to measures of hedonic aspects of mental well-being, the eudaimonic aspects of mental well-being encompass a range of different concepts and related measures. These measures often cover dimensions such as meaningfulness, purpose, and belongingness (e.g., Ryan and Deci 2001; Ryff and Singer 1998). Although there are several different operationalizations of eudaimonic well-being (Kashdan et al. 2009), sense of coherence (Antonovsky 1985, 1987) and Ryff's psychological well-being scales (Ryff 1989; Ryff and Keyes 1995) stand out as the conceptualizations that offer the most solid frameworks for the empirical investigation of linkages to physiological indicators and physical health.

Sense of Coherence and Its Physiological Correlates

Sense of coherence (SOC) refers to the level of stability in an individual's confidence in structure, predictability, and intelligibility (Antonovsky 1985, 1987). These three dimensions are considered to characterize resilient individuals who manage to deal successfully with life, find meaning, and grow by facing adversity. This means that SOC can be considered a global orientation that influences the individual's perception and interpretation of various situations. As a global orientation, SOC involves taking into consideration whether everyday life is demanding and challenging, whether these demands and challenges need to be dealt with, and whether there are resources available for dealing with these challenges and demands. In keeping with Antonovsky (1985, 1987, 1993), an individual's SOC may modify a stress reaction in various ways at various stages of the stress reaction. For example, individuals with a stronger SOC are less likely to experience stimuli as stressful and consequently do not suffer from the stress and strain that burden individuals with a weaker SOC. Thus, the constant ongoing and lifelong interplay between SOC and stress is assumed to influence physical health. While it is known that SOC is associated with various health outcomes (Surtees et al. 2002), less is known about the actual physiological correlates of SOC that underlie these associations.

Physiological Correlates of Sense of Coherence

Much of the research on physiological underpinnings of SOC is cross-sectional and has compared physiological correlates in individuals with distinct profiles of SOC. When it comes to cardiovascular indicators, middle-aged women with a weak SOC have been found to have higher systolic blood pressure than women with a strong SOC; diastolic blood pressure follows the same pattern, albeit not statistically significantly (Lindfors et al. 2005). Yet another study (Konttinen et al. 2008) which included a larger sample of women and men showed no associations between SOC and blood pressure. As for metabolic markers such as blood lipids, middle-aged women with a weak SOC have been shown to exhibit poorer lipid profiles in terms of lower levels of high-density lipoproteins (HDLs) and higher levels of triglycerides than do women with a strong SOC (Svartvik et al. 2000). Another study failed to replicate theses results for HDL and triglycerides, mainly due to a lack of statistical power (Lindfors et al. 2005). However, in showing that women with a weak SOC had higher levels of total cholesterol than women with a strong SOC, the association between blood lipids and SOC was replicated. Yet, a recent study that included analyses of SOC and total cholesterol in women and men showed no differences in the associations between total cholesterol and SOC for subgroups with distinct SOC profiles (Konttinen et al. 2008).

The associations of cumulative load, in terms of allostatic load and SOC, have also been investigated longitudinally in women (Lindfors et al. 2006). The findings have shown that allostatic load in terms of cardiovascular, metabolic, and lung function was a significant predictor of SOC in middle-aged women with no previous diagnosis of pathology. Interestingly, analyses of the different components included in SOC (i.e., manageability, meaningfulness, and comprehensibility) revealed significant associations between allostatic load and the meaningfulness component, but not for the manageability component. These findings suggest that the relationships between cumulative physiological load not only result from the fact that control, in terms of manageability, is associated with physiology but also underscore the importance of meaningfulness (Lindfors et al. 2006).

Looking across the research on physiological correlates of SOC, it becomes clear that research has focused on peripheral physiological correlates and that studies of central physiological correlates are lacking. Moreover, the existing findings relating to peripheral correlates are mixed. Cohort studies that include only women suggest an association between both cardiovascular and metabolic indicators and SOC (Lindfors et al. 2005). More specifically, the preliminary findings on women show that a stronger SOC is associated with a more favorable physiological profile, while a weaker SOC is associated with a less favorable but also a more exhaustive, physiological profile. In contrast, a recent large-scale study that included adult women and men showed no associations between physiological indicators and SOC (Konttinen et al. 2008). As regards the physiological correlates of SOC, additional research is needed to clarify whether the relationships between physiological indicators and SOC hold for women only and whether these associations are restricted to cardiovascular and metabolic indicators or also include endocrine and immune system parameters. The mixed findings may also result from methodological differences between studies. Among these are different measures of SOC and, as a result, different cutoff points for distinguishing individuals with a strong and a weak SOC, respectively. But current empirical evidence allows for no firm conclusions as regards the physiological correlates of SOC.

Psychological Well-Being

The lifespan developmental approach to mental well-being formulated by Ryff (1989; Ryff and Keyes 1995) describes psychological well-being in terms of six dimensions, including autonomy, environmental mastery, personal growth, positive relations with others, purpose in life, and self-acceptance. These dimensions are considered to characterize well-functioning individuals who manage to deal successfully with daily life, find meaning, and grow from experiences. Importantly, psychological well-being profiles across the different dimensions have been found to vary with respect to age, which underscores natural but dynamic changes in psychological well-being over a lifetime. In keeping with this perspective on psychological well-being, eudaimonic aspects of mental well-being are assumed to be linked to health (Ryff and Singer 1998). This reasoning is based on a view of a good life being associated with a health-promoting lifestyle and behaviors but also with physiological processes linked to the six dimensions of psychological well-being. This means that high levels of growth, mastery, meaning, positive relations, and so on, are important for maintaining physical health and increased resilience.

Physiological Correlates of Psychological Well-Being

Research on physiological correlates of psychological well-being, in terms of the Ryff scales, has been mainly correlational and has examined how the different dimensions of psychological well-being, along with a measure that includes all of the dimensions of well-being, are related to different physiological indicators.

In respect to central mechanisms that focus on how brain activity relates to psychological well-being, greater left than right activation of the prefrontal cortex has been associated with higher levels of psychological well-being, including total scores and five of the dimensions included in Ryff's well-being scales (i.e., environmental mastery, personal growth, positive relations with others, purpose in life, and self-acceptance). Associations have also been found between activation of the left prefrontal cortex and total scores of psychological well-being, as well as for all of the separate dimensions of psychological well-being, excluding autonomy. Importantly, these associations with psychological well-being remain stable when the effects of positive affect are statistically removed. Although the relationships between central physiological indicators and psychological well-being were small, the associations were robust, which indicates that psychological well-being is linked to individual behavioral engagement. There were, however, no linkages between right hemisphere activation and psychological well-being, which supports previous research that showed that the left hemisphere is more involved in processes involving positive affect (Urry et al. 2004).

When it comes to cardiovascular indicators, the findings have shown no associations between blood pressure and the different dimensions of well-being included in the Ryff scales (Lindfors and Lundberg 2002; Ryff et al. 2006). This holds for blood pressure assessments from both health checkups and measurements taken in settings of daily life (Lindfors and Lundberg 2002).

As for endocrine markers such as catecholamines and cortisol, findings suggest that some of the well-being dimensions are associated with endocrine functioning. Regarding catecholamines, Ryff and colleagues (2006) studied older women and found that adrenaline and noradrenaline, respectively, were associated with one of the six dimensions of psychological well-being included in the Ryff scales. In particular, adrenaline was associated with higher levels of positive relations, while noradrenaline was associated with higher levels of autonomy. In contrast, a study including a smaller group of middle-aged women and men found no relationships between catecholamines and psychological well-being (Lindfors and Lundberg 2002). However, this study did show that cortisol was associated with psychological well-being: individuals with high levels of psychological well-being had lower levels of cortisol output throughout the day than did individuals with low levels of psychological well-being. These differences were particularly pronounced for morning cortisol. Looking at the different dimensions of psychological well-being, high cortisol levels in the morning were associated with lower levels of environmental mastery and self-acceptance. Moreover, high levels of cortisol throughout the day were associated with low environmental mastery and purpose in life. In part, these findings have been replicated by Ryff and colleagues (2006) who found that cortisol was associated with high personal growth and purpose in life. Again, higher scores on these two dimensions of psychological well-being were associated with lower levels of cortisol throughout the day, including morning cortisol levels. However, no associations were found for any of the other four dimensions of well-being.

Research focusing on metabolic indicators, including blood lipids and HbA1c, has shown that higher levels of HDL are associated with personal growth and purpose in life, while a high total cholesterol/HDL ratio is associated with lower personal growth (Ryff et al. 2004, 2006). However, other studies report no associations between blood lipids (HDL, LDL, total cholesterol, and triglycerides) and psychological well-being (Lindfors and Lundberg 2002). As for HbA1c, no associations with psychological well-being have been found (Tsenkova et al. 2007).

Focusing on associations between immune system markers and psychological well-being, one study has shown that psychological well-being was associated with a strong vaccine-induced cytokine production (Hayney et al. 2003). Another study on cytokines, albeit a different type of cytokines, found associations with some of the well-being dimensions. Specifically, and in line with the study's hypothesis, higher levels of positive relations with others and with purpose in life were associated with cytokines. Importantly, these relationships remained after statistically controlling for potential confounding variables, such as depression (Friedman et al. 2007).

As regards the multisystems approach of allostatic load, one study has explored the associations between allostatic load and positive relations with others. The research findings of this study revealed that positive relations with others were associated with a lower allostatic load and with less dysregulation within bodily systems (Seeman et al. 2002).

To summarize, the findings on physiological correlates of psychological well-being, in terms of the Ryff scales, are preliminary and show mixed results for different physiological systems and their respective indicators. The findings are promising for central indicators and allostatic load, but since only a few studies on these indicators have been carried out, more research is needed to assess the validity of these findings. In regard to cardiovascular indicators, preliminary findings suggest no associations, and additional research on more diversified groups is needed to clarify any potential associations with metabolic markers. Also, the findings relating to catecholamines are mixed. However, the preliminary research on cortisol and immune system markers suggests a link to psychological well-being. As for the immune system, research has focused on different indicators, and these findings need to be replicated in other groups in order to assess their validity. When it comes to cortisol, individuals with high psychological well-being have cortisol levels within an optimal or moderate range which suggests that the cortisol output is more moderate. Although the findings differ between studies with regard to the dimensions of psychological well-being having an association with cortisol, lower cortisol levels have been linked with purpose in life. This, in turn, suggests that lower cortisol levels and purpose in life may be crucial to maintaining health.

Integrating Findings on Physiological Correlates of Mental Well-Being

Looking across the research on physiological correlates of mental well-being makes it clear that most studies relate to the hedonic orientation and investigate associations between positive affect and different physiological indicators. The recent systematic reviews of positive affect and physical health and potential physiological correlates (e.g., Steptoe et al. 2009; Pressman and Cohen 2005) illustrate clearly that positive emotions and affect are associated with physiology. The fact that there are systematic reviews also suggest that it should be both possible and useful to procure summaries of current findings, in order to consolidate and refine the research with respect to different research designs and their relation to different physiological indicators (in terms of acute and chronic physiological functioning). In addition, the research often includes and controls for spurious relationships of other factors, including psychosocial and demographic factors such as age, gender, social status, and ethnicity (Pressman and Cohen 2005). In contrast to the research on affect and emotions, the knowledge of physiological correlates of other hedonic measures (e.g., life satisfaction) is very limited. However, some studies, including the parallel investigation of hedonic and eudaimonic well-being, have explored life satisfaction (e.g., Urry et al. 2004). Although the existing findings suggest that more complex measures of hedonic well-being have different physiological correlates than do eudaimonic measures of well-being and positive affect, the findings are still preliminary and do not cover different physiological systems.

While the research on hedonic measures that focus on positive emotions and affect clearly show an association with physiology, the existing research on physiological correlates of eudaimonic measures is, at best, promising. Specifically, the studies on eudaimonic measures, such as sense of coherence and psychological well-being, suggest an association between physiological functioning and meaning (e.g., Lindfors and Lundberg 2002; Lindfors et al. 2006; Ryff et al. 2006). Such associations between experiences of meaning and physiology also point to potential linkages between positive psychological functioning, physiology, and increased improvement of long-term health. In addition, the findings underscore one of the central aspects of the eudaimonic orientation, namely, the aspect of leading a meaningful life (Ryff and Singer 1998). However, the preliminary findings on eudaimonic well-being should not be regarded as conflicting with findings on hedonic well-being. Instead, research including the parallel investigation of hedonic and eudaimonic measures of well-being with the same study participants and in the same setting suggests that the physiological correlates of hedonic and eudaimonic well-being, respectively, are distinct, yet somewhat overlapping (e.g., Ryff et al 2006; Urry et al. 2004). This, in turn, suggests that there are physiological correlates of both hedonic and eudaimonic well-being but that these have different roles. Following Fredrickson's (1998, 2004) line of reasoning, experiences of hedonic well-being in terms of positive affect and positive emotions, and their broadening of thought-action repertoires, are necessary for an individual to build and achieve eudaimonic well-being, including a meaningful life. This view suggests that there is a constant interplay between hedonic and eudaimonic aspects of well-being. Such interplay between different levels of mental well-being could partly explain variations in physiological correlates. However, at the same time, such associations also underscore the need to distinguish between acute and chronic physiological functioning and their associations with hedonic and eudaimonic well-being, respectively. Ideally, further research into the physiological correlates of mental well-being should include repeated assessment of physiological indicators across different bodily systems in a laboratory setting and in real-life situations among women and men taking part in a longitudinal study. This would allow for the disentanglement of acute and chronic physiological patterns and for the investigation of single physiological indicators and cumulative physiological functioning in terms of allostatic load (as related to hedonic and eudaimonic well-being). However, it is not always possible to bring about certain research designs, and since many groups are not included in longitudinal research programs, additional cross-sectional laboratory and real-life studies are needed in order to look at fine-grained patterns in different groups, including, for instance, children and adolescents. In studying physiological correlates of mental well-being in different groups, it is important to make expectations clear in terms of physiology in healthy individuals without chronic disease or other major health problems. Importantly, the flexibility of bodily systems varies according to health status but also with age (e.g., McEwen and Seeman 1999). When it comes to optimal physiological functioning, healthy and younger individuals more often exhibit ideal physiological patterns with moderate levels of activity, adequate recovery, and so on, than do older individuals with chronic disease. This means that it can be difficult to distinguish physiological correlates of mental well-being in groups, including younger and/or older individuals. Specifically, trends may not become statistically significant. Or, perhaps other, nontraditional statistical methods are needed to adequately measure physiological correlates of healthy individuals. In contrast, the bodily systems of older or sick individuals have started to wear down, meaning that these individuals typically have higher levels of allostatic load than do other individuals. Therefore, it is easier to distinguish unfavorable patterns of bodily functioning and link these to mental well-being. Yet, in addition to physiological functioning, patterns of mental well-being also seem to vary by age and health status. However, such associations underscore the need to investigate additional and alternative ways of explaining the physiological patterns related to hedonic and eudaimonic measures of mental well-being.

Although the research suggests that there is a direct pathway between physiology and mental well-being (e.g., Dockray and Steptoe 2010), other factors may also affect this relationship, such as the influence of more favorable lifestyle choices and health behavior patterns, genetics, early childhood development, and psychosocial factors including social status and resources available for dealing with daily stress and strain. It is vital that future research explores the impact of such factors on variations in mental well-being and physiology across the course of life.

Conclusions

This chapter has summarized research findings on commonly studied central and peripheral bodily systems and their relations with hedonic and eudaimonic aspects of mental well-being. While findings show clear associations between different physiological systems and hedonic well-being in terms of positive affect, findings related to eudaimonic well-being are inconclusive but seem to suggest that there are physiological correlates of meaning. However, additional research is needed to further clarify how physiological underpinnings of various aspects of mental well-being vary in different groups of individuals across the course of life. To make such clarification possible, future research designs need to encourage the parallel study of bodily functioning associated with hedonic and eudaimonic well-being while taking into account health behaviors and psychosocial factors. Ultimately, findings linking mental well-being and physiological functioning may help tailor interventions that can promote and build positive health.

References

Andreassi, J. L. (2006). *Psychophysiology: Human behavior and physiological response* (5th ed.). Mahwah: LEA.

Antonovsky, A. (1985). The lifecycle, mental health and sense of coherence. *Israeli Journal of Psychiatry and Related Sciences, 22*, 273–280.

Antonovsky, A. (1987). *Unraveling the mystery of health: How people manage stress and stay well.* San Francisco: Jossey-Bass.

Antonovsky, A. (1993). Complexity, conflict, chaos, coherence, coercion and civility. *Social Science and Medicine, 37*, 969–981.

Chida, Y., & Steptoe, A. (2008). Positive psychological well-being and mortality: A quantitative review of prospective observational studies. *Psychosomatic Medicine, 70*, 741–756.

Cohen, S., & Pressman, S. D. (2006). Positive affect and health? *Current Directions in Psychological Science, 15*(3), 122–125.

Danner, D. D., Snowdon, D. A., & Friesen, W. V. (2001). Positive emotions in early life and longevity: Findings from the nun study. *Journal of Personality and Social Psychology, 80*(5), 804–813.

Davidson, R. J. (2004). Well-being and affective style: Neural substrates and biobehavioral correlates. *Philosophical Transactions of the Royal Society of London, Series B, 359*, 1395–1411.

Deci, E. L., & Ryan, R. M. (2008). Hedonia, Eudaimonia and well-being: An introduction. *Journal of Happiness Studies, 9*, 1–11.

Diener, E. (1984). Subjective well-being. *Psychological Bulletin, 95*, 542–575.

Dockray, S., & Steptoe, A. (2010). Positive affect and psychobiological processes. *Neuroscience and Biobehavioral Reviews, 35*(1), 69–75.

Fredrickson, B. L. (1998). What good are positive emotions? *Review of General Psychology, 2*, 300–319.

Fredrickson, B. L. (2004). The broaden-and-build theory of positive emotions. *Philosophical Transactions of the Royal Society of London, Series B, 359*, 1367–1377.

Fredrickson, B. L., Manusco, R. A., Branigan, C., & Tugade, M. M. (2000). The undoing effect of positive emotions. *Motivation and Emotion, 24*, 237–258.

Friedman, E. M., Hayney, M., Dienberg Love, G., Singer, B. H., & Ryff, C. D. (2007). Plasma interleukin-6 and soluble IL-6 receptors are associated with psychological well-being in older women. *Health Psychology, 26*(3), 305–313.

Ganzel, B. L., Morris, P. A., & Wethington, E. (2010). Allostatis and the human brain: Integrating models of stress from the social and life sciences. *Psychological Review, 117*(1), 134–174.

Glaser, R., & Kiecolt-Glaser, J. K. (2005). Stress-induced immune dysfunction: Implications for health. *Nature Reviews Immunology, 5*, 243–251.

Hayney, M. S., Dienberg Love, G., Buck, J. M., Ryff, C. D., Singer, B., & Muller, D. (2003). The association between psychosocial factors and vaccine-induced cytokine production. *Vaccine, 21*, 2428–2432.

Kashdan, T. B., Biswas-Diener, R., & King, L. A. (2009). Reconsidering happiness: The costs of distinguishing between hedonics and eudaimonia. *Journal of Positive Psychology, 3*(4), 219–233.

Keyes, C. L. M. (2002). The mental health continuum: From languishing to flourishing in life. *Journal of Health and Social Behavior, 43*, 207–222.

Keyes, C. L. M., Shmotkin, D., & Ryff, C. D. (2002). Optimizing well-being: The empirical encounter of two traditions. *Journal of Personality and Social Psychology, 82*(6), 1007–1022.

Kiecolt-Glaser, J. K. (2009). Psychoneuroimmunology psychology's gateway to the biomedical future. *Perspectives on Psychological Science, 4*(4), 367–369.

Konttinen, H., Haukkala, A., & Uutela, A. (2008). Comparing sense of coherence, depressive symptoms and anxiety, and their relationships with health in a population-based study. *Social Science and Medicine, 66*, 2401–2412.

Lindfors, P., & Lundberg, U. (2002). Is low cortisol release an indicator of positive health? *Stress and Health, 18*, 153–160.

Lindfors, P., Lundberg, O., & Lundberg, U. (2005). Sense of coherence and biomarkers of health in 43-year-old women. *International Journal of Behavioral Medicine, 12*(2), 98–102.

Lindfors, P., Lundberg, O., & Lundberg, U. (2006). Allostatic load and clinical risk as related to sense of coherence in middle-aged women. *Psychosomatic Medicine, 68*, 801–807.

Lundberg, U. (2005). Stress hormones in health and illness: The roles of work and gender. *Psychoneuroendocrinology, 30*(10), 1017–1021.

McEwen, B. S. (2007). Physiology and neurobiology of stress and adaptation: Central role of the brain. *Physiological Review, 87*(3), 873–904.

McEwen, B. S., & Seeman, T. (1999). Protective and damaging effects of mediators of stress: Elaborating and testing the concepts of allostasis and allostatic load. *Annals of the New York Academy of Sciences, 896*, 30–47.

Pressman, S. D., & Cohen, S. (2005). Does positive affect influence health? *Psychological Bulletin, 131*(6), 925–971.

Ryan, R. M., & Deci, E. L. (2001). On happiness and human potential: A review of research on hedonic and eudaimonic well-being. *Annual Review of Psychology, 52*, 141–166.
Ryff, C. D. (1989). Happiness is everything, or is it? Explorations on the meaning of psychological well-being. *Journal of Personality and Social Psychology, 57*, 1069–1081.
Ryff, C. D., & Keyes, C. L. (1995). The structure of psychological well-being revisited. *Journal of Personality and Social Psychology, 69*, 719–727.
Ryff, C. D., & Singer, B. H. (1998). The contours of positive human health. *Psychological Inquiry, 9*(1), 1–28.
Ryff, C. D., & Singer, B. H. (2008). Know thyself and become what you are: A eudaimonic approach to psychological well-being. *Journal of Happiness Studies, 9*(1), 13–39.
Ryff, C. D., Singer, B. H., & Dienberg Love, G. (2004). Positive health: Connecting well-being with biology. *Philosophical Transactions of the Royal Society of London, Series B, 359*, 1383–1394.
Ryff, C. D., Dienberg Love, G., Urry, H. L., Muller, D., Rosenkranz, M. A., Friedman, E. M., Davidson, R. J., & Singer, B. (2006). Psychological well-being and ill-being: Do they have distinct or mirrored biological correlates? *Psychotherapy and Psychosomatics, 75*, 85–95.
Seeman, T. E., Singer, B. H., Ryff, C. D., Dienberg Love, G., & Levy-Storms, L. (2002). Social relationships, gender and allostatic load across two age cohorts. *Psychosomatic Medicine, 64*(3), 395–406.
Seligman, M. E. P. (1998). *Learned optimism*. New York: Simon and Schuster.
Steptoe, A., Wardle, J., & Marmot, M. (2005). Positive affect and health related neuroendocrine, cardiovascular and inflammatory processes. *Proceedings of the National Academy of Sciences, 102*, 6508–6512.
Steptoe, A., Dockray, S., & Wardle, J. (2009). Positive affect and psychobiological processes relevant to health. *Journal of Personality, 77*(6), 1747–1775.
Surtees, P., Wainwright, N., Luben, R., Khaw, K. T., & Day, N. (2002). Sense of coherence and mortality in men and women in the EPIC-Norfolk United Kingdom Prospective Cohort Study. *American Journal of Epidemiology, 158*, 1202–1209.
Svartvik, L., Svartvik, L., Lidfeldt, J., Nerbrand, C., Samisoe, G., Schersteń, B., & Nilsson, P. M. (2000). Dyslipidaemia and impaired well-being in middle-aged women reporting low Sense of Coherence. The Women's Health in the Lund Area (WHLA) Study. *Scandinavian Journal of Primary Health Care, 18*(3), 177–182.
Tsenkova, V. K., Dienberg Love, G., Singer, B. H., & Ryff, C. D. (2007). Socioeconomic status and psychological well-being predict cross-time change in glycosylated hemoglobin in older women without diabetes. *Psychosomatic Medicine, 69*, 777–784.
Urry, H. L., Nitschke, J. B., Dolski, I., Jackson, D. C., Dalton, K. M., Mueller, C. J., Rosenkranz, M. A., Ryff, C. D., Singer, B. H., & Davidson, R. J. (2004). Making a life worth living: Neural correlates of well-being. *Psychological Science, 15*(6), 367–372.

Part III
Toward the Application of Positive Mental Health Internationally

Chapter 13
Recovery: A Complete Mental Health Perspective

Helene L. Provencher and Corey L.M. Keyes

Interventions and research surrounding mental health treatment are oriented toward the alleviation of mental illness symptoms and functional impairments. This approach reflects the pathogenic paradigm in which mental health is conceived of as the absence of psychopathology. Until recently, mental health as something positive (e.g., Jahoda 1958) remained undefined, unmeasured, and therefore largely ignored. In 1999, the US Surgeon General defined good mental health as "a state of successful performance of mental function resulting in productive activities, fulfilling relationships with people, and the ability to adapt to change and to cope with adversity" (U.S. Public Health Service 1999).

This definition coincides with social scientists' views of mental health, which has come to be known as individuals' quality of life in the domain of subjective well-being. Reviews (Keyes 2006b; Ryan and Deci 2001) have acknowledged as many as 13 specific dimensions of subjective well-being that, when factor analyzed, represent the latent structure of emotional well-being and positive functioning in adults (Keyes 2002) and adolescents(Keyes 2005b, 2006a) (see Table 13.1). Whereas emotional well-being refers to positive emotions toward one's own life, such as happiness and life satisfaction, positive functioning is measured as psychological and social well-being, which reflect a sense of engagement and fulfillment in one's private and social life (Keyes 1998; Ryff and Singer 1996).

Positive mental health is a core construct for mental health promotion (Barry 2009) and the salutogenic paradigm (Antonovsky 1979) because it requires the study and implementation of the causes of good health in order to prevent disease and promote recovery. Until recently, positive mental health was defined and

H.L. Provencher, Ph.D. (✉)
Faculty of Nursing, Laval University, Pavilion Ferdinand-Vandry, local 3495, 1050, Medecine Street, Quebec City, QC, Canada G1V 0A6
e-mail: helene.provencher@fsi.ulaval.ca

C.L.M. Keyes, Ph.D.
Department of Sociology, Emory University, Atlanta, GA, USA

C.L.M. Keyes (ed.), *Mental Well-Being: International Contributions to the Study of Positive Mental Health*, DOI 10.1007/978-94-007-5195-8_13,

Table 13.1 Factors and 13 dimensions reflecting mental health as flourishing

Hedonia (i.e., emotional well-being)
1. *Positive affect*: Cheerful, interested in life, in good spirits, happy, calm and peaceful, full of life
2. *Avowed quality of life:* Mostly or highly satisfied with life overall or in domains of life
Positive psychological functioning (i.e., psychological well-being)
3. *Self acceptance:* Holds positive attitudes toward self, acknowledges, likes most parts of personality
4. *Personal growth:* Seeks challenge, has insight into own potential, feels a sense of continued development
5. *Purpose in life:* Finds own life has a direction and meaning
6. *Environmental mastery:* Exercises ability to select, manage, and mold personal environs to suit needs
7. *Autonomy:* Is guided by own, socially accepted, internal standards and values
8. *Positive relations with others:* Has, or can form, warm, trusting personal relationships
Positive social functioning (i.e., social well-being)
9. *Social acceptance:* Holds positive attitudes toward, acknowledges, and is accepting of human differences
10. *Social actualization:* Believes people, groups, and society have potential and can evolve or grow positively
11. *Social contribution:* Sees own daily activities as useful to and valued by society and others
12. *Social coherence:* Interest in society and social life and finds them meaningful and somewhat intelligible
13. *Social integration:* A sense of belonging to, and comfort and support from, a community

measured piecemeal, with a focus on specific and often only emotional aspects of well-being rather than including positive functioning in life (Zubrick and Kovess-Masfety 2005). There is a growing consensus on the heuristic value of hedonic and eudaimonic well-being for further developing knowledge about positive aspects of mental health (Barry 2009). Here, the *mental health continuum long* (Keyes 2002) and *short* (Keyes 2006a) *forms* are used not only as a guide to build new instruments for—but also as a measure of—positive mental health, such as the Warwick-Edinburgh Mental Well-being Scale (Tennant et al. 2007).

Another important distinction between mental health promotion and mental illness treatment concerns the complete state model of mental health (Keyes 2005a, 2007). Such a distinction has been represented in the scientific literature for more than half a century (Jahoda 1958; World Health Organization 1948) and posits that mental health is not only the absence of mental illness but also the presence of subjective well-being. More recently, the availability of a research methodology for assessing states of complete mental health has provided specific criteria for combining indicators of mental illness and positive mental health (i.e., subjective well-being). This was developed and used to study the model of complete mental health, which is also called the two (or the *dual*) continua model (Keyes 2005a, 2007).

Since the mid-1980s, persons with psychiatric disabilities have highlighted that it was possible to recover from mental illness, here corresponding to the achievement of a full and meaningful life in spite of enduring psychiatric symptoms or impairments. Consistent with this view, phenomenological and other qualitative approaches (Silverstein and Bellack 2008), and numerous personal accounts (e.g., Ridgway 2001; Spaniol and Koehler 1994), have provided a better understanding of personal and environmental factors that hinder or facilitate recovery, as well as valuable insight about key dimensions (e.g., hope, empowerment, positive sense of identity) and phases underlying this experience (Onken et al. 2007). The voices of persons with psychiatric disabilities are thus viewed as the *royal road* to advance knowledge on recovery, and the acquisition and use of experiential knowledge (e.g., critical analysis of personal experiences) is especially targeted in peer support interventions (Mead et al. 2001).

A large number of researchers and clinicians have endorsed consumers' viewpoints on recovery. Provencher (2002), for instance, has defined recovery as the transcendence of symptoms, functional limitations, and social handicaps attached to mental illness, from which emerges a new sense of existence, the performance of meaningful roles in society, and a better sense of well-being and quality of life. However, consumers' definition of recovery has challenged a more traditional view of this phenomenon that is still largely represented in the scientific community, which conceives of recovery through the lens of the disease and focuses on the extent, or the level, of remission from mental illness (Silverstein and Bellack 2008). In this vein, several long-term follow-up studies have reported significant improvement in psychiatric symptoms and deficits—or even complete recovery—from schizophrenia over time, in contrast to the deteriorating course that is typically assumed for this disorder (Calabrese and Corrigan 2005).

Distinct conceptions of recovery may be viewed as desirable and as providing enriching perspectives and stimulating multidisciplinary work in order to better understand this phenomenon. However, such diversity remains problematic until theoretical approaches are developed to clearly address how they can complement each other. Potential attempts to resolve this issue may reduce ongoing tensions, encourage a dialogue, and foster collaboration among proponents, whereas neglect of this issue may perpetuate the confusion that prevails about recovery and may possibly carry the risk of decreased interest in the delivery of recovery-oriented services over the long run. What has been overlooked so far has been the fact that those proposed conceptions of recovery rely on distinct approaches of mental health: the search and engagement in a pleasant and fulfilling life in alignment with the salutogenic vision and the alleviation of mental illness outcomes with the pathogenic vision. This stresses the relevance of theoretical approaches that bring together mental illness and positive mental health.

This chapter proposes that the study and process of recovery from mental illness can be augmented by adopting the model of complete mental health. The first part presents a brief overview of Keyes' model. Current definitions of recovery are then reexamined based on their underlying conceptions of mental health. Third, recovery is redefined as a complete mental health experience, relying on two complementary processes and outcomes, restoration from mental illness, and optimization of positive mental health. An emphasis is placed on outcomes, which are viewed as pathways to complete mental health over the recovery process. Finally, some concluding remarks are made about how the complete view of mental health recovery extends previous conceptions, and some future directions for research in order to advance knowledge in this area are proposed.

Complete Mental Health

Positive mental health, like mental illness, is a syndrome of symptoms that consist of an individual's subjective well-being. Previous research on subjective well-being (Keyes 2005b; Ryan and Deci 2001) yielded latent factors that are the converse of the cluster of symptoms used in the DSM-IV-TR (American Psychiatric Association 2000) to diagnose major depressive episode (MDE). Depression requires symptoms of *an*hedonia, and positive mental health consists of symptoms of hedonia, or emotional well-being; depression consists of symptoms of *mal*functioning, and positive mental health consists of symptoms of eudaimonia, or positive functioning.

Table 13.1 presents clusters of symptoms of positive mental health, and the diagnosis of states of positive mental health is modeled after the DSM-III-R approach to diagnosing MDE. In order to be diagnosed as *flourishing* in life, individuals must exhibit high levels (*every day* or *almost every day* during the past 2 weeks) on at least one measure of hedonic well-being and high levels on at least six measures of positive functioning. Individuals who exhibit low levels (*never* or *once or twice* during the past 2 weeks) on at least one measure of hedonic well-being and low levels on at least six measures of positive functioning are diagnosed as *languishing* in life. Adults who are *moderately mentally healthy* do not fit the criteria for either flourishing or languishing in life. A continuous assessment sums up all measures of positive mental health, and conclusions have not varied between the categorical and the continuous assessment of positive mental health.

The following findings come from papers using the 1995 Midlife in the United States (MIDUS) survey, a random-digit-dialing sample of noninstitutionalized English-speaking adults between the ages of 25 and 74 living in the 48 contiguous states. The MIDUS used DSM-IV-TR (APA 2000) criteria to diagnose four mental disorders (i.e., major depressive episode, panic, generalized anxiety, and alcohol dependence) using the Composite International Diagnostic Interview Short Form (CIDI-SF) scales. Four separate summary measures served as indicators of mental illness, operationalized as the number of symptoms of major depressive episode, generalized anxiety, panic disorder, and alcohol dependence. Three scales served as indicators of positive mental health: the summed scale of emotional well-being (i.e., single item of satisfaction with life + a six-item scale of positive affect), the summed scale of psychological well-being (i.e., Ryff's six scales summed together), and the summed scale of social well-being (i.e., Keyes' five scales summed together).

Confirmatory factor analysis was used to test the complete state model of mental health. The single factor model hypothesizes that the measures of mental health and mental illness reflect a single latent factor, support for which would indicate that the absence of mental illness implies the presence of mental health. The two-factor model hypothesizes that the measures of mental illness represent the latent factor of mental health that is distinct from, but correlated with, the latent factor of mental illness that is represented by the measures of mental illness. The data strongly supported the two-factor model (Keyes 2005a), and the two continua model has been recently confirmed in US adolescents (Keyes 2009b).

Across studies, the latent factor of mental illness correlates with the latent factor of mental health ($r = -.55$). Although level of good mental health tends to increase as mental illness symptoms decrease, the association is moderate. Data support the argument that the absence of mental illness does not imply the presence of mental health; too, the presence of mental illness does not imply the absence of some level of mental health. Complete mental health is a state in which individuals are free of mental illness and are flourishing. Of course, flourishing may sometimes occur with an episode of mental illness, and moderate mental health and languishing can occur both with and without a mental illness.

With regard to states of positive mental health, languishing adults reported the highest prevalence of any of the four mental disorders, as well as the highest prevalence of two or more mental disorders during the past year. In contrast, flourishing individuals reported the lowest prevalence of any of the four 12-month mental disorders or their comorbidity. Compared with languishing or flourishing, moderately mentally healthy adults were at intermediate risk of any of the mental disorders, or two or more mental disorders, during the past year. The modest correlation between the latent continua reflects the tendency for the risk of mental illness to increase as mental health decreases. For example, the 12-month risk of major depressive episode was over five times greater for languishing than flourishing adults.

In addition, previous findings on Keyes' model revealed that level of mental health differentiated the level of functioning for those with, and for those free of, a mental disorder. Of the 77% MIDUS adults free of any of the four mental disorders, the 16.6% who were flourishing functioned better than the 50.6% with moderate mental health: those who were flourishing reported the fewest workdays missed, the fewest workdays cutback by one-half, the lowest rate of cardiovascular disease, the lowest level of health limitations of activities of daily living, the fewest chronic physical conditions at all ages, the lowest healthcare use (medical visits, hospitalizations, and medications), and the highest levels of psychosocial functioning. In terms of psychosocial functioning, this meant that completely mentally healthy adults reported the lowest level of perceived helplessness, the highest level of knowing what they want from life, the highest level of self-reported resilience (e.g., that they try to learn from adversities), and the highest level of intimacy (e.g., that they have very close relationships with family and friends). Using the same criterion measures, the 9.8% who were languishing and free of mental disorder functioned worse than adults with moderate mental health (Keyes 2007). Of the 23% MIDUS adults with at least one of the four mental disorders, the 1.5% who were flourishing functioned better than the 14.5% who had moderate mental health and who, in turn, functioned better than the 7.0% who were languishing. In other words, level of mental health differentiates levels of impairment and disability, even among adults who have had a mental illness in the past year; just over two-thirds of adults with a mental disorder in the past year had at least moderate or flourishing mental health. In short, previous research on Keyes' model has provided evidence that anything less than complete mental health results in increased impairment and disability (Keyes 2007).

Recovery from Mental Illness

Over the last two decades, recovery has become the overarching aim of mental health services systems in many countries: Australia, New Zealand, England, Scotland, and the United States, to name a few (Slade et al. 2008). Current definitions of recovery, as a process and as an outcome, are now revisited in light of their underlying conceptions of mental health.

A Pathogenic View of Recovery

As mentioned before, the vision of recovery as an outcome corresponds to the traditional or clinical view of this phenomenon and falls under the umbrella of *scientific-oriented definitions* (Silverstein and Bellack 2008). Outcomes of recovery here are defined from a pathogenic perspective which views mental health as improvements in typical indicators of mental illness, such as psychiatric symptoms and impairments in cognitive, role, and social functioning. However, there is still an ongoing debate about the requirements for declaring someone recovered. Some authors (Andreasen et al. 2005) have proposed that the full remission of symptoms and the return to premorbid levels of function are necessary, whereas others (Liberman and Kopelowicz 2005; Torgalsboen 2005) have suggested that partial remission of symptoms and role restoration that are sustained over two consecutive years are sufficient.

The pathogenic view of recovery is also represented in the literature that focuses on key dimensions, or process elements, that are involved in the minimization of mental illness and that have been particularly documented in *consumer-oriented definitions* (Silverstein and Bellack 2008). More specifically, this side of the recovery experience targets the building of protective factors against relapse, functional deterioration, and handicap, which has been traditionally addressed in the field psychiatric rehabilitation (Anthony et al. 2002). Those protective elements refer to personal and environmental resources that contribute to the reduction of mental illness and its negative social consequences (e.g., stigma, discrimination). At the individual level, they involve the restoration of skills that had been altered by the illness and the learning of illness management strategies, such as strategies for preventing relapse or coping with enduring symptoms, as well as advocacy skills for getting needed services (Mueser et al. 2006; Salyers et al. 2009). At the environmental level, they include the provision of accommodations for supporting the performance of social roles, such as parents, students, or workers (e.g., later start times or flexible break times as work adjustments). They also rely on the use of community interventions for restoring civil rights and reducing barriers to social exclusion, such as educating potential employers and other members of the community about mental illness (Corrigan et al. 2008). In addition, several subjective changes take place throughout this process, such as the development of a positive identity based on restored abilities (Brown and Kandirikirira 2007), a renewed sense of hope for better prevention of illness relapses, or the development of a sense of empowerment, which encompasses increased self-efficacy in coping with mental illness, active participation in the planning of individualized services (Adams and Drake 2006; Drake et al. 2009), and advocacy for defending rights as consumers (Onken et al. 2007). In short, the building of protective factors against mental illness and their related subjective processes are aligned with a pathogenic view of recovery and with the use of mental illness indicators as outcomes.

A Salutogenic Perspective of Recovery

In addition to the pathogenic view, consumer-oriented definitions emphasize another side of the recovery experience in which the pursuit of positive emotions (e.g., happiness, life satisfaction) and the engagement in fulfilling activities are highlighted despite the presence of mental illness. Positive mental health is at the center of this view of recovery and underlies a salutogenic conception of mental health, although never recognized as such. The dimensions of flourishing (see Table 13.1) are used as a framework to propose linkages between recovery and positive mental health, drawing on three lines of literature.

First, qualitative research and personal accounts (Ridgway 2001; Spaniol and Koehler 1994) call attention to consumers' experiences and aspirations that are aligned with positive mental health (see Table 13.1). Brown and Kandirikirira (2007), for instance, found that persons in recovery require and strive for a positive identity, which reflects *self-acceptance*. Individuals also said they require and seek to engage in meaningful activities and to develop positive relationships with other people and with their environments, which reflect *purpose in life*, *positive relations with others*, and *social acceptance*. Narratives of persons in recovery also reveal their need and aspiration for living in communities where they are seen as more than their illness and where their contributions are valued, which are signs of positive mental health called *social integration* and *social contribution*. Persons in recovery also need and strive to manage their lives, stay healthy, and be resilient to setbacks, which reflect *environmental mastery* and, to some extent, *autonomy* (i.e., confidence to express personal opinions, needs).

Several dimensions of positive mental health are indeed targeted in recovery interventions. Consistent with hedonic well-being, having pleasure, fun, and happiness in life through involvement in leisure and social activities is promoted in supported socialization (Davidson et al. 2003, 2004, 2006). With regard to positive functioning, psychological well-being is enhanced in a self-development program (Oades 2008) and other treatment programs, for example, Well-Being Therapy (WBT) (Fava and Ruini 2003) for persons with recurrent depression or functional Cognitive Behavioural Therapy (fCBT) (Cather et al. 2005) for those with schizophrenia. In line with social well-being, peer support encourages those individuals who want to contribute to social changes and to engage in pro-social behaviors, such as using political strategies to increase access to resources (e.g., housing, paid work) (Mead et al. 2001). In this vein, capabilities approaches (Nussbaum 2000; Sen 1999) are increasingly used as guides to promote measures of social inclusion, such as securing access to participatory structures in local organizations in order to join collective efforts oriented toward the welfare of the whole community (Ware et al. 2007).

Finally, several dimensions that are assessed in recovery instruments strongly resemble the dimensions of subjective well-being that make up the assessment and diagnosis of positive mental health. For instance, subjective quality of life, as indexed by life satisfaction, reflects hedonic well-being and has been widely used in clinical practice and evaluation research. The Recovery Assessment Scale (Corrigan et al. 2004) is a self-report questionnaire that is widely used and relies on five dimensions—personal confidence and hope, willingness to ask for help, goal and success orientation, reliance on others, and no domination by symptoms—which all somewhat overlap with purpose in life, environmental mastery, autonomy, and positive relations with others. The RAS reflects psychological well-being, for the most part (see Table 13.1), and is even stronger for post-traumatic growth. This latter concept refers to positive shifts in personality schema and assumptive worlds following significant life crises (e.g., bereavement, chronic disability) (Tedeschi et al. 1998) and captures the process of thriving in recovery or becoming better off than before mental illness (Onken et al. 2007). The three dimensions of post-traumatic growth overlap with those of psychological well-being: changes in philosophy are aligned with the dimensions of purpose in life and with autonomy; changes in perceptions reflect those of environmental mastery, personal growth, and self-acceptance; and changes in relationships mirror the dimension of positive relationships with others (see Table 13.1). In this vein, the evaluation of psychological well-being (Ryff and Singer 1996) has been particularly recommended for tracking changes in growth in longitudinal studies (Joseph and Linley 2008). However, it should be emphasized that flourishing implies thriving and also directs attention to other meaningful experiences, such as positive emotions and a sense of fulfillment in social life. Finally, a special focus has been recently placed on the need for a better understanding of changes in self-experience over the recovery process, and the Scale to Assess Narrative Coherence (STAND) (Lysaker et al. 2006) has been developed to measure the extent of a coherent story about self-experience based on personal narratives of persons with schizophrenia. Four specific dimensions of self-experience are evaluated, namely, social worth, connectedness with others, agency, and illness conception. *Social worth* concerns a positive view about oneself in private and public life, reflecting the dimensions of self-acceptance and social contribution. *Connectedness with others* refers to a fulfilling and intimate relationship with at least one person, in line with the dimension of positive relationships with others. *Agency* corresponds to the perceived ability to affect one's own destiny and to engage meaningfully with others and reflects the dimensions of mastery and positive relationships with others. Finally, *illness conception* refers to the ability to address and face diverse personal challenges, including those related to the management of schizophrenia, and overlaps with the dimensions of mastery and personal growth. Those four aspects of self-experience are thus aligned with several dimensions of positive functioning (see Table 13.1).

In summary, personal and environmental changes contributing to the improvement of psychiatric symptoms and illness impairments represent an important side of recovery and underlie a pathogenic view of this experience. A salutogenic perspective is also represented, as other transformations target the achievement of optimal levels of emotional well-being and positive functioning. The ability to function well in a life, toward which one also feels good, is the *sine qua non* of good mental health (i.e., flourishing) and, therefore, of complete recovery.

Recovery of Complete Mental Health

The two continua model (Keyes 2007) incorporates the pathogenic and salutogenic perspectives into a unitary, complete view of recovery. Here, this experience is redefined as two complementary processes and outcomes: restoration from mental illness and optimization of positive mental health. Keyes's model underscores the need to better understand and intervene in factors and conditions that help persons, with and without mental illness, to flourish in life. Several of them have been previously discussed as key elements related to the pathogenic and salutogenic views of recovery, respectively, underlying the processes of restoration and optimization. A brief overview of strategies for promoting those two processes is now presented.

Through restoration, persons in recovery take steps to manage, and make the most of, the limitations imposed by mental illness. At the individual level, peer and psychiatric rehabilitation interventions (Copeland 2000; Corrigan et al. 2008; Drake et al. 2005) may provide support for the development of illness management skills, the reduction of deficits in a variety of domains (e.g., cognitive, social, and role functioning), and the restoration of roles, including those performed in normative settings. At the environmental level, strategies are oriented toward the alleviation of stress in the family (e.g., reduction of expressed emotions) and other milieus (e.g., provision of work accommodations) (Becker and Drake 2005; Glynn et al. 2006). In addition, other interventions are provided for decreasing stigma and discriminatory behaviors within surrounding environments and the general population (Corrigan and Gelb 2006; Corrigan et al. 2005).

Through optimization, persons in recovery take steps to move up the continuum of positive mental health. As previously mentioned, this may involve the use of supported socialization (Davidson et al. 2004), WBT (Fava and Ruini 2003) or fCBT (Cather et al. 2005) for enhancing positive emotions or positive functioning.

Building on personal strengths represents another strategy for promoting positive mental health. For instance, a self-report measure has been developed to assess a series of character strengths that are classified into six broad virtues: wisdom and knowledge (e.g., love of learning), courage (e.g., perseverance), humanity (e.g., kindness), justice (e.g., citizenship), temperance (e.g., self-control), and transcendence (e.g., spirituality) (Peterson and Seligman 2004). This survey instrument has been used as a tool for helping people with severe mental illness to identify their top five character strengths, also called signature strengths. Such activity was perceived as enjoyable and as having contributed to an increase in a sense of pride and self-esteem in participants (Resnick and Rosenheck 2006). At the environmental level, optimization strategies are oriented toward the provision of support for interpersonal flourishing (Ryff and Singer 2000), which includes opportunities to develop intimate and reciprocal relationships (Mead et al. 2001; Ware et al. 2007). Actions directed at community development are also undertaken to promote social inclusion. They entail initiatives for encouraging civic and social participation, such as those that increase access to participatory structures within mental health and nonmental health organizations (Ware et al. 2007). Other community-level interventions aim to reduce poverty and to improve access to basic resources (e.g., education, employment, affordable housing), such as those documented in the field of mental health promotion (Barry 2009). It is also worthwhile to mention the Strengths Model (Rapp and Goscha 2006)—a case management program targeting the maximization of personal and environmental strengths—and its potential efficacy for enhancing positive mental health.

Of additional relevance are strategies that are likely to promote positive changes in both restoration and optimization processes. For instance, supported approaches in employment (Becker and Drake 2005), education (Mowbray et al. 2003), and housing (Fakhoury et al. 2002) tailor activities, roles, or living environments based on the person's deficits, strengths, and aspirations. Other combined strategies can be found in helping processes that promote recovery (Anthony et al. 2003; Drake 2005). These include developing relationships with peers or professionals in which learning from illness relapse is emphasized, focusing on the optimal use of strengths, and promoting shared decision-making in the planning of individualized services (Adams and Drake 2006; Drake et al. 2009). Spiritual (e.g., meditating, praying) and wellness strategies (e.g., exercising) are also used to overcome difficulties in dealing with mental illness and for living as fully as possible (Russinova and Cash 2007). Finally, the recovery-oriented system of services (Anthony 2000) is concerned with the alleviation of mental illness and the promotion of positive mental health. Whereas treatment and crisis services specifically target the alleviation of mental illness, enrichment services support the maximization of personal strengths and wellness/prevention services aim at the enhancement of positive mental health and physical health (e.g., healthy life styles). Self-help services also sustain the development of personal empowerment over the management of mental illness and positive mental health. Another example is case management, which coordinates and secures access services across several intervention programs, including mental health promotion services.

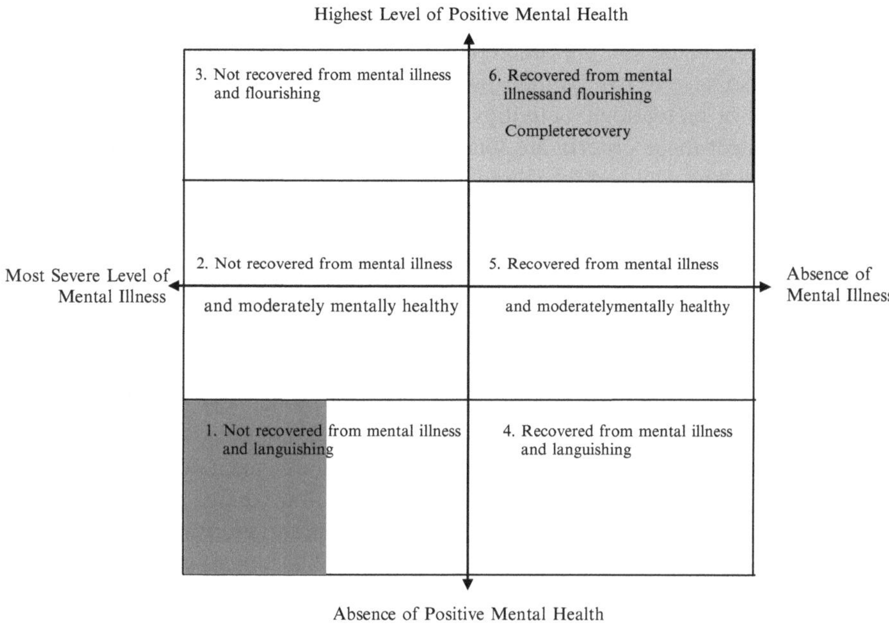

Fig. 13.1 Pathways to complete mental health in recovery

Pathways to Complete Mental Health in Recovery

Recovery is a nonlinear and highly individualized process (Spaniol et al. 2002), and changes in complete mental health occur throughout this journey and are viewed as recovery outcomes. To illustrate such dynamics, a categorical approach is proposed for evaluating pathways in recovery along two continua: mental illness and positive mental health. With regard to the mental illness continuum, Liberman and Kopelowicz's (2005) criteria are used to distinguish among those who are recovered and those who are nonrecovered from mental illness, with schizophrenia as an example of psychiatric disorder. With regard to the positive mental health continuum, Keyes's (2005a, 2007) criteria are used to differentiate between persons who are flourishing, who are moderately mentally healthy, or who are languishing.

Figure 13.1 shows two perpendicular axes that are used to illustrate pathways in complete mental health over the recovery process. Based on the criteria proposed by Liberman and Kopelowicz (2005), the horizontal axis represents the presence or absence of recovery: individuals who are located at the right of the midpoint are considered as recovered from mental illness, whereas those who are at the left are viewed as not recovered. More specifically, the midpoint indicates moderate levels of symptoms (i.e., score of four or less on each of the positive and negative symptom items of the Brief Psychiatry Rating Scale) and the restoration of roles in normative settings. In addition, individuals who are located at the right side of the midpoint hold a part-time or full-time competitive work, whereas those who have other work status are located at the left (e.g., unemployment, prevocational training). Recovered individuals also have to live on their own (without supervision) and be involved in weekly social or recreational activities with persons without mental illness; those who do not meet these criteria are located at the left. From the pathogenic view, individuals are thus declared recovered when they fulfill all of the above criteria for at least two consecutive years. Based on the criteria proposed by Keyes, the vertical axis represents the diagnoses of positive mental health, namely, languishing, moderate mental health, and flourishing. From the salutogenic view, individuals are thus declared recovered when they meet the requirements for flourishing.

Six states of recovery emerge from the combination of mental illness and positive mental health outcomes: (1) nonrecovered from mental illness and languishing, (2) nonrecovered from mental illness and moderately mentally healthy, (3) nonrecovered from mental illness and flourishing, (4) recovered from mental illness and languishing, (5) recovered from mental illness and moderately mentally healthy, and (6) recovered from mental illness and flourishing. Altogether, these six states of complete recovery highlight that the route to recovery lies not in the alleviation of mental illness exclusively but in the enhancement of positive mental health as well.

Persons who are viewed as *nonrecovered from mental illness and languishing* (recovery state 1) have little hope or motivation for making their lives better. They may not be engaged in the exploration of personal strengths and opportunities within their environments that would allow them to build on their potential. They may also see themselves as psychiatric patients and as having a "career" in mental illness. Involvement in roles and activities is likely to be perceived as ways of passing time and keeping oneself busy. At the extreme bottom left of Fig. 13.1, the shaded area corresponds to the initial phase of recovery, where the individual is overwhelmed by the disability (Spaniol et al. 2002). These individuals have little control over the mental illness or of life in general, lack self-confidence, and feel disconnected from the self and others.

Persons who are viewed as *nonrecovered from mental illness and moderately mentally healthy* (recovery state 2) are struggling to build a meaningful and satisfying life. In contrast to those who are languishing, they have a more positive outlook on their lives and their own potential to better enjoy and function in life. They may be in the process of discovering that they possess positive assets and strengths and may be engaged in activities in which they can further develop. They may also place more importance on who they *want to be* rather than who they *no longer are* (Pettie and Triolo 1999). Being active and doing things that bring joy and pleasure are important to them, such as participating in social activities, volunteering, or working in sheltered settings. Such activities help them to realize that they have the potential for playing a more active role in society. Among persons belonging to this profile, individuals who have reached some illness stability bear some resemblance to those who are involved in the second phase of the recovery process where individuals struggle with the disability (Spaniol et al. 2002). Building a sense of confidence in being able to act in their own interests characterizes their journey.

Persons who are viewed as *nonrecovered from mental illness and flourishing* (recovery state 3) have not reached partial symptomatic remission but are involved in nonnormative activities and roles that are perceived as enjoyable, satisfying, and fulfilling. This highlights the fact that consumers differ a great deal in their choice of meaningful and challenging activities; some value normative activities while others do not. Several reasons may account for preferences in nonnormative activities (e.g., volunteering, transitional work) or occasional self-employment, such as having control over work hours, pacing the reentry to the regular market, or prioritizing creative or independent work over other types of jobs (e.g., Brown and Kandirikirira 2007). Individuals who are flourishing and performing those activities may see their impairments as part of a positive identity through disability pride. In line with the social model of disability (Sayce 2000), they may reject the sick role, perceive social oppression as the main source of disability, advocate for their rights and entitlements as disabled persons (e.g., housing and benefits services), and request supportive and socially inclusive measures for living their lives as fully as possible (e.g., vocational or educational opportunities, peer support, leisure activities). On the other hand, other individuals belonging to state 3 may have built a sense of positive identity apart from impairments, no longer viewing them as core aspects of their selves. This may have emerged from the cultivation of personal strengths and positive assets through volunteering or self-employment which provided a less-structured work pattern that allowed them to flourish alongside other preferential activities, such as leisure or artistic work (e.g., painting, writing) (e.g., Brown and Kandirikirira 2007). Peers, acting as role models, may help individuals who want to move from nonnormative to normative roles, strengthening their sense of hope and personal empowerment in the pursuit and the achievement of those goals (Russinova 1999).

Persons who are viewed as *recovered from mental illness and languishing* (recovery state 4) have been successful in at least partially restoring what has been altered by the illness, but they remain quite unsatisfied with their lives and are involved in normal activities and roles that are not perceived as self-fulfilling. As recovery is a nonlinear process, it is possible that those individuals experience setbacks from the fifth or the sixth state (see Fig. 13.1). For instance, a person who is recovered from mental illness and moderately mentally healthy (state 5) decides to quit a job for another one that is believed to be more challenging. After a short enrollment in this new position, the person realizes that it does not fit with previous expectations in that the tasks are quite repetitive and dull, provide few opportunities for self-actualization, and generate an overall sense of dissatisfaction. As a result, this person may show a lower level of positive mental health, possibly moving from the state of being moderately mentally healthy to languishing.

Persons who are viewed as *recovered from mental illness and moderately mentally healthy* (recovery state 5) are similar to those who are living with the disability, the third phase of the recovery process (Spaniol et al. 2002). They look for normal and meaningful activities and roles that help them to build on their personal strengths and improve their quality of life. Although some still may feel limited by the illness, they value themselves as persons of worth and become more and more able to use environmental resources to meet their personal goals. Those individuals perceive that they are making progress in finding their real places (or niches) in society. They are proud of their accomplishments and are optimistic about their futures.

Persons who are viewed as *recovered from mental illness and flourishing* (recovery state 6) shared characteristics with those who are living beyond the disability, the final and fourth phase of the recovery process (Spaniol et al. 2002). This profile corresponds to the shaded area located at the top right of Fig. 13.1. Individuals who belong to this category have reached optimal levels of subjective well-being. They look for opportunities to challenge themselves and to reach a sense of serenity and peace of mind. They are involved in diverse normal roles and activities, such as work or parental and intimate relationships, and are more self-accepting and like who they are or who they have become. They see their futures as promising, and the pursuit of personal goals is viewed as a challenging experience. Roles and activities are perceived as concrete means of self-actualization and as ways of contributing to society (Provencher et al. 2002). Some individuals may be involved in advocacy activities not only to defend their own rights but also the rights of others. Apart from the illness, a healthy sense of self is now well established, which results from successful efforts to maximize personal strengths and from the optimal use of experiential knowledge that has been acquired throughout the recovery process. When deficits are still present, individuals are well aware of them and take them into consideration in the pursuit of challenging goals, knowing how to best use them while continuing to grow and optimize their own potential. For example, a person who has sleeping problems at night will look for jobs during evening or night shifts. Finally, individuals feel well connected to their pasts and accept former aspects of themselves. With regard to social connectedness, they have learned how to build positive relationships with others and how to resolve conflicts when they occur. They both receive and provide support to others.

Additional Reflections on Complete Mental Health Recovery

Whether recovery should be viewed as an outcome or as a process is still being debated in the literature (Davidson et al. 2010; Roe et al. 2007). Proponents of recovery as a process (Davidson et al. 2010) argue that the restoration of altered capacities leading to *recovery as an outcome* (e.g., symptoms, impaired functioning) is rather incomplete, as personal and social transformations that sustain pleasant and fulfilling experiences in recovery are still being overlooked. We endorse those views. However, having a good life is not an outcome of recovery for those proponents, and we do not hold this view. As previously mentioned, more than 40 years of research have contributed to the definition of what constitutes a good or flourishing life, and we have proposed several linkages between dimensions of positive mental health and recovery. Unlike previous conceptions, our model posits positive mental health as an outcome of recovery and uses the view of mental health as a complete state to reframe recovery. Complete mental health recovery thus involves two independent but complementary experiences—restoration from mental illness and optimization of positive mental health—and each one is defined both as a process and an outcome. What is differentiated here is the mental health approach that underlies each experience: mental illness outcomes that result from the process of restoration (e.g., a disease-oriented view) and positive mental health from the optimization process (e.g., a good mental health view). Our model does not reject a pathogenic conception of recovery but views it as insufficient to define recovery in that it requires the addition of a salutogenic conception that focuses on the promotion of positive mental health.

Subjective process elements may act as protective factors against mental illness and the achievement of positive mental health. Although their detailed discussion is beyond the scope of this chapter, they include self-redefinition, hope, empowerment, and connectedness with others (Noordsy et al. 2002; Onken et al. 2007) and are redefined within the specific contexts of restoration and optimization. For instance, the development of personal empowerment over mental illness (e.g., strategies for preventing relapses) complements the acquisition of skills used for coping with languishing states, as learned in WBT (Fava and Ruini 2003). Another example concerns the development of a positive identity, along with the reduction of self-engulfment (e.g., viewing oneself only as a schizophrenic) (Lally 1989), self-stigma (i.e., negative view of oneself resulting from the internalization of social prejudices against persons with mental illness) (Corrigan et al. 2008), and the building of a health-oriented sense of self that is based on personal strengths and assets (Davidson and Strauss 1992). In addition, several objective or illness-related dimensions are viewed as playing an important role in moderating or mediating recovery, including substance abuse, duration of untreated psychosis, good initial response to neuroleptics, adherence to treatment, and premorbid history (Liberman and Kopelowicz 2005). How they may interact with subjective factors remains unclear as well as how their separate and interactive influences work to reduce mental illness and maximize positive mental health.

Our model draws attention to individuals who are flourishing, regardless of their involvement in nonnormative (state 3) or normative (state 6) activities, which is consistent with consumers' viewpoints on recovery. It can be inferred that both types of activities provide opportunities for optimal experiences, which are characterized by full absorption (i.e., when an awareness of time disappears), high involvement in the task regardless of external rewards (e.g., paid work), enjoyment, sense of accomplishment, and perceived control over the task although still viewed as challenging and as one that maximizes competencies (Della Fave and Massimini 2004). In particular, more research is needed to further determine the profile of individuals who perceive optimal experiences when doing nonnormative activities (Frese et al. 2009). A variety of factors may be explored, such as illness-related factors (e.g., premorbid functioning, cognitive, and functional deficits), personal factors (e.g., values, life goals, meaning of recovery), and how they interact with environmental factors (e.g., support for the person's own choice and pursuit of activities).

Discussion

Keyes' model has been of heuristic value in drawing attention to the alleviation of mental illness and the promotion of positive mental health as two independent but related goals in recovery. However, limitations of the proposed methodology for assessing pathways to complete mental health in recovery still have to be addressed, as well as proposals for the direction of future clinical interventions and research.

Limitations

The proposed typology of complete recovery states should be seen as a first attempt at bridging mental illness and positive mental health indicators. Liberman and Kopelowicz's operational criteria for recovery have been used for three main reasons: It allows for both symptomatic and functional recovery to be assessed, it provides clear guidelines that are proposed for evaluating each criterion, and it provides support for its discriminant and predictive validity (Liberman and Kopelowicz 2005). However, the most controversial aspect is, without a doubt, the return to normal roles as a recovery criterion, which is particularly disputed by consumers (Deegan 1996). For them, roles and activities that bring a sense of satisfaction in life, pleasure, and fulfillment are crucial issues, whatever their performance in normative or nonnormative settings. With regard to domains of recovery, previous research has demonstrated that improvements in symptoms are relatively independent from the restoration of cognitive and psychosocial functions in persons with schizophrenia, in contrast to those with anxiety disorders for whom mild symptoms coexist with mild disability (Andreasen et al. 2005). For instance, a person with schizophrenia who holds a competitive job may still show moderate levels of psychiatric symptoms. Therefore, criteria for evaluating specific domains of recovery have been strongly recommended, such as recovery of symptoms, cognitive functioning, or psychosocial functioning (i.e., recovery of vocational functioning) (Lieberman et al. 2008; Lysaker et al. 2010). The operational definition of functional recovery remains a controversial topic (Wunderink et al. 2009). The ongoing debate needs to clarify issues that are related to both the level (e.g., attempts, progress, and success in normative and nonnormative activities) and the breadth (e.g., independent living, productivity, and social activities) of accomplishment (Harvey and Bellack 2009). For instance, there is considerable variation in the social life of healthy individuals, which raises the question of what exactly are the minimal standards for determining whether individuals with mental illness have recovered in this area. That is to say, is it necessary to have an active social life in addition to employment and independent living?

The three states of positive mental health—languishing, moderate, and flourishing—have been mainly studied in persons with depression and anxiety disorders. There is a strong need to further validate existing measures of subjective well-being in persons with severe mental illness (e.g., schizophrenia, bipolar disorders), including the Mental Health Continuum-Short Form (Keyes 2009a). This scale offers the advantage of measuring positive functioning rather than mere emotional well-being (i.e., satisfaction with life). In addition, hedonic and eudaimonic well-being may be used as a framework to develop new scales on subjective recovery outcomes. Additional research has to be done to validate the diagnostic criteria of positive mental health and to determine the prevalence of the three states in persons with severe mental illness. Future research should also translate the list of assessment criteria into expert clinical assessment in order to track changes in positive mental health and to compare self-reports with clinical assessments. This refinement is particularly needed as the assessment of positive mental health relies on the use of self-report instruments, which can be questionable in persons with poor insight and severe cognitive deficits. Duration criterion also needs to specify how long minimal requirements are to be and how long they must be maintained for flourishing, moderately mentally healthy, and languishing states.

Directions for Future Research

An important area of future research is the study of mechanisms that will allow us to better understand how the experience of restoration from mental illness can contribute to the optimization of positive mental health and vice versa. One hypothesis concerns both the resources developed during the restoration process (e.g., empowerment over the illness) and the role they may possibly play in promoting positive mental health in addition to preventing exacerbation of the illness. Another hypothesis involves the possibility that a flourishing mental state may counteract the reappearance of the illness, acting as a buffer (Keyes 2007). Additional work is required to determine whether individuals who are recovered from mental illness and have moderate or flourishing mental health are more likely to counteract the detrimental effects of stress, and to even grow from it, as compared to those who are recovered from mental illness but languishing. A final hypothesis deals with the potential role of languishing as a risk factor in the recurrence of mental illness (Keyes 2007). For instance, individuals with mental illness who are languishing may be more likely to deal with stressors in an ineffective way, having at their disposals a more limited set of coping options.

The study of flourishing in persons recovering from mental illness also calls for additional theories to better understand turning points from which may emerge positive emotions and a sense of growth. For instance, previous research on meaning-based coping (e.g., redefining priorities in life in a more meaningful way) has shown that this type of coping triggers positive emotions and sustains efforts to overcome chronic stress (Folkman and Moskowitz 2000). Its role as a potential mechanism underlying the promotion of positive mental health in recovery deserves more attention (Provencher 2007).

Finally, longitudinal data are required to better understand the evolution of individuals within each state and among the six states of recovery over time, including the process of moving from one state to another. The six states may represent specific stepping stones in the recovery process.

Conclusion

The purpose of this chapter has been to elevate the place of positive mental health and complete mental health when attempting to understand the experience of recovery. Restoration from mental illness and optimization of positive mental health are viewed as two complementary processes and outcomes in recovery. Individuals who are flourishing in life and who show low functioning in the pathogenic sense deserve more research attention, which would entail a better understanding of the nature and the meanings given to their optimal experiences. Additional efforts are needed to further develop and test interventions that enable persons with mental illness to achieve a flourishing life.

References

Adams, J. R., & Drake, R. E. (2006). Shared decision-making and evidence-based practice. *Community Mental Health Journal, 42*(1), 87–105.

American Psychiatric Association. (2000). *Diagnostic and statistical manual of mental disorders: DSM-IV-TR* (4th ed.). Washington, DC: American Psychiatric Association.

Andreasen, N. C., Carpenter, W. T., Kane, J. M., Lasser, R. A., Marder, S. R., & Weinberger, D. R. (2005). Remission of schizophrenia: Proposed criteria and rationale for consensus. *The American Journal of Psychiatry, 162*, 441–449.

Anthony, W. A. (2000). A recovery-oriented service system: Setting some system level standards. *Psychiatric Rehabilitation Journal, 24*(2), 159–168.

Anthony, W. A., Cohen, M., Farkas, M., & Gagne, C. (2002). *Psychiatric rehabilitation* (2nd ed.). Boston: Center for Psychiatric Rehabilitation, Sargent College of Health and Rehabilitation Sciences, Boston University.

Anthony, W. A., Rogers, E. S., & Farkas, M. (2003). Research on evidence-based practices: Future directions in an era of recovery. *Community Mental Health Journal, 39*(2), 101–114.

Antonovsky, A. (1979). *Health, stress, and coping*. San Francisco: Jossey-Bass.

Barry, M. (2009). Addressing the determinants of positive mental health: Concepts, evidence and practice. *International Journal of Mental Health Promotion, 11*(3), 4–17.

Becker, D. R., & Drake, R. E. (2005). *A working life for people with severe mental illness*. New York: Oxford University Press.

Brown, W., & Kandirikirira, N. (2007). *Recovering mental health in Scotland. Report on narrative investigation of mental health recovery*. Glasgow: Scottish Recovery Network.

Calabrese, J. D., & Corrigan, P. W. (2005). Beyond dementia praecox: Findings from long-term follow-up studies of schizophrenia. In R. Ralph & P. W. Corrigan (Eds.), *Recovery in mental illness: Broadening our understanding of wellness* (pp. 63–84). Washington, DC: American Psychological Association.

Cather, C., Penn, D. L., Otto, M. W., Yovel, I., Mueser, K. T., & Goff, D. C. (2005). A pilot study of functional Cognitive Behavioral Therapy (fCBT) for schizophrenia. *Schizophrenia Research, 74*(2–3), 201–209.

Copeland, M. E. (2000). *Wellness recovery action plan*. West Dummerston: Peach Press.

Corrigan, P. W., & Gelb, B. (2006). Three programs that use mass approaches to challenge the stigma of mental illness. *Psychiatric Services, 57*, 393–398.

Corrigan, P. W., Salzer, M., Ralph, R., Sangster, Y., & Keck, L. (2004). Examining the factor structure of the recovery assessment scale. *Schizophrenia Bulletin, 30*(4), 1034–1041.

Corrigan, P. W., Watson, A. C., Heyrman, M. L., Warpinski, A., Gracia, G., Slopen, N., & Hall, L. L. (2005). Structural stigma in state legislation. *Psychiatric Services, 56*, 557–563.

Corrigan, P. W., Mueser, K. T., Bond, G. R., Drake, R. E., & Solomon, P. (2008). *Principles and practice of psychiatric rehabilitation: An empirical approach*. New York: Guilford Press.
Davidson, L., & Strauss, J. S. (1992). Sense of self in recovery from severe mental illness. *British Journal of Medical Psychology, 65*(2), 131–145.
Davidson, L., Haglund, K. E., Stayner, D. A., Rakfeldt, J., Chinman, M. J., & Tebes, J. K. (2003). "It was just realizing … that life isn't one big horror": A qualitative study of supported socialization. *Psychiatric Rehabilitation Journal, 24*(3), 275–292.
Davidson, L., Shahar, G., Stayner, D. A., Chinman, M. J., Rakfeldt, J., & Kraemer Tebes, J. (2004). Supported socialization for people with psychiatric disabilities: Lessons from a randomized controlled trial. *Journal of Community Psychology, 32*(4), 453–477.
Davidson, L., Shahar, G., Staeheli Lawless, M., Sells, D., & Tondora, J. (2006). Play, pleasure, and other positive life events: "Non-specific" factors in recovery from mental illness. *Psychiatry, 69*(2), 151–163.
Davidson, L., Tondora, J., & Ridgway, P. (2010). Life is not an "outcome": Reflections on recovery as an outcome and as a process. *American Journal of Psychiatric Rehabilitation, 13*(1), 1–8.
Deegan, P. E. (1996). Recovery as journey of heart. *Psychiatric Rehabilitation Journal, 19*(3), 91–97.
Della Fave, A., & Massimini, F. (2004). Bringing subjectively into focus: Optimal experiences, life themes, and person-centered rehabilitation. In P. Linley & S. Joseph (Eds.), *Positive psychology in practice* (pp. 581–597). Hoboken: Wiley.
Drake, R. E. (2005). How evidence-based practices contribute to community integration: A commentary on Bond et al., Community Ment Health J. 2004 Dec; 40 (6):569–588. *Community Mental Health Journal, 42*, 87–90.
Drake, R. E., Merrens, M. R., & Lynde, D. W. (2005). *Evidence-based mental health practice: A textbook*. New York: Norton.
Drake, R. E., Wilkniss, S. M., Frounfelker, R. L., Whitley, R., Zipple, A. M., McHugo, G. J., & Bond, G. R. (2009). The Thresholds-Darmouth partnership and research on shared decision making. *Psychiatric Services, 60*(2), 142–144.
Fakhoury, W. K. H., Murray, A., Shepherd, G., & Priebe, S. (2002). Research in supported housing. *Social Psychiatry and Psychiatric Epidemiology, 37*, 301–315.
Fava, G. A., & Ruini, C. (2003). Development and characteristics of a well-being enhancing psychotherapeutic strategy: Well-being therapy. *Journal of Behavior Therapy and Experimental Psychiatry, 34*(1), 45–63.
Folkman, S., & Moskowitz, J. T. (2000). Stress, positive emotion, and coping. *Current Directions in Psychological Science, 9*(4), 115–118.
Frese, F., Knight, E., & Saks, E. (2009). Recovery from schizophrenia: With views of psychiatrists, psychologists, and others diagnosed with this disorder. *Schizophrenia Bulletin, 35*(2), 370–380.
Glynn, S., Cohen, A. N., Dixon, L. B., & Noosha, N. (2006). The potential impact of the recovery movement on family interventions for schizophrenia: Opportunities and obstacles. *Schizophrenia Bulletin, 32*(3), 451–463.
Harvey, P. D., & Bellack, A. S. (2009). Toward a terminology for functional recovery in schizophrenia: Is functional remission a viable concept? *Schizophrenia Bulletin, 35*(3), 300–306.
Jahoda, M. (1958). *Current concepts of positive mental health*. New York: Basic Books.
Joseph, S., & Linley, P. A. (2008). *Trauma, recovery, and growth: Positive psychological perspectives on post-traumatic stress*. Hoboken: Wiley.
Keyes, C. L. M. (1998). Social well-being. *Social Psychology Quarterly, 61*(2), 121–140.
Keyes, C. L. M. (2002). The mental health continuum: From languishing to flourishing in life. *Journal of Health and Social Behavior, 43*(2), 207–222.
Keyes, C. L. M. (2005a). Mental illness and/or mental health? Investigating axioms of the complete state model of health. *Journal of Consulting and Clinical Psychology, 73*(3), 539–548.
Keyes, C. L. M. (2005b). The subjective well-being of America's youth: Toward a comprehensive assessment. *Adolescent and Family Health, 4*(1), 3–11.
Keyes, C. L. M. (2006a). Mental health in adolescence: Is America's youth flourishing? *The American Journal of Orthopsychiatry, 76*(3), 395–402.

Keyes, C. L. M. (2006b). Subjective well-being in mental health and human development research worldwide: An introduction. *Social Indicators Research, 77*(1), 1–10.
Keyes, C. L. M. (2007). Promoting and protecting mental health as flourishing. *American Psychologist, 62*(2), 95–108.
Keyes, C. L. M. (2009a). *Brief description of the Mental Health Continuum Short Form (MHC-SF).* Retrieved on-line November 22, 2009, from http://www.sociology.emory.edu/ckeyes/
Keyes, C. L. M. (2009b). The nature and importance of positive mental health in America's adolescents. In R. Gilman, E. S. Huebner, & M. J. Furlong (Eds.), *Handbook of positive psychology in schools* (pp. 9–23). New York: Routledge.
Lally, S. J. (1989). Does being in here mean there is something wrong with me? *Schizophrenia Bulletin, 15*(2), 253–265.
Liberman, R. P., & Kopelowicz, A. (2005). Recovery from schizophrenia: A criterion-based definition. In R. O. Ralph & P. W. Corrigan (Eds.), *Recovery in mental illness: Broadening our understanding of wellness* (pp. 101–129). Washington, DC: American Psychological Association.
Lieberman, J. A., Drake, R. E., Sederer, L. I., Belger, A., Keefe, R., Perkins, D., & Stroup, S. (2008). Science and recovery in schizophrenia. *Psychiatric Services, 59*(5), 487–496.
Lysaker, P. H., Buck, K. D., Hammound, K., Taylor, A. C., & Roe, D. (2006). Associations of symptom remission, psychosocial function and hope with qualities of self-experience in schizophrenia: Comparisons of objective and subjective indicators of recovery. *Schizophrenia Research, 82*, 241–249.
Lysaker, P. H., Roe, D., & Buck, K. D. (2010). Recovery and wellness amidst schizophrenia: Definitions, evidence, and the implications for clinical practice. *Journal of the American Psychiatric Nurses Association, 16*(1), 36–42.
Mead, S., Hilton, D., & Curtis, L. (2001). Peer support: A theoretical perspective. *Psychiatric Rehabilitation Journal, 25*(2), 134–141.
Mowbray, C. T., Megivern, D., & Holter, M. C. (2003). Supported education programming for adults with psychiatric disabilities: Results from a national survey. *Psychiatric Rehabilitation Journal, 27*(2), 159–167.
Mueser, K. T., Meyer, P. S., Penn, D. L., Clancy, R., Clancy, D. M., & Salyers, M. P. (2006). The illness management and recovery program: Rationale, development, and preliminary findings. *Schizophrenia Bulletin, 32*(1 Suppl), S32–S43.
Noordsy, D. L., Torrey, W., Mueser, K. T., Mead, S., O'Keefe, C., & Fox, L. (2002). Recovery from severe mental illness: An intrapersonal and functional outcome definition. *International Review of Psychiatry, 14*(4), 318–326.
Nussbaum, M. C. (2000). *The capabilities approach*. Cambridge, UK: University of Cambridge Press.
Oades, L. (2008). Helping people with mental illness flourish through self-development program. Retrieved on line November 22, 2009, from http://media.uow.edu.au/releases/UOW042499.html
Onken, S. J., Craig, C. M., Ridgway, P., Ralph, R., & Cook, J. A. (2007). An analysis of the definitions and elements of recovery: A review of the literature. *Psychiatric Rehabilitation Journal, 31*(1), 9–22.
Peterson, C., & Seligman, M. E. P. (2004). *Character strengths and virtues*. New York: Oxford University Press.
Pettie, D., & Triolo, A. M. (1999). Illness as evolution: The search for identity and meaning in the recovery process. *Psychiatric Rehabilitation Journal, 22*(3), 255–262.
Provencher, H. L. (2002). L'expérience du rétablissement: perspectives théoriques. *Santé Mentale au Québec, 27*(1), 35–64.
Provencher, H. L. (2007). Role of psychological factors in studying recovery from a transactional stress-coping approach: Implications for mental health nursing practices. *International Journal of Mental Health Nursing, 16*(3), 188–197.
Provencher, H. L., Gregg, R., Mead, S., & Mueser, K. T. (2002). The role of work in the recovery of persons with psychiatric disabilities. *Psychiatric Rehabilitation Journal, 26*(2), 130–142.
Rapp, C. A., & Goscha, R. (2006). *The strengths model: Case management with people with psychiatric disabilities* (2nd ed.). New York: Oxford University Press.

Resnick, S. G., & Rosenheck, R. A. (2006). Recovery and positive psychology: Parallel themes and potential synergies. *Psychiatric Services, 57*(1), 120–122.
Ridgway, P. (2001). ReStorying psychiatric disability: Learning from first person narratives. *Psychiatric Rehabilitation Journal, 24*(4), 343–353.
Roe, D., Rudnick, A., & Gill, K. J. (2007). The concept of "being in recovery". *Psychiatric Rehabilitation Journal, 30*(3), 171–173.
Russinova, Z. (1999). Providers' hope-inspiring competence as a factor optimizing psychiatric rehabilitation outcomes. *Journal of Rehabilitation, 65*(4), 50–57.
Russinova, Z., & Cash, D. (2007). Personal perspectives about the meaning of religion and spirituality among persons with serious mental illness. *Psychiatric Rehabilitation Journal, 30*(4), 271–284.
Ryan, R. M., & Deci, E. L. (2001). On happiness and human potentials: A review of research on hedonic and eudaimonic well-being. In S. Fishe (Ed.), *Annual review of psychopathology* (pp. 141–166). Palo Alto: Annual Reviews, Inc.
Ryff, C. D., & Singer, B. (1996). Psychological well-being: Meaning, measurement, and implications for psychotherapy research. *Psychotherapy and Psychosomatics, 65*(1), 14–23.
Ryff, C. D., & Singer, B. (2000). Interpersonal flourishing: A positive health agenda for the new millennium. *Personality and Social Psychology Review, 4*(1), 30–44.
Salyers, M. P., Godfrey, J. L., McGuire, A. B., Gearhart, T., Rollins, A. L., & Boyle, C. (2009). Implementing the illness management and recovery program for consumers with severe mental illness. *Psychiatric Services, 60*(4), 183–190.
Sayce, L. (2000). *From psychiatric patient to citizen: Overcoming discrimination and social exclusion.* London: Macmillan.
Sen, A. (1999). *Development as freedom.* New York: Anchor Books.
Silverstein, S., & Bellack, A. S. (2008). A scientific agenda for the concept of recovery as it applies to schizophrenia. *Clinical Psychology Review, 28*(7), 1108–1124.
Slade, M., Amering, M., & Oades, L. (2008). Recovery: An international perspective. *Epidemiologia e Psichiatria Sociale, 17*(2), 128–137.
Spaniol, L., & Koehler, M. (1994). *The experience of recovery.* Boston: Center for Psychiatric Rehabilitation, Sargent College of Health and Rehabilitation Sciences, Boston University.
Spaniol, L., Wewiorski, N. J., Gagne, C., & Anthony, W. A. (2002). The process of recovery from schizophrenia. *International Review of Psychiatry, 14*(4), 327–336.
Tedeschi, R. G., Park, C. L., & Calhoun, L. G. (1998). *Posttraumatic growth: Positive changes in the aftermath of crisis.* Mahwah: Lawrence Erlbaum.
Tennant, R., Hiller, L., Fishwick, R., Platt, S., Joseph, S., Weich, S., Parkinson, J., Secker, J., & Stewart-Brown, S. (2007). The Warwick-Edinburgh Mental Well-being Scale (WEMWBS): Development and UK validation. *Health and Quality of Life Outcomes, 5*, 63.
Torgalsboen, A. K. (2005). What is recovery from schizophrenia? In L. Davidson, C. Harding, & L. Spaniol (Eds.), *Recovery from severe mental illnesses: Research evidence and implications for practice* (Vol. 1, pp. 302–315). Boston: Center for Psychiatric Rehabilitation, Sargent College of Health and Rehabilitation Sciences, Boston University.
U.S. Public Health Service. (1999). *Mental health: A report of the Surgeon General.* Rockville: Author.
Ware, N. C., Hopper, K., Tugenberg, T., Dickey, B., & Fisher, D. (2007). Connectedness and citizenship: Redefining social integration. *Psychiatric Services, 58*(4), 469–474.
World Health Organization. (1948). *World Health Organization constitution Basic documents.* Geneva: Author.
Wunderink, L., Sytema, S., Nienhuis, F. J., & Wiersma, D. (2009). Clinical recovery in first-episode schizophrenia. *Schizophrenia Bulletin, 35*(2), 362–369.
Zubrick, S., & Kovess-Masfety, V. (2005). Indicators of mental health. In H. Herman, S. Saxena & R. Moodie (Eds.), *Promoting mental health: Concepts, emerging evidence, practice* A report of the World Health Organization, Department of Mental Health and Substance Abuse in collaboration with the Victorian Health Promotion Foundation and University of Melbourne. Geneva: World Health Organization.

Chapter 14
The Significance of Salutogenesis and Well-Being in Mental Health Promotion: From Theory to Practice

Eva Langeland and Hege Forbech Vinje

Salutogenesis (*salute*—of health, and *genesis*—the origins, or coming into existence) has its origin in Greek writings and was actualized in modern times by humanistic psychologists such as Carl Rogers, Abraham Maslow, and the late sociologist Aaron Antonovsky (1923–1994). It was Antonovsky (1979) who coined the term and developed the theory of salutogenesis as a neologism to pathogenesis and the emphasis in medicine on risk factors and diseases. He posed the question "What explains movement towards the health pole of the ease/dis-ease continuum?" (Antonovsky 1996a, p. 15). His answer to this salutogenic question was formulated in terms of the sense of coherence (SOC) and general resistance resources (GRR). The salutogenic model suggests how SOC may be strengthened and how it contributes to coping with the trials and tribulations of life, thereby contributing to health and well-being.

In considering mental illness treatment and recovery, traditional therapy has focused mainly on pathogenesis in connection with adverse life circumstances which have been dealt with by diagnosis and medication. Too little attention has been paid to salutogenesis, mental health promotion, and individuals' potential for recovery based on their resources. From the perspective of positive psychology, treatment should not be synonymous with fixing what is broken; it also requires nurturing what is best within us (Seligman 2002), since well-being *is* possible for people experiencing mental illness (Slade 2010).

As a result of research and theorizing on health as a positive state, and in addition to the search for a complement to traditional therapy, new orientations and concepts have emerged, including positive psychology (Snyder and Lopez 2007), empowerment (Wallerstein 2006), resilience (Friedli 2009), recovery (Slade 2010), and of course, salutogenesis (Antonovsky 1979, 1987, 1996a, b). These understandings

E. Langeland (✉)
Health and Social Sciences, Bergen University College, Bergen, Norway
e-mail: eva.langeland@hib.no

H.F. Vinje
Health Sciences, Vestfold University College, Horten, Norway
e-mail: hege.f.vinje@hive.no

C.L.M. Keyes (ed.), *Mental Well-Being: International Contributions to the Study of Positive Mental Health*, DOI 10.1007/978-94-007-5195-8_14,

challenge health professionals to facilitate peoples' movement toward higher levels of health. This includes a focus on macro-level factors, such as the promotion of social inclusion, which challenges stigma and discrimination and promotes societal well-being. In the twenty-first century, this orientation became the norm rather than the exception for mental health professionals (Slade 2010).

This chapter describes a talk-therapy intervention program which is based on a salutogenic approach (Langeland et al. 2007). This intervention has been evaluated in a randomized controlled trial study, showing positive effects on SOC. In addition, an evaluation performed by the group's participants revealed that between 85 and 95% experienced their participation as being greatly, or very greatly, contributive to better mental health, and had been useful, or very useful, to their everyday life (Langeland et al. 2006). Talk-therapy groups that have been conducted afterward (Langeland and Vinje 2010) have shown corresponding results in relation to strengthening SOC, mental health, well-being, and utility in everyday life. The knowledge base for the program is research, theory, and data from the participants' evaluation of the program.

Salutogenesis

The underlying assumptions which form the philosophical basis of salutogenesis are, for the most part, explicitly identified, although some must be inferred. Salutogenesis has an organic perspective, rather than the mechanistic perspective, of pathogenesis. The human being is viewed as an open system that contains social, psychological, and genetic subsystems, but it is the integration of the whole which is emphasized in the concept of SOC (Antonovsky 1979; Sullivan 1989). The theory of salutogenesis represents a broader perspective on health than does pathogenesis orientation. It does not view health as a dichotomous variable but instead as movement along a continuum. It focuses on the story of the whole person rather than on specific problems and diagnoses. It sees people as biological, psychological, social, and spiritual beings who are both proactive and reactive and who make choices. Persons are seen as actively involved in health seeking and self-actualization. Further, salutogenesis understands tension and strain as potentially health promoting, rather than as inevitably health damaging. The theory stresses the use of potential and/or existing resistance resources to enhance coping and not primarily on minimizing risk factors, as well as emphasizing active adaptation as the ideal in treatment (Antonovsky 1987). Table 14.1 contrasts and compares the basic assumptions and main concepts of salutogenesis and pathogenesis, as the assumptions and concepts of salutogenesis form the foundation of the talk-therapy intervention program described in this chapter.

Antonovsky (1987) explains that SOC is a global orientation that expresses the extent to which one has a pervasive, enduring, though dynamic feeling of confidence that the stimuli experienced in the course of living are structured, predictable, and explicable (i.e., have a comprehensibility), in addition to the extent to which the

Table 14.1 An overview of the basic assumptions and main concepts of the pathogenic and salutogenic models[a]

Assumptions regarding	Pathogenesis	Salutogenesis
Self-regulation of the system	Homeostasis	Overcoming heterostasis
	Mechanistic	Organic
Definition of health and disease	Dichotomy	Continuum
Scope of the concept of health	Pathology of disease	Resistance resources
	Diagnosis	Person's history
	Reductionism	Holism
		Sense of coherence
Causes of health and disease	Risk factors	Health-promoting factors
	Negative stressors	Person's history
Effect of stressors	Potentially causing disease	Potentially causing disease or promoting health
Intervention	Implementing effective remedies ("magic bullets")	Active adaptation, risk reduction, appropriate challenges, and resource development

[a]Adapted from Noack's work (as cited in Bengel et al. 1999, p. 32)

resources are available to meet the demands posed by these stimuli (i.e., a manageability) and the extent to which the demands are seen as challenges worthy of investment and engagement (i.e., meaning). To have a strong SOC is to be motivated to cope with stress, to believe that the challenge is understood, and to believe that coping resources are available.

The salutogenic orientation emphasizes four spheres in human life in which people must invest if they do not want to lose resources and meaning over time: inner feelings, immediate personal relationships, major activity, and existential issues (Antonovsky 1987). This means, as Lindstrøm (2001) explains, that it is important to be able to form a view of life (ideological, religious, or political), to know people one perceives to be supportive (the function of social support), to have mental stability, and to be involved in rewarding everyday activities, such as work, sports, and education.

Salutogenesis identifies perceived individual and collective GRRs that may promote the effective management of tension in demanding situations. Higher levels of GRRs are associated with a stronger SOC. Because the interaction between a person and the environment will always be in flux, it is not possible to identify all possible GRRs. Therefore, Antonovsky (1979) formulated the following definition that provides a criterion to identify GRRs: "every characterization of a person, group or environment that promotes effective management of tension" (p. 99).

In addition, he identifies the following GRRs as exemplars:

- *Culture* gives people a place in the world. SOC may be enhanced in a culture that enables social participation (e.g., participation in social decision-making, the visual arts, handicrafts, song, music, outdoor life, garden work, and different kinds of athletic sports).

- *Social support* is a crucial GRR. People who have close ties to others resolve tension more easily than those who lack that quality in their relationships. The perceived certainty about the availability of social support is often sufficient for this to be an effective component of GRR, with the quality of social support, such as intimate emotional ties, being especially important. The concept of *emotional closeness* refers to the degree to which a person experiences emotional ties and social integration in different groups (Sagy and Antonovsky 2000).
- *Religion and values* give direction and meaning to life.
- *Physical and biochemical* resources, such as a strong physique, good genes, and a strong immune system, are key GRRs.
- *Material goods,* such as money, food, clothing, and accommodation, are of obvious significance.
- *Continuity, overview, and control* are macro-sociocultural coping resources that are decided by the culture and society that a person is part of.
- Good *coping strategies* are characterized by rationality, flexibility, and foresight, including the ability to regulate emotions.
- *Knowledge and intelligence.*
- *Self-identity* is a resource on the emotional level and is a crucial coping resource.

The relationship between GRR and SOC is reciprocal. GRRs, such as social support, lead to a stronger SOC, and it is SOC that makes a person able to mobilize and make use of social support (Antonovsky 1979; Landsverk and Kane 1998). When people experience concordance between their use of GRRs and their expectations, wishes, and demands, life's challenges are experienced as *appropriate*. The experience of appropriate challenges in daily life strengthens SOC.

A Positive Mental Health Concept

Mental health may be conceptualized in either negative or positive terms. A negative conceptualization of mental health is based on an understanding that the absence of symptoms indicates good mental health. A positive mental health concept focuses on the presence of health-promoting factors, such as meaningful work and good relationships. Mental health is more than the absence or minimization of mental symptoms, since states and capacities have value in themselves. According to the WHO's definition of mental health, it is "a state of well-being in which the individual realizes his or her own abilities, can cope with the normal stresses of life, can work productively and fruitfully, and is able to make a contribution to his or her community" (WHO 2001, p. 1).

In salutogenesis, the primary focus is on the dynamic interaction between health-promoting factors and stressors in human life and on how people can move to the healthier end of the health continuum. A sense of coherence is proposed to be a significant variable in affecting this movement (Antonovsky 1985). Mental health refers to a person's position at any point in the life cycle on "… a continuum that

		MENTAL PROBLEMS	
		MANY	FEW
PLEASURES	MANY	1. Many pleasures and many problems	2. Many pleasures and few problems
	FEW	3. Few pleasures and many problems	4. Few pleasures and few problems

Fig. 14.1 Mental health in relation to mental well-being

ranges from excruciating emotional pain and total psychological malfunctioning, at one extreme, to a full, vibrant sense of psychological well-being at the other" (Antonovsky 1985, p. 274).

Antonovsky describes the movement on the continuum toward better mental health as shifting:

> [F]rom the use of unconscious psychological defense mechanisms toward the use of conscious coping mechanisms; from the rigidity of defensive structures to the capacity for constant and creative inner readjustment and growth; from a waste of emotional energy toward its productive use; from emotional suffering toward joy; from narcissism toward giving of oneself; and from exploitation of others to reciprocal interaction. (Antonovsky 1985, p. 274)

The concept of mental health has developed over time, becoming more and more directed toward well-being. To a larger extent, newer research in psychiatry focuses on well-being by strengthening positive experiences rather than by limiting treatment to reducing or removing the illness or symptoms. Quality-of-life assessments for people with sustained mental health problems have increasingly taken an overall well-being perspective by assessing multiple life domains, including measures of functional status, access to resources and opportunities, and a *sense* of well-being.

Næss and Eriksen (2006, p. 39) reveal what mental health is comprised of in relation to *quality-of-life* (defined as mental well-being) measurements in the figure above (Fig. 14.1).

Quality-of-life research searches for knowledge that may contribute to the reduction of problems and the increase of pleasures. Traditional mental health research has not made a distinction between boxes 1 and 3 or 2 and 4. It has aimed primarily at getting people out of boxes 1 and 3, typically by conflating disease and quality of life and by including symptom scales within the measures used to assess quality of life (Rapley 2003). The aim of the salutogenic perspective may be understood as bringing as many people as possible into box 2 with many pleasures and few problems, whereas a sense of coherence is theorized to enhance coping and adaptation by the use of general resistance resources (GRR), which effectively mediate the tension caused by omnipresent stressors and ultimately reduce the number of stressful experiences (Antonovsky 1979, 1987; Landsverk and Kane 1998), thereby increasing overall well-being. This is compatible with the salutogenic definition of mental health.

Mental Health Promotion

Although health promotion is a central focus in society in general, this concept has had a minimal presence in psychiatric services (Berger 2003; Langeland 2007b). Mental health promotion and well-being perspectives allow for the evaluation of people's broader life situations, as opposed to just narrowly focusing on disease. These perspectives are rooted in postmodern public health and the realization of the Ottawa Charter in terms of salutogenesis and well-being (Lindstrøm and Eriksson 2006). In the Ottawa Charter (WHO 1986), health promotion is defined as the process of enabling people to both increase control over, and improve their health, and health is seen as a resource for daily life. The charter underscores that health promotion action aims at enabling all people to achieve their fullest health potential, including a secure foundation in a supportive environment as well as access to information, life skills, and opportunities for making healthy choices. The main understanding is that people cannot achieve their fullest health potential unless they are able to take control of those things that determine their health. The core component of the principles of health promotion is suggested to be a combination of salutogenesis and well-being, in which salutogenesis is the process that leads to well-being (Lindstrøm and Eriksson 2006). Mental health promotion often refers to positive mental health and involves adopting an approach based on a positive view of mental health, instead of emphasizing mental illness and deficits. It considers mental health as a resource, as valuable, and as a basic human right, which implies the need to create individual, social, and cultural conditions that enable optimal psychological development.

Realizing that mental health is more than the absence of illness can be helpful to people with mental health problems and to their careers. Protective health resources and positive mental health can coexist with occasional severe mental symptoms, such as in people living with schizophrenia. This highlights the value of developing more comprehensive clinical approaches with an additional focus on people's positive mental health, such as their strengths, capabilities, and personal effort in the recovery process. Assessing and building on strengths help people to cope with mental health problems in order to avoid being further diminished by them (Schmolke 2003). Three health-promoting factors have been identified as important to the recovery process (Anthony et al. 1994; Strauss 1996), which are that people (a) perceive themselves as something other than just a diagnosis and a disease, (b) explore themselves with respect to their whole person, and (c) take control over their own lives. Additional factors such as hope, identity, meaning, and personal responsibility have emerged as central in the recovery process (Slade 2010).

Moreover, data from 40 years of research provides strong empirical support for the benefits of privileging participants to their role in the process of change. As a result, treatment should be organized around participants' resources, perceptions, experiences, and ideas (Duncan et al. 2010).

The Salutogenic Model Applied in Clinical Settings

Research shows the significance of the salutogenic approach in mental health promotion, including various mental health problems (Langeland 2007b; Langeland and Vinje 2010; Griffiths 2009), schizophrenia (Schmolke 2003; Bengtsson-Tops and Hansson 2001; Landsverk and Kane 1998) and depression (Skärsäter et al. 2005; Carstens and Sprangenberg 1997). The Sense of Coherence Questionnaire (Antonovsky 1987) has been used in many intervention studies in mental health to measure outcome (Blomberg et al. 2001; Kørlin and Wrangsjø 2002; Lundqvist 1995; Sack et al. 1997; Weissbecker et al. 2002). To the best of our knowledge, however, the entire salutogenic model of health (including all the basic assumptions and core concepts about health) developed as salutogenic therapy principles and interventions has not previously been applied in either a research or clinical setting and is not described in the literature. Nevertheless, there is some literature on the different aspects of the application of salutogenesis. For example, one study has attempted to adapt the core concept of SOC as a theoretical basis of previously established psychological education in schizophrenia (Landsverk and Kane 1998). Other studies have used elements of salutogenic thinking, such as the creation of empowering dialogues in general practice (Malterud and Hollnagel 1999), in the treatment of depression in schizophrenia (Menzies 2000), in the treatment of conduct disorder (Hansson et al. 2004), and in couples therapy (Lundblad and Hansson 2005), and a salutogenic framework of family members' experiences with palliative home care staff has been developed (Milberg and Strang 2007). Others have developed models with elements of salutogenic thinking, such as an assets model (Morgan and Ziglio 2007) and the Red Lotus Health Promotion model (Gregg and O'Hara 2007).

Based on this, one may conclude that there is a need for intervention studies in which the primary outcome sought is SOC, coping, and health (defined as a person's subjective experience of being in a positive state of well-being). Furthermore, it has been suggested that the most immediate research of the salutogenic model of health should now be implemented as a guide to mental health promotion initiatives and research (Erikson and Lindstrøm 2005). Bengel et al. (1999) emphasized that developing salutogenic therapy principles and intervention programs is of great importance for the future development of salutogenesis in the recovery framework.

Theoretical Framework for Salutogenic Talk-Therapy Groups

Theory is a frame of reference that is crucial in research and in program evaluation. An intervention is not ready to be evaluated unless the theoretical basis of the intervention has been developed and implemented, given that the judicious use of a theoretical framework can illuminate areas that might otherwise not be visible (Taylor 2004). An intervention may serve as a guide to mental health practice when better coping, well-being, and positive mental health are the main targets.

The salutogenic talk-therapy group intervention program has been developed for people with different mental health problems and consists of 16 talk-therapy meetings which last for 2 h and 15 min each, with additional homework, for a period of 16 weeks. Although the intervention program described in this chapter has been specifically developed for people with mental health problems, we will argue that it may also be adapted to people with different health problems, as the salutogenic approach primarily gives a general description of how SOC, health, and well-being may be strengthened. Additionally, anyone whose aim is increased coping and thriving in everyday life should focus on mental health.

Acquiring and applying this knowledge about salutogenesis in one's practice may be used as a tool for shedding light on people's strengths and raise people's consciousness about their health and well-being. All knowledge that may help implement a salutogenic approach in the best possible way is therefore relevant for practitioners, researchers, and other professionals. In addition to the salutogenic model of health, the approach in our research consists of knowledge from positive psychology (Snyder and Lopez 2007), which includes mental health as flourishing (Keyes 2007a, b), flow as optimal experience (Csikszentmihayi 1997; Lutz 2009), authentic happiness (Seligman 2002), recovery processes (Slade 2010), and the self-tuning model of self-care (Vinje and Mittelmark 2006; Vinje 2007). One theory of social support (Weiss 1974) supports the operationalization of social support, which Antonovsky regards to be a vital resistance resource. Both Weiss and Antonovsky emphasize the importance of the quality of social support. Rogers' experience of person-centered therapy (Rogers 1957) corroborates the fact that the attitudes of unconditional positive regard, accurate empathy, and genuineness perceived by participants in their helpers are necessary for therapeutic progress. Bandura's (1991) self-efficacy theory points to various ways of strengthening in a group process, whereas Antonovsky's other vital resistance resource, self-identity, uses the five unique capacities through which he claims a person learns: self-regulation, symbolizing, vicarious learning, forethought, and self-reflection (Antonovsky 1991). Narrative therapy (Anderson and Goolishian 1988, 1992) provides tools to encourage participants' awareness of their coping histories, thus increasing their consciousness in relation to their internal and external resources. Interventions drawn from solution-focused therapies can be effective when the aim is to increase participants' insight into their coping ability (de Shazer 1991; Watkins 2001). These theories and knowledge support, supply, and emphasize the interpretation and operationalization of a salutogenic approach.

Implementation of Theoretical Perspectives

Aim of the Salutogenic Approach

The main aim of a salutogenic approach is to increase participants' awareness of and confidence in their potential, their internal and external resources, and their ability to use these to increase their SOC, coping, and level of mental health and well-being. Accordingly, the focus is on how to enter into a good circle or positive feedback loop. The intervention has been developed for people with various, but relatively stable, mental health problems who are able to have a dialogue and live in their private homes, but need some support from the health system. The concept of mental health problems used here typically encompasses mental suffering, mental illness, mental disorders, mental problems, and psychosocial problems.

Salutogenic Talk-Therapy Groups

In salutogenic talk-therapy groups, the leaders arrange for participants to acquire experiences that strengthen and increase SOC and well-being. It has been suggested that experiences which are characterized by consistency, emotional closeness, load balance, a sense of belonging, and participation in shaping outcomes contribute in promoting SOC (Antonovsky 1991; Sagy and Antonovsky 2000). These experiences may enable the participants to stay well or get well, and are sought within the groups.

The intervention is specially developed for talk-therapy groups, with mental health professionals as the group leaders. The intervention consists of the salutogenic therapy principles that reflect the attitudes desired and the focus of the program, illustrating what the topics and homework in the sessions might look like. In talk-therapy groups, a central ideal is that conversations are characterized as a therapeutic *dialogue* (Egan 2002), while the groups are characterized by mutual, egalitarian relationships, in which the tenor of conversations between the group leaders and participants is similar to those between the participants themselves (Antonovsky 1990; Gilligan and Price 1993; Rogers 1980). Traditionally, mental health professionals learn to maintain their distance and stay in control. This is important, though research demonstrates that intimacy, spontaneity, and personal engagement may have therapeutic effects (Borg 2007; Langeland and Wahl 2009).

The reason for choosing a group as the best method is the beneficial effect of *symbolic interactionism* (Blumer 1969). Further, Yalom (1975) identifies 11 interdependent therapeutic group aims: to give hope, to encourage universalization, to share information, to engender altruism, to try new approaches, to develop social competence, to promote vicarious learning, to promote learning between people, to encourage group solidarity, to achieve catharsis, and to encourage existential viewpoints.

The Role of the Group Leader

The group leader focuses on creating a conversational and interactional climate that will promote a desirable change in the participants. By acknowledging one's inability to know the participants' *truth*, the group leader conveys a combination of unconditional positive regard, empathy, and genuineness by respecting that the participants are experts on themselves and their unique situations and experiences, including their pain, suffering, and concerns (Rogers 1957). From a salutogenic perspective, the group leader functions more as a dialogue partner, achieving a balance between listening empathetically to participants' difficulties while taking into account their strengths and resources (Duncan et al. 2010). It is the attitude and confidence in people's innate potential for growth and development that is in focus. The group may function as a *facilitator of self-definition*, and a considerable onus is placed on providers and consumers to build the type of relationship that can inspire hope that will help bolster positive thoughts against the negative impact of societal stigma and marginalization (Stanhope and Solomon 2008).

To be qualified as a group leader, the leaders participate in a 3-week training program containing the theoretical framework of salutogenesis, the supporting theories, and implementation of the salutogenic therapy principles (see the next chapter), including how to be a good group leader and dialogue partner (Langeland 2007b).

The Mental Health Promotion Process: A Salutogenic Approach

The basic assumptions and core concepts in salutogenesis, including supporting theories, may be operationalized into a salutogenic approach, as illustrated in Table 14.2.

The five basic components or therapy principles in this intervention are as follows: (1) the health continuum model, (2) the story of the person, (3) health-promoting (salutary) factors, (4) the understanding of tension and strain as potentially health promoting, and (5) active adaptation (Antonovsky 1987).

Health as Two Continua

Movement Toward Health

To promote health from a salutogenic perspective, the primary focus must be on the dynamic interaction between resistance resources and stressors in human life and how to help the participants to move toward the healthy end of that continuum. For example, this can be done by asking a rating question: "On a

Table 14.2 A mental health promotion process in talk-therapy groups based on a salutogenic approach

Salutogenesis	Salutogenic therapy principles	Desired outcomes
1. Health as two continua	– Movement toward health	– *Increasing tolerance for various feelings*
	– Universalizing mental health problems	– *Improving active adaptation*
	– Introducing the metaphor of the stream of life	
2. The story of the participant	– Diagnosis as a narrow description	– *Experiencing oneself as a person*
	– Listening to the participant's narrative identity: shedding light on individual coping ability	– *Structuring life experiences that reinforce sense of coherence*
		– *Increasing perception of coping in the narrative identity*
3. Health-promoting (salutary) factors	– Extending coping resources	– *Improving self-identity*
	– Paying attention to what is currently functioning well and asking questions to increase the awareness of resources	– *Increasing perception of the quality of social support such as attachment, social integration, opportunity for nurturing, reassurance of worth, reliable alliance, and guidance*
	– Promoting resistance resources, particularly social support and self-identity	
4. Stress, tension, and strain as potentially health promoting	– Discussing appropriate challenges	– *Increasing acceptance of one's own potential and coping ability*
	– Universalizing the feelings of tension	– *Experiencing one's resources*
5. Active adaptation	– Promoting a climate of unconditional positive regard, empathy, and genuineness	– *Experiencing motivation for change*
	– Developing participants' unique capacities	– *Thinking more salutogenic and developing positive patterns for health promotion*
	– Developing crucial spheres in human existence	– *Increasing perceptions of comprehensibility, manageability, and meaning; improving SOC*
	– Stimulating flow experiences	– *Increasing emotional, psychological, and social well-being; positive mental health*

scale of 0–10, in which 0 is the worst and 10 is the best you have ever felt, how do you rate yourself today?" If the answer is 7, you may ask why the answer is 7 and not 5. By the use of such a solution-focused question, one may increase a person's attention on coping possibilities, on good experiences, and on the

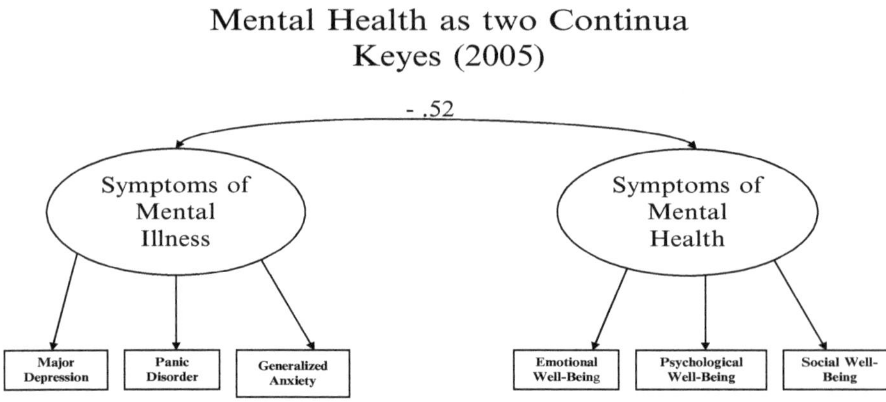

Fig. 14.2 Mental health as two continua

perceptions of health-promoting factors. The next question may be "What do you need to do to move yourself up to an 8?" This may be a method of increasing the participant's awareness of coping, of positive experiences, and/or of different health-promoting factors. In this way, one's attention is focused on possibilities, and the attention is placed on adding resources and on what is functioning well in their lives.

Newer research reveals that it is clinically relevant to define mental health as a two continua model because people may have symptoms of both mental health *and* mental illness, thereby indicating the need for health professionals to support a reduction of the symptoms of mental illness and an improvement in the symptoms of mental health (Keyes 2007a). Keyes' study documents that symptoms of mental health and of mental illness are two different dimensions that have a relationship which, together, constitute the overall level of mental health. Confirmatory factor analysis reveals that the latent factors of mental health and mental illness are correlated at --.52. From a clinical standpoint, this means that although there is a tendency for mental health to improve when mental illness decreases, this connection is moderate (see Fig. 14.2, Keyes 2005, 2007b).

The mere absence of the symptoms of mental illness does not necessarily mean a happy life, whereas the presence of these symptoms does not necessarily mean an unhappy life (Keyes 2007a, b; Hyland 1992). It is necessary to experience the presence of salutogenic factors in order to thrive and attain well-being. Symptoms do not always cause problems because the relationship between these two variables is moderated by other psychological factors (Hyland 1992). These factors may be various coping strategies (Bandura 1991) and the experiencing of *flourishing* as emotional, psychological, and social well-being (Keyes 2007a).

The clinical relevance of this view of health became obvious in one of the talk-therapy groups when a participant discovered that she could be healthy, even though she had an illness. It was a good "aha" experience for her to think that she could be both depressed and in a good mood, but not at the same time. Although she had a diagnosis of depression, she could feel healthy. This is an example of how a person is influenced by the concepts we describe ourselves with and in how we define each other. By defining herself in a more constructive way, one that she acknowledge as meaningful, she experienced a more encouraging self-image.

Accordingly, knowledge about how to promote good mental health may yield important therapeutic insights on how to strengthen health-promoting competence among people with long-term mental health problems. From a salutogenic perspective, Keyes argues that the signs of mental health may be emotional, psychological, and social well-being. Emotional well-being is characterized by being happy, interested, and satisfied with life. Signs of psychological well-being are self-acceptance, environmental mastery, positive relationships with others, personal growth, autonomy, and purpose in life. Social well-being includes making a contribution to society, social integration, social growth, acceptance of others, social interest, and coherence (Keyes 2007a).

Universalizing Mental Health Problems

People have different levels of health, but on the same two continua. This universalism is a precondition to understanding and judging another participant's expression. Some examples of topics that the participants and leaders may recognize as universal in daily life are existing and possible new relationships, how to organize the day, how to receive criticism and praise, how to balance activity and rest, how to practice self-care, and how to cope with sleeping problems. To illustrate universalism and health development, Antonovsky uses the following metaphor, which can be presented to a salutogenic talk-therapy group.

Introducing the Metaphor of the Stream of Life

All human beings are in a river that is the stream of life, and nobody stays on the shore. It is not enough to promote health by avoiding stress or by building bridges to keep people from falling into the river. Instead, people have to learn to swim. There are forks in the river that can lead to gentle streams or to dangerous rapids and whirlpools. The crucial, salutogenic question is "Wherever one is in the stream, what shapes and promotes one's ability to swim well?" (Antonovsky 1987). This way of looking at life may be useful in group work because the participants can easily identify with it, thus acknowledging and accepting their own ups and downs and focusing on adaptive behavior (how to swim well) in everyday life.

The Story of the Participant

Mental health professionals can help people to structure life experiences in such a way that may enhance and reinforce SOC. A person's individual story is important because only in the awareness of one's life situation can the resources that contribute to recovery be found, understood, and fostered. The pathways to recovery are uniquely defined by each person individually and need to be holistic in scope since mental health problems are complex interactions of mind, body, spirit, and social environment that are unique to each individual. Accordingly, the focus in the groups is on each participant as a whole and on their own experiences. Participants use their own words and describe their inner lives. Stories about recovery processes may reduce stigma by illustrating that people with mental health problems are as ordinary and human as others; consequently, such stories may represent good, vicarious learning. It is often a challenge to get people out of their diagnosis (*the diagnostic box*), but only when they do so will they experience and increase the consciousness of their own individuality and identity.

Diagnosis as a Narrow Description

Salutogenesis underpins the importance of acknowledging the participant primarily as a person and mobilizing his or her strengths so that the person's resistance resources are given the best possible conditions in the fight against illness and suffering (Malterud and Solvang 2005). Receiving a diagnosis influences people's self-understanding in that they experience themselves as psychiatric patients and/or a diagnosis. Identifying the whole person by one characteristic reduces people to a label, which functions as a barrier to recovery. Ahern and Fisher (2001) state that people in a recovery process may view every expression of emotion or change in mood as a symptom of an illness in remission that can return at any time. Accordingly, a person with a psychiatric diagnosis may experience being deprived of the right to be a normal human being with various normal feelings because what this person says and does is interpreted as related to the diagnosis (being within the diagnostic box). Taking responsibility for one's life may disappear together with the feeling of self when a diagnosis is identified. In this context, it may be helpful to encourage the perception of a diagnosis as a narrow description of reality (White 1991, 1997). As a result, the aim of the participant is to rediscover the self as a person beyond the diagnosis, by looking at various feelings as parts of being a normal human being, and to accept the experiences as positive, all of which are important parts of becoming a person (Rogers 1961). Each participant is given assistance in rediscovering the self as a whole person. In this rediscovery process, the group leader acts more as a *facilitator of self-definition* (Stanhope and Solomon 2008). In this respect, leaders have an important task as a role model. When the therapist expresses feelings that are genuine and from the heart, it can be pivotal because the therapist then contributes to universalizing various feelings. This process of discovery may be defined as recovery. The utility of diagnosis in relation to treatment and prognosis may be limited (Duncan et al. 2010). Included in the group of depressed people, there are large variations with regard to the level of suffering and motivation for treatment. Depression comprises both deeper depression and a more general depression as an answer to normal loss and disappointment. Not knowing about the diagnosis and case history may be an advantage, making it possibly easier to meet participants in a freer, more open, and less prejudiced manner. Rogers (1961) confirms this experience when he claims that a diagnosis may be more of an obstacle than a help. Our group leaders experienced this as well. At the start of a group, they only needed to know that the participants were struggling on a daily basis with mental health problems and that they needed some type of help and support. We therefore recommend that the inclusion criteria for salutogenic talk-therapy groups be based on the person and on individual levels of functioning, and on the ability to participate in dialogue, and not be based on the diagnosis (Langeland et al. 2006, 2007). As symptom reduction becomes replaced by the more holistic personal goals of the participants, a diagnosis will exert less of an influence on how they perceive themselves (Stanhope and Solomon 2008).

Listening to the Participant's Narrative Identity: Shedding Light on Individual's Coping Ability

It is decisive to view the participants as persons who are signified as the bearers of stories of heroic effort (everyday heroes) that exceed their stories about their suffering. It is important to see the significance of acknowledging and exhibiting respect for the power that exists in gaining control over the difficulties in individuals' lives (Duncan et al. 2004).

Stories, however, are gross simplifications. To illustrate this, one may use the following figure or ground metaphor: A story may be perceived as a figure that appears based on a certain background. When a participant's story is saturated with problems, it may be important to ask for alternative stories, out of which another figure may appear that is unique to the situation, and in which the person perceives meaning, motivation, energy, and the ability to cope (White and Epston 1990). Consequently, the person's narrative identity is changed through new stories as a result of the dialogue (Anderson and Goolishian 1988). The salutogenic perspective focuses on how to activate, emancipate, and increase participants' perceptions of their resources and potentials that are, to say it with Rogers (1961), on the edge of their awareness. It can be said that this process can shed light on other parts of participants' experiences. All experience is real, but nevertheless we cannot gain insight into the entire experience at the same time. Hence, one may say that this therapy is insight-oriented, as it reveals the person's ability to actively adapt (Antonovsky

1987) and to self-tune, with the aim of achieving active coping (Vinje and Mittelmark 2006). The participants have little insight into these abilities when they are standing in the shadow of the history of their dominant problem. Even so, it is important to stress that participants' experiences should be acknowledged and validated before they can begin to open up to new possibilities and directions (Gilligan and Price 1993; Rogers 1957). Subsequently, from an empathetic stance, the leader may encourage participants to create an identity that has coherence and meaning for them, though it is the participants themselves who must choose whether they want to integrate an alternative story as part of their identity.

Health-Promoting (Salutary) Factors

Extending Coping Resources

The salutogenic orientation leads to thinking in terms of factors which promote participants' movement toward the healthy end of the continuum. We cannot limit the promotion of health to being low on risk factors because health-promoting factors actively contribute to health in a direct manner (Antonovsky 1996a, b). This approach can be operationalized in the groups by focusing on adding resources in contrast to revealing the causes of problems. Causes of the problems do not need to be found before possibilities for promoting health are found. One example may be a man who is suffering from voices in his head. A central question may concern what other voices he can add instead of how he can dispel the existing voices. The critical skill needed in controlling the voices would be the man's ability to obtain a sufficient voice of his own in his social environment, and consequently feeling stronger than the voices both inside and outside his head (Romme and Escher 1993).

Another example is when a person with alcohol problems in treatment perceives a one-sided focus to stop drinking. However, what will the person do to thrive in life, and what will this person fill life with if not drinking? This illustrates that less "bad stuff" is not compatible with increased thriving. Health and well-being are more than the absence of negative influences. A focus on the factors that shape how well a person thrives, as well as the "good stuff," may increase the experience of meaning and well-being. A perception of meaning creates energy and motivation.

Paying Attention to What Is Currently Functioning Well in Participants' Lives and Asking Questions to Increase the Awareness of Resources

From a salutogenic viewpoint, it is essential to pay attention to what is functioning well in participants' lives and to the good experiences, as opposed to the bad experiences, and to draw out the optimistic potential from stories saturated with problems (de Shazer 1991). The main point is to ask questions that stimulate the person to think of resources or possible resources, or to invite that person to "conjure up" or wishfully think such resources into being. In addition, people may be helped to identify current strategies by asking solution-focused questions (Watkins 2001). For example, the leader may ask a participant who suffers from depression: "How do you manage to endure despite your suffering?" Such a question may increase that person's consciousness of available resources and current coping strategies. The next question may be whether the participant can apply these experiences to new situations. Another example is of a woman who talks about suffering from anxiety. She may be asked what is occurring when her symptoms of anxiety are fewer and whether she can describe situations in which she has feelings of well-being and is not suffering from anxiety. In that way, her experience of her own coping resources and well-being can be increased. Another description of what may be in focus in a salutogenic talk-therapy group can be seen in the example where the participant describes how a rather difficult day has been managed. The participant answers by saying it was accomplished by simply focusing on and working on different everyday activities, despite a feeling of heaviness. The participant divides the duties into partial aims, and the whole thing gradually becomes easier; in this way, a sense of coping appears.

Yet another example is to ask a question that takes the problem away—the miracle question (de Shazer 1991). The group leader may say: "Now I will come with a curious question. It's evening and you've gone to bed. While you are sleeping, your suffering disappears without you knowing it. When you wake up—how will you recognize that your problems are gone? How will your environment recognize it?" A question such as this allows the person to bring more of the previous unproblematic experiences into the conversation; thus, the goals developing from the miracle question are not limited to just eliminating the problem.

Promoting Resistance Resources, Particularly Social Support and Self-Identity

Social support and self-identity appear as the most direct GRRs (Antonovsky 1979). Social support is a crucial GRR, with a key aim of the groups being the establishment of a good climate so that participants can develop positive connections to their natural supports. Thus, self-isolation is actively challenged within the groups.

Weiss (1974) supports Antonovsky's view on social support and has identified six social functions, or *provisions*, that may be obtained from relationships with others. An attempt could be made to apply these six relational provisions in the groups to better facilitate health-promoting interaction and communication. These provisions are attachment, social integration, opportunity for nurturing, reassurance of worth, reliable alliance, and guidance. The leaders may focus on those whom the participants refer to as helpful in their daily life and/or those things they do to get people to help them. One may also try to increase the awareness of opportunities for nurturing. An example of the latter is when participants reflect on their ability to nurture and when one of the participants says to another: "I experience that you are such a positive person." The participant then demonstrates having appreciation for the positive feedback. Focusing on this will increase awareness of their resources and of who they are, which, in turn, strengthens their manageability and self-identity.

Newer research reveals that the ability to give nurturance is especially important in raising consciousness among people with mental health problems because they are often recipients of care; accordingly, their coping may be strengthened (Langeland and Wahl 2009). Their strengthened social competence may subsequently be applied in settings outside the group.

Action and choice enhances self-identity and confirms who the participants are. If a participant carries out an action that represents a new, good experience, it will weaken this participant's particular problematic history, thereby changing and improving self-identity. Being encouraged toward constructive action is a basic step in the gradual process of changing one's self-identity, while undertaking choices is yet another factor that enhances self-identity and mental health. Increasing participants' consciousness of their own possible choices is therefore key in the groups. Choice may be defined as an active, reflected decision with respect to the alternatives. Nonetheless, reflection seems to be a process intertwined with introspection, which are both two key elements in the skill of self-tuning (Vinje and Mittelmark 2006).

Within the groups, the participants are stimulated to engage in self-examination and the contemplation of their own thoughts, feelings, desires, dreams, and the meaningfulness of life (introspection), in addition to comparing this inner comprehension with the outer world, available resources, and the possibilities of living in accordance with it (reflection). Vital to this process is the strengthening of one's *sensibility,* referring to the participants' self-sensitivity and awareness (Vinje and Mittelmark 2006). Vinje and Mittelmark (2006) show that when people become adept at self-care, a relatively constant introspection takes place in the form of sensibility, which is a prereflective, preverbal ability used to receive and read signals from our own bodies, emotions, existential depths, and social environment. This triggers reflection, and a key element of reflection is self-monitoring, through which one may gain an appreciation of how events and feelings are interrelated. In the groups, we found that this process enabled self-tuning to be accomplished through changes in one's situation and/or in the self, which seemed to enhance the participants' health-promoting recovery processes (Langeland and Vinje 2010).

Self-regulation by setting limits may be an important issue for many participants, such as how to decline an invitation. Because of this, a key topic is proposing alternatives on how participants can regulate themselves to choose among different proposals and to take responsibility for their choices. Responsibility emancipates resources and thus creates hope for the future (intentionality). To move from doing *depressive activities* to doing *pleasurable activities* is an example of a result of constructive and conscious self-development and identity (Laitinen et al. 2007).

Stressors, Tension, and Strain as Potentially Health Promoting

Implicit in the salutogenic model is the view that stressors, tension, and strain are potentially health promoting.

Discussing Appropriate Challenges

In the groups, the participants are challenged to adapt to a variety of stressful circumstances because exposure to stress factors (such as new people and experiences) is a necessary part of maturation, growth, and development (Ahern and Fisher 2001). The salutogenic model distinguishes between tension and stress. When demands exceed a person's resources or, more precisely, a person's ability to use resources, then the tension created by the stressor leads to stress, and the person moves toward a lower level of health. Accordingly, setting appropriate challenges is of great importance in creating life experiences that promote SOC and enable coping.

In this model, health is considered a process in which people learn to identify resources which contribute to health and to use these resources (a) to experience life as being consistent, (b) to find an appropriate overload/underload balance, and (c) to participate in making decisions that are relevant to one's own life. Over time, a person with many such experiences comes to see the world as one that makes sense (Antonovsky 1987). Thus, a measure for what is an appropriate challenge is whether the challenge in question is experienced as consistent, is contributing to an overload/underload balance, and is one whereby the participants are invited to decide on whether what is taking place in the group is relevant to their life.

Universalizing the Feelings of Tension

This view of tension and stress is reflected in the leader's attitude, for example, by acknowledging that the feeling of tension the participants may often feel in a group, particularly in the beginning, can be generalized by emphasizing that this is a normal feeling. Leaders can also admit that they sometimes feel tension within a group. Such admissions may contribute to universalism and become a release for the participants.

Active Adaptation

A basic argument in the salutogenic approach is the therapists' attitude toward treatment. An active adaptation is considered the ideal in treatment, and the focus is on the person with a unique history and overall problem of active adaptation to an inevitably stressor-rich environment. Each person needs to be treated based on individual positions in life and on individual perceptions of this.

Promoting a Climate of Unconditional Positive Regard, Empathy, and Genuineness

A combination of the basic, general, active attitudes of unconditional positive regard, accurate empathy, and genuineness offered by the helper and perceived by the participants is necessary for creating a climate in the group that fosters therapeutic progress (Rogers 1957).

People with mental health problems usually feel vulnerable, though in itself vulnerability does not necessarily create motivation for change. Research shows that clients are motivated to change primarily by their perception of the quality of the group leader's or co-participants' empathic positive regard (Braaten 1999). Accordingly, a person's readiness for change, and for revealing one's vulnerability, is based on their perceived unconditional positive regard, accurate empathy, and genuineness from significant others, which gives energy to their emotional, psychological, social, and behavioral preparation for implementing change.

The provider of care must be highly empathetic and sensitive to the process of relating to the participants as whole persons. Antonovsky (1987, p. 9) maintains: "When one searches for effective adaptation of the organism, one can move beyond post-Cartesian dualism and look to imagination, love, play, meaning, will, and the social structure that foster them." Our experience from teaching self-tuning to students of health promotion is that activating and developing introspection, sensibility, and reflection involves being vulnerable in the sense of opening up to life and becoming aware of feelings, bodily sensations, relationships, patterns of thought, and signals from existential depths (Vinje 2007). In the talk-therapy groups, it is particularly apparent that it is the trustful climate of the group that stimulates the opening up to oneself and to other group members. This process of becoming aware helps one to become increasingly more in tune with one's self and to express one's strengthened self-identity in real life. Hence, a sense of coherence may be enhanced from inside and out, so to speak. The willingness to show one's vulnerability due to a caring, accepting, and trustful atmosphere seems to be a characteristic of these groups and seems to be an important resource that stimulates the health-promoting process.

Developing Participants' Unique Capabilities

An important element in people's motivation to change is the expectation that their actions will produce the desired results. A belief in themselves determines their initial decision to work on their problems, to expend effort, and to be persistent in the face of adversity (Bandura 1991). This underscores the importance of people's most significant others, such as the group leader and co-participants, having a belief in their possibilities for recovery.

The five unique capacities through which a person learns are self-regulation, self-reflection, symbolizing, forethought, and vicarious learning (Antonovsky 1991). These potentialities may be used consciously when working with active adaptation within the groups. The salutogenic approach views the human being as an open self-regulating system. A person with a high level of health manages self-regulation. Additionally, Antonovsky highlights self-reflection as an essential tool for constructing coping stories and for people helping each other to find external and internal resources in the active adaptation to various challenging situations through creative processes. Rogers (1961) also emphasizes self-reflection as being basic to all personal development and as an important tool in the process of emancipating people's autonomy and actualizing tendencies inherent in humans. Self-reflection strengthens self-identity and self-worth. The aim is to increase consciousness and symbolization by grasping the knowledge that exists on the edge (*the hazy area*) of a person's awareness (*subceptions*). Moreover, increased consciousness strengthens forethought in that a person becomes more able to influence their own development and outcome.

Sense in SOC includes both perceptions and subceptions. When working with increased consciousness, the subceptions become perceptions. In this way, SOC may be strengthened by increased knowledge and comprehensibility. For that reason, people's experiences may be more conscious and extended.

Participants may also learn by listening to each other and learning vicariously through not only other's experiences but from those of the group leaders as well. One participant says that on several occasions when she felt bad, she had gotten an inner picture from another participant who had told a coping story. She then thought that she could do the same. She succeeded, and it became a good coping experience for her. To be each other's role models in the group may thus be an important change factor. Our experience is in accordance with these arguments, although we also find it valuable to emphasize introspection and sensibility in order to more fully explain the process at play. It is not reflection, per se, that is important, but the reflection that is triggered by introspection and the contemplation of one's own thoughts, feelings, desires, dreams, and meaning of life. Reflection is also dependent on a sensibility defined as a precognitive apprehension of one's inner state (Vinje 2007). Sensibility therefore represents a vital part of the participant's self-communication, in which the signals from the self are captured by the participant and made the object of reflection.

Developing Crucial Spheres in Human Existence

An important part of personal development and recovery is that participants themselves take more control of their own development. This is why it may be a primary objective in the groups to try to increase participants' awareness of and investment in the vital topics inner feelings, immediate personal relationships, major activities, and existential issues in their daily living, with the hope of increasing their SOC and coping skills (Antonovsky 1987). The homework is based on these topics, with Table 14.4 giving examples of the content of the homework. The homework may therefore function as an inner voice, much like a continuation of the group, which helps to increase the impact of the group.

Stimulating Flow Experiences

The concept of *flow* (Csikszentmihayi 1997) may shed some light over the significance of appropriate challenges and the strengthening of SOC: "Flow tends to occur when a person's skills are fully involved in overcoming a challenge that is just about manageable. Optimal experiences usually involve a fine balance between one's ability to act, and the available opportunities for action" (Csikszentmihayi 1997, p. 30). Accordingly, the key is to acquire good coping experiences by perceiving appropriate challenges. Lutz (2009) suggests that flow may be SOC experienced in the here and now, while SOC is also a product of flow over time. An important activity in salutogenic talk-therapy groups is to discuss what may or does give each person an experience of flow. The participants exchange ideas about good coping experiences and about how one may intervene in everyday activities to conduct more constructive activities that promote a sense of coping and positive mental health.

The Structure of the Program

The program consists of 16 group meetings and homework assignments. The meetings focus on, and aim to improve, SOC, mental health, and well-being. The first part is relatively nondirective because the participants are simply given the opportunity to discuss challenges which are of importance for them presently, in the context of daily activity. In the last part, homework is the main content. Table 14.3 shows the structure of the program. Homework is based on the crucial spheres in human existence, and the participants are invited to write a reflective note about the given topic (Table 14.3).

The first (1, 2, and 3) and the second part (5, 6, and 7) last 1 h each.

The first meeting is an introductory session in which the focus of the intervention and structure are presented and the participants and group leaders are introduced to one another, whereas the last meeting is a summary session in which the intervention is evaluated as a whole. There are no firm guidelines to indicate how many sessions such a group program should consist of. The most important thing, however, is that there are enough sessions to stimulate the cognitive and emotional processes of positive change among the participants, so as to continue for a long time afterward.

The first time the talk-therapy groups were implemented, each session lasted 1 h and 30 min (Langeland et al. 2006, 2007). However, the participants' evaluation revealed that this was too short. Consequently, in the next talk-therapy groups, each session was expanded to 2 h and 15 min, which has been evaluated from most of the participants as being the appropriate duration. The participants also emphasized the importance of leaders who kept a firm structure, including the salutogenic focus and homework.

Table 14.3 Structure of every session

1	A here-and-now round: each participant is given an opportunity to explain their feelings and with what they are engaged in their daily lives
2	Decide on the basis of the round whether themes have emerged on which to reflect and explore thoroughly
3	Conversation about a chosen topic, situation, or experience
4	15-min break
5	Conversation about the topic based on a reflection note the participants prepare for homework (second and subsequent sessions)
6	Assigning homework for the next session. The participants are encouraged to write a reflection note about a given task (all sessions except the last)
7	Each participant is given the opportunity to discuss their experience with the group

One of the groups continued after the first 16 sessions because the participants asked for it, as the participants wanted this extra time to decide on their homework together and not simply receive it from the leaders. This was evaluated as a positive step because they experienced more influence on the content and ownership of their homework. The next step in the group—after another 16 sessions—is that they wanted to try to be a self-help group without professional leaders but with some professional guidance. This is an example of how group participants gradually mobilize their own power and participate more in their own development and in shaping outcomes.

Table 14.4 illustrates an example of the topics and goals for the 16 sessions, which is based on the structure of the groups shown in Table 14.3, and should be understood in the context of the theoretical framework and mental health promotion process, including the salutogenic therapy principles and the desired outcome (Table 14.2).

Conclusions

This chapter reiterates that mental health professionals must give priority to, and apply a salutogenic approach that aims to improve SOC, mental health, and well-being in people with mental health problems. Although studies reveal that mental symptoms negatively influence well-being, it is important to give assistance, as well as to reduce symptoms, and to help people to nurture what is best within themselves and their social supports by building on their strengths, opportunities, and values, and not just on their problems and limitations (cf. Fig. 14.2: Mental health as two continua).

This chapter displays current information regarding the significance and utility of focusing on mental health and well-being from a salutogenic perspective. The present study has used the salutogenic model and other relevant supporting theories as a theoretical framework for mental health promotion intervention, which has been evaluated and has demonstrated positive effects on SOC, mental health, and

Table 14.4 An example of an intervention program

Session	Content part 1: examples of themes that may emerge at the here-and-now round	Goals	Content part 2: homework	Goals
1	Presentation	Becoming acquainted with the others and familiar with the intervention as a whole	Explaining and discussing the homework and assigning the first homework	Seeing the point and aim of the homework and thus creating meaning and motivation
	Information and conversation about structure and focus	Create a basis for an atmosphere of safety and confidence		
2	How to cope with such feelings as boredom, loneliness, and sadness	Accepting and taking into account various natural feelings Being aware of what happens when these feelings decrease and other feelings occur	What are you doing in everyday life with which you feel comfortable? What do you need to actualize your wishes or needs?	Increasing awareness of activities that create good experiences (flow) and being aware of needs to actualize more of this
3	Discuss opportunities for getting paid work	Experiencing how others may give guidance that may be useful	Describe an event from the last week in which you felt satisfied with yourself	Paying attention to inner feelings of satisfaction and coping
4	Coping stories: a participant tells a story about how she has coped with being afraid of the dark	Paying attention to coping stories and investigate whether these may be utilized in other situations	Think of people whom you nurture during the week	Being aware of the ability to contribute in personal relations
5	How to cope with feelings perceived as symptoms such as anxiety or voices in the head What happens when the symptoms decrease?	Considering the value of taking control of one's own situation and strengthening the feeling that there is a way out of difficulty	If you were given the possibility to choose freely, what would you then want to do?	Being aware of needs and wishes

6	How to cope with a important meeting with the Social Security office	Strengthening the ability to plan and manage a challenge	What would you answer if someone asked you what you are doing in your everyday life?	Being aware of the activities of daily living and being prepared for a imagined situation in a relationship
7	Good relationships: a participant tells about good relationships with his or her grandchildren	Being aware of how social relations may affect coping and quality of life	Describe what you experience on a good day	Paying attention to good inner feelings and being conscious of what creates these feelings
8	How to receive praise from a participant in the group	Daring to open up and perceive positive feedback and thus feel reassurance of worth	Think of something or someone who means a lot to you: what do you appreciate about this contact?	Being aware of strengths and coping resources in existing personal relationships
9	Choice: being aware of options for coping with a difficult situation in a mother–daughter relationship	Considering the value of being active and taking responsibility for one's choices	What is important for you in your life?	Increasing the ability to choose to do things that are meaningful
10	How to set limits toward a friend in a polite but determined manner	Being conscious of the possibility for self-regulation	How do you take care of your needs for activity and rest?	Considering the value of taking control of and confidence in one's own needs and inner feelings
11	How to cope with sleeping problems	Experiencing that other participants may share their own experiences with the same problem	Take yourself on a fantasy trip and ask yourself what you want to do or experience in your everyday life or at least once in your life	Being aware of one's own dreams and reflecting upon whether some can be fulfilled

(continued)

Table 14.4 (continued)

Session	Content part 1: examples of themes that may emerge at the here-and-now round	Goals	Content part 2: homework	Goals
12	How to cope with a family event, such as a wedding	Being aware of the ability to plan in relation to imagined situations	What characterizes people who have or have had a positive influence in your life?	Being aware of strengths and coping resources in personal relationships and discussing the possibility of creating relationships with these qualities
13	How to cope with going to the library	Experiencing taking one's own needs seriously and that active action may increase the sense of coping	How would you go about pleasing another person?	Being conscious of activities that encourage good personal relationships
14	How to organize the day	Reflecting on sources of strength in the activities of daily living	What positive characteristics of yourself do you experience after participating in the group?	Reflecting on and allowing oneself to pay attention to personal strengths and good inner feelings
15	Good experiences: a participant wants to tell about a good experience, such as a trip	Perceiving the importance of paying attention to good feelings	Describe ways in which you could proceed without the group. Eventually discuss whether the group could continue	Reflecting on where to go without the group Eventually discuss in which form and how the group could continue
16	Sum up and reflect on all the meetings	Being aware of whether the participant wants to keep contact with someone in the group	Of what importance has the group been for you?	Being aware of good experiences from the group and thus increasing the possibility that these may be used in new situations

well-being. As a result, this intervention may serve as a guide to mental health practice when the stimulation of health-promoting processes and active adaptation are the main targets. This helps to guide mental health professionals to ask and interpret people's experiences in reference to their health potential and their perception of themselves primarily as a person, thus attempting to (a) maximize their resistance to stress, (b) increase their awareness and use of resources, and (c) help them manage tension in order to consequently promote a stronger SOC, mental health, and experience of well-being. To assist in facilitating the salutogenic process, the relationship between mental health professionals and their clients must be seen as a partnership rather than the traditional hierarchical health care provider–health care receiver relationship.

The salutogenic model can be regarded as a theoretical tool and framework for a positive mental health concept and promotion, especially for mental health professionals, because it has the potential to illuminate how a new ideology and view of mental health can be realized. It yields a robust description of how coping on individual, collective, and interdisciplinary levels may be created by focusing on the availability of salutogenic strengths that enhance SOC and well-being, and includes challenges and engagement as natural parts of life. SOC is considered vital to positive mental health, as it involves the capacity to respond flexibly to stressors. Subsequently, a salutogenic understanding of mental health promotion and coping with mental health problems could contribute to a collaborative approach to its management. The current chapter documents how people with mental health problems can apply salutogenic thinking to help increase participation in their own development and trust in their own potential for coping.

To increase well-being in people with mental health problems, the treatment of symptoms is important, although the outcome may improve if treatment also focuses on other factors, such as GRRs and mental health as a positive state (including emotional, psychological, social, and spiritual/existential well-being). Accordingly, if a person's mental symptoms are targeted while other factors related to well-being are neglected, a poorer treatment outcome could result. However, from a salutogenic perspective, this also includes creating resources—and mental symptoms may be perceived as a resource since they may create an opportunity for self-tuning, which itself offers an opportunity to explore the circumstances around the symptoms, such as the contexts in which the symptoms occur, diminish, or disappear. From this, it may be concluded that in order to improve SOC and well-being, treatment programs should aim to improve, create, and strengthen salutogenic factors, such as social support and ego identity, as well as to reduce symptoms.

SOC and well-being seem to be significant variables in the assessment and treatment of people with mental health problems. In addition, this health-promoting perspective stimulates questions as to how much importance mental health professionals should attach to resource-activating methods and the extent to which they should recognize and foster mental health and life satisfaction aspects among their clients.

Although salutogenesis gives attention to factors that promote increased health, well-being, and recovery, it does not deny phenomena that do not. The psychologist Martin Seligman, for example, moved from research on learned helplessness to learned optimism. Still, that does not mean that he denies the existence of learned helplessness. Salutogenesis takes the existence of negative emotions and resistance into account; the metaphor of health in the river of life documents this, which is the basis for the concept of resistance resources. The key is to create order out of chaos, and health is something one has to work actively and proactively on in order to maintain and increase it. It is also crucial to be aware of the difference between being focused on resources and possibilities and on thinking positively.

Mapping out what makes life worth living is not the same as playing "be happy" games. Care also includes giving respect and attention to people's resources and to what gives life its meaning. This may be particularly important when people have heavy thoughts and negative feelings, because this approach creates hope and positive energy and gives small glimpses of light that can make a crucial difference for people. This could be an important step to overcome the victim role that many people with mental health problems experience. The salutogenic approach focuses on peoples' active adaptation in interplay with their surroundings, which is the ideal in treatment, and should include a focus on health-promoting factors, appropriate challenges, and crucial spheres in order to strengthen SOC, mental health, and well-being.

References

Ahern, L., & Fisher, D. (2001). Recovery at your own pace. *Journal of Psychosocial Nursing, 39*(4), 22–32.

Anderson, H., & Goolishian, H. (1988). Human systems as linguistic systems: Preliminary and evolving ideas about the implications for clinical theory. *Family Process, 27*(4), 371–393.

Anderson, H., & Goolishian, H. (1992). The client is the expert: A not knowing approach to therapy. In S. McNamee & K. Gergen (Eds.), *Therapy as social construction* (pp. 25–39). London: Sage.

Anthony, W., Cohen, M., & Farkas, M. (1994). *Psychiatric rehabilitation*. Boston: Center for Psychiatric Rehabilitation.

Antonovsky, A. (1979). *Health, stress and coping*. San Francisco: Jossey-Bass.

Antonovsky, A. (1985). The life cycle, mental health and the sense of coherence. *Israel Journal of Psychiatry and Related Sciences, 22*(4), 273–280.

Antonovsky, A. (1987). *Unraveling the mystery of health: How people manage stress and stay well*. San Francisco: Jossey-Bass.

Antonovsky, A. (1990). Pathways leading to successful coping and health. In M. Rosenbaum (Ed.), *Learned resourcefulness: On coping skills, self-control, adaptive behavior* (pp. 3–63). New York: Springer.

Antonovsky, A. (1991). The structural sources of salutogenetic strengths. In C. L. Cooper & R. Payne (Eds.), *Personality and stress: Individual differences in the stress process* (pp. 67–104). New York: Wiley.

Antonovsky, A. (1996a). The salutogenic model as a theory to guide health promotion. *Health Promotion International, 11*(1), 11–18.

Antonovsky, A. (1996b). The sense of coherence. A historical and future perspective. *Israel Journal of Medical Sciences, 32*, 170–178.

Bandura, A. (1991). Self-efficacy mechanism in psychological activation and health promoting behavior. In J. Madden (Ed.), *Neurobiology of learning, emotion, and affect* (pp. 229–269). New York: Raven Press Ltd.

Bengel, J., Strittmatter, R., & Willmann, H. (1999). *What keeps people healthy?* The current state of discussion and the relevance of Antonovsky's salutogenic model of health (Vol. 4). Cologne: Federal Centre for Health Education. Retrieved from http://www.bzga.de

Bengtsson-Tops, A., & Hansson, L. (2001). The validity of Antonovsky's sense of coherence measure in a sample of schizophrenic patients living in the community. *Journal of Advanced Nursing, 33*(4), 432–438.

Berger, H. (2003). Gesundheitsförderung–Ein neuer Weg in der Psychatrie. [Health Promotion–a change of paradigm in psychiatry]. *Psychiatric Praxis, 30*, 14–20.

Blomberg, J., Lazar, A., & Sandell, R. (2001). Long-term outcome of long-term psychoanalytically oriented therapies: First findings of the Stockholm outcome of psychotherapy and psychoanalysis study. *Psychotherapy Research, 11*, 361–382.

Blumer, H. (1969). *Symbolic interactionism: Perspective and method*. Englewood Cliffs: Prentice Hall.

Borg, M. (2007). *The nature of recovery as lived in everyday life*. Doctoral dissertation. Trondheim: NTNU.

Braaten, L. (1999). To what extent do clients discriminate among the group leader's basic therapeutic attitudes? A person-centered contribution. *The Person-Centered Journal, 6*(1), 32–45.

Carstens, J. A., & Sprangenberg, J. J. (1997). Major depression: A breakdown in sense of coherence? *Psychological Reports, 80*, 1211–1220.

Csikszentmihayi, M. (1997). *Finding flow: The psychology of engagement with everyday life*. New York: Basic.

de Shazer, S. (1991). *Putting difference to work*. New York/London: W.W. Norton & Company.

Duncan, B. L., Miller, S. D., & Sparks, J. (2004). *The heroic client: A revolutionary way to improve effectiveness through client-directed, outcome-informed therapy*. San Francisco: Jossey-Bass.

Duncan, B. L., Miller, S. D., Hubble, M. A., & Wampold, B. E. (2010). *The heart & soul of change: Delivering what works in therapy* (2nd ed.). Washington, DC: American Psychological Association.

Egan, G. (2002). *The skilled helper: A problem-management and opportunity-development approach to helping* (7th ed.). Pacific Grove: Brooks/Cole.

Erikson, M., & Lindstrøm, B. (2005). Validity of Antonovsky's sense of coherence scale: Systematic review. *Journal of Epidemiology and Community Health, 59*, 460–466.

Friedli, L. (2009). *Mental health, resilience and inequalities*. Retrieved from http://www.euro.who.int/__data/assets/pdf_file/0012/100821/E92227.pdf

Gilligan, S., & Price, R. (1993). *Therapeutic conversations*. New York/London: W.W. Norton & Company.

Gregg, J., & O'Hara, L. (2007). The Red Lotus Health Promotion Model: A new model for holistic, ecological, salutogenic health promotion practice. *Health Promotion Journal of Australia, 18*(1), 12–19.

Griffiths, C. A. (2009). Sense of coherence and mental health rehabilitation. *Clinical Rehabilitation, 23*, 72–78.

Hansson, K., Olsson, M., & Cederblad, M. (2004). A salutogenic investigation and treatment of conduct disorder (CD). *Nordic Journal of Psychiatry, 58*, 5–16.

Hyland, M. E. (1992). A reformulation of quality of life for medical science. *Quality of Life Research, 1*, 267–272.

Keyes, C. L. M. (2005). Mental illness and/or mental health? Investigating axioms of the complete state model of health. *Journal of Consulting and Clinical Psychology, 73*(3), 539–548.

Keyes, C. L. M. (2007a). Promoting and protecting mental health as flourishing. A complementary strategy for improving national mental health. *American Psychologist, 62*(2), 95–108.

Keyes, C. L. M. (2007b, September). *Positive mental health: Why is it different from mental disorders?* Paper presented at European conference on Joining Forces across Europe for Prevention and Promotion in Mental Health European Network for Mental health promotion and mental disorder prevention (IMHPA), Barcelona.

Kørlin, D., & Wrangsjø, B. (2002). Treatment effects of GIM therapy. *Nordic Journal of Music Therapy, 11*, 3–15.

Laitinen, I., Ettorre, E., & Sutton, C. (2007). Gaining agency through healthy embodiment in groups for depressed women. *European Journal of Psychotherapy and Counseling, 9*(2), 209–226.
Landsverk, S. S., & Kane, C. F. (1998). Antonovsky's sense of coherence: Theoretical basis of psychoeducation in schizophrenia. *Issues in Mental Health Nursing, 19*, 419–431.
Langeland, E. (2007b). Sense of coherence and life satisfaction in people suffering from mental health problems. An intervention study in talk-therapy groups with focus on salutogenesis. Doctoral dissertation. Bergen: University of Bergen.
Langeland, E., & Vinje, H. F. (2010, June). *Promoting active adaptation and sense of coherence in people with mental health problems participating in talk-therapy groups: The participants' experiences*. Poster session presented at the 5th European Conference on Positive Psychology (ECPP), Copenhagen.
Langeland, E., & Wahl, A. K. (2009). The impact of social support on mental health service users' sense of coherence: A longitudinal panel survey. *International Journal of Nursing Studies, 46*(6), 830–837.
Langeland, E., Riise, T., Hanestad, B. R., Nortvedt, M. W., Kristoffersen, K., & Wahl, A. K. (2006). The effect of salutogenic treatment principles on coping with mental health problems—randomised controlled trial. *Patient Education and Counseling, 62*, 212–219.
Langeland, E., Wahl, A. K., Kristoffersen, K., & Hanestad, B. R. (2007). Promoting coping: Salutogenesis among people with mental health problems. *Issues in Mental Health Nursing, 28*, 275–295.
Lindstrøm, B. (2001). The meaning of resilience. *International Journal of Adolescent Medicine and Health, 13*(1), 7–12.
Lindstrøm, B., & Eriksson, M. (2006). Contextualizing salutogenesis and Antonovsky in public health development. *Health Promotion International, 21*(3), 238–244.
Lundblad, A. M., & Hansson, K. (2005). Outcomes in couple therapy: Reduced psychiatric symptoms and improved sense of coherence. *Nordic Journal of Psychiatry, 59*, 374–380.
Lundqvist, T. (1995). Chronic cannabis use and the sense of coherence. *Life Sciences, 56*(23/24), 2145–2150.
Lutz, J. (2009). Flow and sense of coherence: Two aspects of the same dynamic? *Global Health Promotion, 16*, 63–67.
Malterud, K., & Hollnagel, H. (1999). Encouraging the strengths of women patients. A case study from general practice on empowering dialogues. *Scandinavian Journal of Public Health, 27*, 254–259.
Malterud, K., & Solvang, P. (2005). Vulnerability as a strength: Why, when, and how? *Scandinavian Journal of Public Health, 33*(Suppl 66), 3–6.
Menzies, V. (2000). Depression in schizophrenia: Nursing care as a generalized resistance resource. *Issues in Mental Health Nursing, 2*, 605–617.
Milberg, A., & Strang, P. (2007). What to do when 'there is nothing more to do'? A study within a salutogenic framework of family members' experience of palliative home care staff. *Psycho-Oncology, 16*(8), 741–751.
Morgan, E., & Ziglio, E. (2007). Revitalising the evidence base for public health: An assets model. *Promotion & Education, 14*, 17–22.
Næss, S., & Eriksen, J. (2006). *Diabetes og livskvalitet.* [Diabetes and quality of life]. Retrieved from http://www.nova.no/asset/2077/1/2077_1.pdf
Rapley, M. (2003). Quality of life with special populations. In M. Rapley (Ed.), *Quality of life research: A critical introduction* (pp. 167–189). London: Sage.
Rogers, C. R. (1957). The necessary and sufficient conditions for therapeutic personality change. *Journal of Consulting Psychology, 21*(2), 95–103.
Rogers, C. R. (1961). *On becoming a person*. Boston: Houghton Mifflin Company.
Rogers, C. R. (1980). *A way of being*. Boston: Houghton Mifflin Company.
Romme, M., & Escher, S. (1993). *Accepting voices*. London: Mind Publications.

Sack, M., Kunsebech, H. W., & Lamprecht, F. (1997). Sense of coherence and psychosomatic treatment outcome. An empirical study of salutogenesis. *Psychotherapie Psychosomatik Medizinische Psychologie, 47*, 149–155.
Sagy, S., & Antonovsky, H. (2000). The development of the sense of coherence: A retrospective study of early life experiences in the family. *Journal of Ageing and Human Development, 51*, 155–166.
Schmolke, M. (2003). Discovering positive health in the schizophrenic patient. A salutogenic oriented study. *Verhaltenstherapie, 13*, 102–109.
Seligman, M. E. P. (2002). *Authentic happiness: Using the new positive psychology to realize your potential for lasting fulfilment*. New York: Free Press.
Skärsäter, I., Langius, A., Ågren, H., Häggstrøm, L., & Dencker, K. (2005). Sense of coherence and social support in relation to recovery in first-episode patients with major depression: A one-year prospective study. *International Journal of Mental Health Nursing, 14*, 258–264.
Slade, M. (2010). Mental illness and well-being: The central importance of positive psychology and recovery approaches. *BMC Health Services Research, 10*, 26.
Snyder, C. R., & Lopez, S. J. (2007). *Positive psychology. The scientific and practical explorations of human strengths*. Thousand Oaks: Sage.
Stanhope, V., & Solomon, P. (2008). Getting to the heart of recovery and their implication for evidence-based practice. *British Journal of Social Work, 38*, 885–899.
Strauss, J. S. (1996). Subjectivity. *Journal of Nervous and Mental Diseases, 184*(4), 205–212.
Sullivan, G. (1989). Evaluating Antonovsky's salutogenic model for its adaptability to nursing. *Journal of Advanced Nursing, 14*, 336–342.
Taylor, J. S. (2004). Salutogenesis as a framework for child protection: Literature review. *Journal of Advanced Nursing, 45*(6), 633–643.
Vinje, H. F. (2007). *Thriving despite adversity: Job engagement and self-care among community nurses*. Doctoral dissertation. Bergen: University of Bergen.
Vinje, H. F., & Mittelmark, M. (2006). Deflecting the path to burn-out among community health nurses: How the effective practice of self-tuning renews job-engagement. *International Journal of Mental Health Promotion, 8*(4), 36–47.
Wallerstein, N. (2006). *What is the evidence on effectiveness of empowerment to improve health*? Retrieved from http://www.euro.who.int/__data/assets/pdf_file/0010/74656/E88086.pdf
Watkins, P. (2001). *Mental health nursing: The art of compassionate care*. Oxford: Butterworth-Heinemann.
Weiss, R. (1974). The provisions of social relationships. In Z. Rubin (Ed.), *Doing onto others* (pp. 17–26). Englewood Cliffs: Prentice Hall.
Weissbecker, I., Salmon, P., Studts, J. L., Floyd, A. R., Deder, E. A., & Sephton, S. E. (2002). Mindfulness-based stress reduction and sense of coherence among women with fibromyalgia. *Journal of Clinical Psychology in Medical Settings, 9*, 297–307.
White, M. (1991). Deconstruction and therapy. *Dulwich Centre Newsletter 3*, 21–40. Adelaide, South Australia: Dulwich Centre Publications.
White, M. (1997). *Narratives of therapists' lives*. Adelaide: Dulwich Centre Publications.
White, M., & Epston, D. (1990). *Narrative means to therapeutic ends*. Adelaide: Dulwich Centre Publications.
WHO. (1986, November). *Ottawa charter for health promotion*. Retrieved from http://www.who.int/hpr/NPH/docs/ottawa_charter_hp.pdf
WHO. (2001). *Strengthening mental health promotion*. (Fact sheet, no. 220). Geneva: World Health Organization, pp. 1–2. Retrieved from https://apps.who.int/inf-fs/en/fact220.html
Yalom, I. D. (1975). *The theory and practice of group psychotherapy*. New York: Basic Books.

Chapter 15
Positive Psychology Interventions: Research Evidence, Practical Utility, and Future Steps

Dianne A. Vella-Brodrick

This chapter will examine various conceptualizations of well-being, how it is measured, and why improving well-being is important. The main focus of this chapter will be on exploring methods for enhancing well-being and examining the empirical evidence for or against their efficacy and practical utility. While this chapter is not intended to be a systematic and exhaustive review of positive interventions, it does aim to give an overview of a range of widely used interventions, particularly those used within the field of positive psychology. This chapter will then critically review some of the factors that impact the success of positive interventions in enhancing well-being and will conclude with a set of recommendations for optimizing the real world application of positive interventions.

What Is Well-Being?

Within the social science literature, well-being has traditionally been operationalized as *subjective well-being*, whereby there are cognitive and affective (positive and negative) components (Diener 1994). Well-being is present when the positive aspects of everyday life considerably outweigh the negative ones. The focus of subjective well-being on life satisfaction and feeling good has resulted in this construct being closely aligned with hedonia. Such a narrow perspective of well-being has raised concern among some well-being scholars (e.g., Delle Fave et al. 2011; Keyes 2002; Ryff 1989). To address this shortcoming, new approaches have been developed, such as Ryff's (1989) model of psychological well-being, which espouses the

D.A. Vella-Brodrick (✉)
Faculty of Medicine, Nursing and Health Sciences,
School of Psychology and Psychiatry, Monash University, Victoria, Australia
e-mail: dianne.vella-brodrick@med.monash.edu.au

C.L.M. Keyes (ed.), *Mental Well-Being: International Contributions to the Study of Positive Mental Health*, DOI 10.1007/978-94-007-5195-8_15,

importance of positive relations with others, environmental mastery, psychological growth, life purpose, autonomy, and self-acceptance for the attainment of well-being. This model is often aligned with the eudaimonic perspective of well-being and has been integrated in therapeutic approaches, such as *well-being therapy* (Fava et al. 1998). Waterman (2008) has also heralded the importance of the eudaimonic perspective of well-being and has recently developed the Questionnaire for Eudaimonic Well-Being (Waterman et al. 2010).

More contemporary perspectives on well-being have, however, underscored the multidimensional nature of well-being by reconciling the two previously disparate schools of thought (hedonic and eudaimonic) into more integrated models (Kashdan et al. 2008; Keyes et al. 2002; Ryan and Deci 2001). Examples include the Orientations to Happiness (OTH) framework originally developed by Seligman (2002) and later extended to the PERMA model (Seligman, 2011) and the Complete State Model of Mental Health (Keyes 2005, 2007).

The OTH framework describes three pathways to achieve happiness, namely, pleasure, which primarily concerns sensory gratification and fostering positive emotions about the past, present, and future; engagement, which involves being fully immersed in life's core activities; and meaning, which revolves around and serving a higher purpose for the greater good. All three pathways have been shown to be significant correlates of well-being, with engagement and meaning of particular importance (Peterson et al. 2005; Vella-Brodrick et al. 2009). The PERMA model (Seligman, 2011) also includes explicit dimensions relating to relationships- the importance of connecting with others, and accomplishment - reflecting on achievements and successes.

Keyes (2005, 2007) has outlined emotional, social, and psychological factors as being fundamental to sound mental health and to flourishing. The Mental Health Continuum, developed by Keyes, is a measure which aligns with his conceptual framework. Another recent measure that adopts this integrated approach to well-being by including items on emotional experiences, interpersonal relationships, and positive functioning is the Warwick-Edinburgh Mental Well-Being Scale (Tennant et al. 2007). Delle Fave et al. (2011) have also developed a qualitative and quantitative approach to measure the full range of well-being. These recent approaches acknowledge the breadth of defining and measuring well-being and respect the subjective nature of well-being, while maintaining that well-being entails key components, such as positive emotions, meaning, engagement, and quality relations.

Is Well-Being Amenable to Change?—The Fading Debate

A key question among scholars interested in health and well-being concerns whether people are destined to a certain level of happiness or whether their level of happiness can be controlled to some extent, and preferably by the benefactors themselves, so as to foster self-management and autonomy. The answer to this question is critical to the central mission of positive psychology, which is to assist individuals, groups, and communities to flourish and reach their full potential (Seligman and Csikszentmihalyi 2000). Hence, some discussion about the malleability of well-being will now follow.

The happiness set point theory, sometimes referred to as the dynamic equilibrium theory, claims that happiness levels remain stable over time despite changes in life circumstances, even major ones (Headey 2006). The happiness set point is thought to operate similarly to other human homeostatic systems. For example, core body temperature, when operating effectively, seeks to maintain a temperature of around 37 degrees Celsius, irrespective of threats from parasites or external conditions. This adaptation is commonly referred to as the hedonic treadmill (Brickman and Campbell 1971) or *homeostatic control* (Cummins 2003). After repeated exposure to a stimulus, sensitivity is reduced, resulting in a need for increased stimulation in order to experience the same level of pleasure that was originally experienced. Often, this perspective is supported by citing research undertaken by Brickman et al. (1978), which found that the happiness of 22 major lottery winners and 29 paralysis accident victims soon returned to the normal range in comparison to a control group of 22 participants. These aforementioned theoretical perspectives challenge the viability of initiatives aimed at increasing individual happiness, which has led some to state that "[i]t may be that trying to be happier is as futile as trying to be taller and therefore is counterproductive" (Lykken and Tellegen 1996, p. 189). However, a noteworthy but often overlooked point is that baseline well-being data for the participants in Brickman et al.'s study were not actually collected, but their post-event well-being was instead compared with a control group. In other words, the temporal aspect, which is critical for interpreting these findings, was not included in this study. More longitudinal research, taking into account participants' actual baseline measures, is needed. Taking into consideration well-being data from panel studies, the variation in well-being across time for individuals becomes more apparent (Headey 2006).

In light of the mounting evidence favoring the malleability of happiness, Diener et al. (2006) have provided several revisions to the original hedonic treadmill theory. These revisions more readily acknowledge individual differences in adaptation, as well as the prospect of different types of well-being having different set points which may vary in the extent of their malleability.

Lyubomirsky et al. (2005b) estimate in their *Architecture of Sustainable Change* model that 50% of the variance in happiness is attributable to genetics, 10% to circumstantial factors, and 40% to intentional activities. In other words, this model proposes that individuals can actively increase their happiness by engaging in certain types of intentional activities that are cognitive (e.g., adopting an optimistic outlook), behavioral (e.g., physical exercise), or volitional (e.g., using signature strengths to help others).

In sum, it would appear that based on more recent discourse and evidence, many scholars, particularly within the field of positive psychology, believe that examining methods for increasing well-being is a worthy pursuit. This support is further pronounced by the multitude of perceived benefits likely to emerge from these volitional strategies for improving well-being.

What Are the Benefits of Improving Well-Being?

There is theoretical support for the premise that positive emotions serve important functions. For example, Fredrickson (2001) asserted, based on her broaden-and-build theory, that positive emotions (e.g., joy, interest, contentment, and love) serve two important functions: broadening and building. Broadening refers to the facilitation of a more diverse range of thought-action repertoires that foster creativity and exploration. Building refers to the accumulation of physical, intellectual, and social resources which ensue from the exploration process. These resources are thought to better equip individuals for coping with adversity. When these theoretical perspectives were empirically tested via a series of studies, they were supported. For example, Waugh and Fredrickson (2006) found with 247 first-year college students that there was an association between positive emotions and increased assimilation with and understanding of others, namely, their roommate, suggesting that those with higher levels of positive affect tend to form new relationships more readily with others than those with low levels of positive affect. In addition, experimentally induced positive affect has been shown to hasten recovery from cardiovascular reactivity to stressful situations, supporting the notion that positive emotions can serve to "undo" negative states and therefore individuals to cope more effectively with the physiological responses to negative emotions (Fredrickson and Levenson 1998).

Consistent with the broaden-and-build theory, Lyubomirsky King et al. (2005a), in their meta-analysis of 225 studies, found that individuals with higher levels of positive affect were more successful in a number of significant life domains, such as health, work, and relationships. It is noteworthy that these studies were cross-sectional and did not enable causality to be established. In other words, it was not known whether happiness led to success or success led to happiness. However, when Lyubomirsky et al. examined the results of experimental studies which induced positive states (often through showing film clips), they found that participants who were in positive states were more sociable and were better able to resolve conflicts than their less positive counterparts. Moreover, their study also included a review of a limited number of longitudinal studies undertaken in naturalistic settings and found that happiness does lead to successful work and relationship outcomes. Such positive outcomes included an increased likelihood of marriage and stronger social support (see Harker and Keltner 2001) and greater income, creativity, productivity, and quality of work (see Estrada et al. 1994). Furthermore, subjective well-being has been shown to play an important role in mental and physical health (Pressman and Cohen 2005). Also, happy individuals are more likely to self-regulate and cope with adversities (e.g., Aspinwall 1998), have healthier immune function (e.g., Davidson et al. 2003), and live longer (e.g., Danner et al. 2001) than less happy individuals. Moreover, happier people have been shown to be more cooperative, charitable, prosocial, and other-centered compared to control participants (e.g., Williams and Shiaw 1999). Therefore, the benefits of positive emotions are not exclusively confined to the individual involved, but permeate more broadly to others.

Clearly, the benefits to be derived from being in a positive state are significant and numerous and serve to underscore the necessity of a full range of emotions spanning the negative/positive spectrum. Therefore, systematically enhancing individual happiness should be an important scientific endeavor. The question now turns to *how* well-being can best be enhanced.

How Can Well-Being Best Be Enhanced?

Although many philosophers have speculated and advised on methods for enhancing well-being, Fordyce (1977) was among the first to formally examine the effects of what are now commonly termed positive psychology interventions (PPIs). It should be noted that not all of these interventions originated under the auspices of positive psychology, but this term serves as a broad label for a range of positive interventions. PPIs are volitional activities that aim to improve well-being by targeting feelings, cognitions, and behaviors (Sin and Lyubomirsky 2009). Participants in Fordyce's research (comprising three studies) included over 200 college students who were led to believe that these positive activities were part of their "Psychology of Adjustment" subject. Participants were assigned to one of three happiness intervention groups (the *insight*, *fundamentals*, or *activities* program), or to a *suggestion* (control) group, and were informed that their participation in the subject would bring them happiness (thus controlling for expectations). All students were instructed to apply their specific program daily over 2 weeks. The fundamentals and activities groups significantly increased their happiness relative to the control group.

In subsequent studies (a series of four studies were undertaken), Fordyce (1983) evaluated the "14 fundamentals for happiness" program, which was developed based on reviews of the happiness literature focusing on malleable methods rather than on personality and objective indicators of happiness and on what worked best in his previous research (Fordyce 1977). The 14 fundamentals for happiness were:

(a) Keep busy and be more active.
(b) Spend more time socializing.
(c) Be productive at meaningful work.
(d) Get better organized and plan things out.
(e) Stop worrying.
(f) Lower your expectations and aspirations.
(g) Develop positive, optimistic thinking.
(h) Become present oriented.
(i) Work on a healthy personality.
(j) Develop an outgoing, social personality.
(k) Be yourself.
(l) Eliminate negative feelings and problems.
(m) Close relationship is the number one source of happiness.
(n) Put happiness as your most important priority. (Fordyce 1983, p. 484)

These fundamental principles were the essence of a course in which detailed explanations with accompanying cognitive and behavioral actualization techniques were provided for each principle. The course also included an overview of work undertaken in the area of psychological happiness. Across the seven studies undertaken by Fordyce (1977, 1983), participants exposed to the fundamentals program demonstrated increased happiness compared to participants from a range of placebo and control conditions. Moreover, 81% of intervention group participants claimed happiness gains, and 38% reported being "much happier" or "extremely happy" as a result of the happiness program. The program fostered "the development of new behaviors and attitudes, changes in lifestyle, new insights and understandings, better copings with bad moods, enhancement of happy moods, to a better awareness of happiness itself" (p. 495). Moreover, 96% of participants indicated that the program had educational merit. Fordyce's (1977, 1983) work provided promising signs that happiness could be improved with deliberate effort.

Despite Fordyce's (1977, 1983) initiatives to incite interest in happiness research, very little work on happiness interventions was undertaken in the 1980s and 1990s. Instead, the focus remained largely on examining the antecedents and predictors of well-being (e.g., Diener et al. 1999). It was not until the inception of positive psychology in the late 1990s that more attention was invested specifically in developing and systematically evaluating PPIs. Research by Seligman et al. (2005) was at the forefront in this respect. Their study was a randomized controlled trial (RCT) involving 577 adult participants who were recruited via the Internet. Five happiness interventions (the gratitude visit, three good things in life, you at your best, using signature strengths in a new way, and identifying signature strengths) were trialed and compared with a placebo control group instructed to write about early memories. See Table 15.1 for descriptions of these interventions. While all participants, including those from the placebo control group, reported gains in happiness and decreased depression immediately after undertaking their respective activities, participants completing the gratitude visit showed gains up to 1 month post-intervention, and participants from the three good things in life and the using signature strengths in a new way interventions showed increases for up to 6 months post-intervention in comparison to the placebo control group. This study provided preliminary evidence that not only can PPIs increase well-being, but they also have the potential to decrease depression.

Research by Seligman et al. (2006) provided additional support for the ability of PPIs to reduce depression by increasing positive emotion, engagement, and meaning as opposed to working directly on depressive symptoms. This research involved two studies, the first focusing on a group of individuals with mild to moderate symptoms of depression as measured by the BDI-II and the second study focusing on a group of individuals with unipolar depression who were seeking treatment at a psychology service provider (and needed to meet the inclusion criteria of having a major depressive disorder). The first study involved 40 students who were randomly assigned to either the positive psychotherapy (PPT) intervention or to a no treatment condition. The PPT intervention involved 2 h per week for 6 weeks of a group-based intervention program (two groups of 8–11 participants) and included activities such

Table 15.1 Descriptions of interventions in Seligman et al.'s (2005) study

*Gratitude visit – 1 week to write a letter to someone who had been kind to them and then to deliver the letter
*Three good things in life – every night for a week, write down three things that went well that day and to provide a causal explanation for each
*You at your best – write about a time when they were at their best and to reflect on the personal strengths displayed in the story. Reflect on the story every day for a week
*Using signature strengths in a new way – identify their strengths and select one of the top 5 strengths to use in new ways every day for a week
*Identifying signature strengths – to take the survey and note their five highest strengths
*Placebo (early memories) – write about early memories every night for a week

Copied from Seligman et al. (2005)

as using signature strengths, three blessings, writing an obituary, a gratitude visit, active-constructive responding, and savoring. See Table 15.2 for a description of these activities.

After 1 year, the PPT group moved to the nondepressed range, whereas the control group stayed in the mild to moderate range. Satisfaction with life also increased for the PPT group; however, the control group also reported increases. In the second study involving 46 clients with unipolar depression, the PPT entailed 14 sessions addressing clients' immediate clinical needs and included homework exercises (selected to suit the participant's specific needs from a pool of 14 exercises). This intervention was compared with a treatment as usual and a treatment as usual plus medication group. Relative to the comparison groups, PPT participants experienced decreased depression and higher remission rates (i.e., absence of depressive symptoms), once again supporting the efficacy of PPT.

Numerous other intervention studies focusing on specific PPIs, such as forgiveness (Reed and Enright 2006), kindness (Otake et al. 2006), and gratitude (Sergeant and Mongrain 2011), have also been undertaken, with many showing favorable outcomes (such as increased hope, positive affect, satisfaction with life, and decreased depression). Emmons and McCullough (2003) examined the effects of a gratitude intervention on well-being over a series of three studies, with participants ranging from students to individuals with neuromuscular disease. Participants were randomly assigned to either the hassles, gratitude, or placebo control group (life events or social comparison). They were instructed to complete their assigned activity either daily or weekly for 2 or 3 weeks (this varied across the three studies). Refer to Table 15.3 for specific instructions. Participants reported their mood states, coping behaviors, health behaviors, physical symptoms, and global life appraisal pre- and post-intervention. In comparison to the placebo control groups, participants who were in the gratitude condition reported improved well-being (e.g., more optimistic appraisals of life, increased level of exercise, decreased reporting of physical symptoms, and increased positive affect). However, not all findings were consistent across the three studies, and not all the outcome variables included in the study demonstrated improvements. Others have also questioned the use of comparison groups which induce negative affect, such as the daily hassle condition (Froh et al. 2009).

Table 15.2 Descriptions of interventions from Seligman et al.'s (2006) study

Session	Description
1	*Using your strengths*: Take the VIA (values in action) strengths questionnaire to assess your top 5 strengths and think of ways to use those strengths more in your daily life
2	*Three good things/blessings*: Each evening, write down three good things that happened and why you think they happened
3	*Obituary/biography*: Imagine that you have passed away after living a fruitful and satisfying life. What would you want your obituary to say? Write a 1–2-page essay summarizing what you would like to be remembered for the most
4	*Gratitude visit*: Think of someone to whom you are very grateful, but who you have never properly thanked. Compose a letter to them describing your gratitude and read the letter to that person by phone or in person
5	*Active/constructive responding*: An active-constructive response is one where you react in a visibly positive and enthusiastic way to good news from someone else. At least once a day, respond actively and constructively to someone you know
6	*Savoring*: Once a day, take the time to enjoy something that you usually hurry through (e.g., eating a meal, taking a shower, walking to class). When it is over, write down what you did, how you did it differently, and how it felt compared to when you rush through it

Table 15.3 Descriptions of interventions from Emmons and McCullough's (2003) study

Condition	Instructions
Gratitude	*There are many things in our lives, both large and small, that we might be grateful about. Think back over the past week and write down on the lines below up to five things in your life that you are grateful or thankful for* (Emmons and McCullough 2003, p. 379)
Hassles	*Hassles are irritants—things that annoy or bother you. They occur in various domains of life, including relationships, work, school, housing, finances, health, and so forth. Think back over today and, on the lines below, list up to five hassles that occurred in your life* (Emmons and McCullough 2003, p. 379)
Life events	*What were some of the events or circumstances that affected you in the past week? Think back over the past week and write down on the lines below the five events that had an impact on you* (Emmons and McCullough 2003, p. 379)
Social comparison (downward)	*It is human nature to compare ourselves to others. We may be better off than others in some ways and less fortunate than other people in other ways. Think about ways in which you are better off than others, things that you have that they do not have, and write these down in the spaces below* (Emmons and McCullough 2003, p. 381)

Cheavens et al. (2006) designed a hope intervention involving 8 × 2-h group sessions. The hope intervention covered aspects such as setting realistic and meaningful goals, developing various pathways for achieving these goals, identifying motivational sources and counteracting motivational challenges, monitoring goal progress, and modifying goals and pathways, as required. Homework tasks were also assigned to intervention group participants. Examples of goals selected by study participants included exercising more often, working on interpersonal relationships, and changing jobs. Participants comprised 32 members from the community who were randomly assigned to either the hope condition or a wait-list control condition. Improvements from pre- to post-intervention and relative to the wait-list control group were found for agency hope (but not pathways hope), anxiety, self-esteem, and purpose in life.

Sin and Lyubomirksy's (2009) meta-analysis provides an efficient overview of the efficacy of 51 different positive psychology interventions ($N = 4{,}266$), including forgiveness (Freedman and Enright 1986; Reed and Enright 2006), positive writing (King 2001), and well-being therapy (Fava et al. 1998). Essentially, this meta-analysis found that PPIs are effective in increasing well-being and decreasing depression, with effect sizes of .29 and .31, respectively. While these results generally support the use of PPIs, at best, these effect sizes are moderate and should not be overestimated. Consequently, gaining insight into methods for improving the efficacy of PPIs is an important next step and will now be explored.

Which Positive Psychology Interventions Work, and for Whom?

With an increasing focus on evidence-based practice, cost-effectiveness, efficient distribution of limited resources, and treatment success, gaining an understanding of the underlying mechanisms behind PPIs—and not just the main effects on well-being—is imperative. This means that at least two fundamental criteria need to be met. First, that there is sound research (including RCTs and meta-analyses) supporting the efficacy of PPIs, and second, that there is sufficient ecological validity demonstrating that PPIs possess real world applicability for a variety of people and outcomes, as intended. Hence, the circumstances under which the interventions are beneficial need to be elucidated. This will enable the selection of appropriate interventions to suit individual needs while concurrently accommodating contextual factors. For example, there is little point in recommending online interventions to individuals who do not have computer access or who are not sufficiently skilled to use a computer.

Lyubomirsky (2008) refers to *person-activity fit* as being important for the selection of PPIs or volitional activities. Person-activity fit is believed to occur when the activity feels natural, enjoyable, and valuable. Ideally, the requirements (or nature) of the activity should align with the skill set, interests, needs, disposition, values, and personal resources of the individual. In addition, the context (or environmental) conditions should also fit the task at hand, in terms of time demands, special equipment, and level of support from significant others.

Research examining the direct effects of an intervention on well-being without considering any potential moderating or mediating factors, while important in the initial stages of determining the broad effects of an intervention, has limitations from a long-term perspective. Although not always consistent, evidence—including RCTs and meta-analyses supporting the efficacy of PPIs—is steadily accumulating, and thus more attention is being directed to understanding interaction effects. As a starting point, Sin and Lyubomirsky (2009), in their meta-analysis, examined interaction effects and found that higher levels of depression, increased age, one-on-one interventions (in contrast to group administration), and interventions of longer duration, heighten the efficacy of PPIs. This information provides some direction for exploring mediating and moderating factors. These types of factors can be divided into three broad categories: (1) participant characteristics, (2) nature of intervention, and (3) contextual factors.

Participant Characteristics

Numerous individual difference factors are plausible mediators or moderators of the efficacy of PPIs. An endless range of state and dispositional factors may be relevant, but some of the most obvious ones include personality, motivation levels, mental health status, character strengths, and sociodemographic factors. Some of these will now be discussed.

Motivation

Sheldon and Lyubomirsky (2006) found that self-concordant motivation, which refers to a commitment to pursue goals that are interesting and align with one's core values, moderates the efficacy of PPIs. Study participants were assigned to either the counting blessings (CB), visualizing best possible selves (BPS), or life events (placebo control) condition. Descriptions of the counting blessings (gratitude) and life events activities were similar to those used in Emmons and McCullough's (2003) study, as outlined in Table 15.2. BPS participants were asked to

> [i]magine yourself in the future, after everything has gone as well as it possibly could. You have worked hard and succeeded at accomplishing all of your life goals. Think of this as the realization of your life dreams, and of your own best potentials. In all of these cases you are identifying the best possible way that things might turn out in your life, in order to help guide your decisions now. You may not have thought about yourself in this way before, but research suggests that doing so can have a strong positive effect on your mood and life satisfaction. So, we'd like to ask you to continue thinking in this way over the next few weeks, following up on the initial writing that you're about to do. (p. 77)

Participants were asked to rate their level of engagement and motivation to continue with the assigned activity. They also reported on how often they did the assigned activity. Of the three groups, self-concordant motivation was found to be highest for the BPS group. Consistent with predictions that the intervention which aligned most closely with the participants' interests and values would be the most effective in improving mood, the BPS participants reported greater increases in positive affect relative to the CB and life events participants. Interestingly, however, participants from all conditions, including life events, reported immediate decreases in negative affect. The most pertinent finding was that an individual's motivational level to undertake an activity influenced the efficacy of the activity. Hence, the use of wait-list control groups would help balance out issues related to motivational factors and should be used where relevant and possible.

Wants Versus Needs

Schueller (2010) found that preference for undertaking a PPI is positively related to adherence to the activity. More recently, Schueller (2011) found no significant difference between participants assigned to activities based on preference compared to those who were randomly assigned an activity. It would seem, then, that determining person-activity fit based on preference is not always straightforward. Giannopoulos and Vella-Brodrick (2011) found that assigning individuals to an intervention which differed from, rather than matched, their dominant orientation to happiness (pleasure, engagement, and meaning) was most effective in enhancing well-being. In other words, participants with, for example, a high-pleasure orientation to happiness, who were assigned to either the three engaging or three meaningful things writing activity, rather than the three pleasurable things writing activity, reported greater well-being benefits. Similarly, Silberman (2007) found with 72 undergraduate psychology students that self-selection into four PPIs (three good things, you at your best, using signature strengths, and the gratitude visit) did not increase the benefits to be gained from undertaking the interventions. These study findings illuminate the situation, whereby activities may match needs but not preferences (wants), and raise the issue of which of these criteria should take precedence when determining person-activity fit. At present, there is insufficient evidence-based research to guide these decisions.

Positive Affect and Personality

Froh et al. (2009), in their study of 89 adolescents, explored positive affect as a moderator of the efficacy of the gratitude visit. As gratitude interventions have not shown consistent well-being benefits in comparison to control conditions, it was thought that the gratitude intervention may only benefit a subgroup of individuals with specific characteristics, such as low positive affect. It was predicted that those already high in positive affect may have experienced an emotional ceiling whereby additional emotional gains are unlikely. Hence, those lower in positive affect may have more scope to improve their positive emotions through the gratitude intervention. They found that adolescents low in positive affect in the gratitude condition reported higher levels of both gratitude and positive affect immediately after the intervention and positive affect at the 2-month follow-up, compared to adolescents in the daily event condition. Hence, positive affect did moderate the efficacy of the gratitude visit.

Personality is another participant characteristic that could influence how well PPIs work. Personality factors have received considerable research attention, with extroversion and emotional stability being particularly identified as strong correlates of well-being (See Diener et al. 1999). However, personality has seldom been examined as an individual difference factor potentially influencing the efficacy of specific PPIs. Yet, it is conceivable that personality may play a large role in determining what interventions will work for specific individuals. For example, do certain interventions, such as the gratitude visit, require high levels of extroversion or openness for them to be effective in enhancing well-being? One study, which has focused on the "depressive personality styles" of being self-critical and needy, found with 772 adults who were assigned to either a gratitude, music, or control exercise for 1 week that those in the gratitude and music conditions reported increased happiness over time in comparison to control participants (Sergeant and Mongrain 2011). Noteworthy in this study, however, is that self-critics reported the most favorable outcomes if they were assigned to a gratitude condition, whereas needy individuals did not benefit from the intervention and indeed decreased with regards to self-esteem. Clearly, the interactive role of personality in relation to PPIs is another area that warrants further investigation.

Mental Imagery

Given that many of the PPIs involve recalling situations (e.g., three good things) or imagining future events (e.g., BPS), there appears to be some reliance on mental imagery skills in the execution of these tasks. Mental imagery is defined as the occurrence of quasisensory or quasiperceptual experiences despite the absence of any real sensory stimuli (Richardson 1969). Mental imagery ability is evident when individuals can immerse themselves in and respond to the mental images, as if they were really occurring.

Researchers of PPIs are beginning to explore the role of mental imagery for increasing happiness and well-being. For example, Peters et al. (2010) examined whether a 15-min BPS condition followed by a further 5 min of mental imagery was more effective at increasing optimism than a control condition in which participants were asked to write about and imagine a typical day in their life. The BPS plus mental imagery condition was more effective at increasing optimism than the control condition. While it is not known whether mental imagery per se was the active ingredient of the PPI (particularly as there was no comparison group without the explicit mental imagery instructions), this finding is consistent with evidence that mental imagery activates emotional systems (more readily than verbal methods) and is therefore an effective tool for amplifying positive emotions (Holmes and Mathews 2010; Holmes et al. 2008).

Just as mental imagery training has been shown to enhance sporting performance (Martin et al. 1999), some competency with mental imagery may be helpful to participants when undertaking PPIs that involve the recall or reexperiencing of events and projecting into the future to imagine what life would be like. A study by Odou and Vella-Brodrick (2011) examined the influence of mental imagery prompts while undertaking the three good things and best possible self-interventions and found there was no difference in intervention efficacy for those with the mental imagery prompts compared to those without the prompts. However, mental imagery ability was positively correlated with well-being, suggesting that by improving mental imagery skills such as controllability and vividness, well-being may be enhanced (or well-being may improve mental imagery ability). Extending on this work, more targeted and controlled studies examining mental imagery ability as a possible moderator or mediator variable, rather than as a component of an intervention, are warranted.

Mindfulness

Mindfulness can be operationalized as both a trait and state and involves heightened awareness of, and attention to, stimuli as well as personal emotions, thoughts, and motives (Brown and Ryan 2003; Thomas 2006). Aspects of mindfulness also seem relevant to the successful undertaking of many PPIs. For example, high levels of awareness and attention are relevant to PPIs, such as savoring and three good things, as these interventions require individuals to be aware of positive events and experiences as they are occurring so that they can be recalled at a later point in time. Given that there are training programs to increase mindfulness (Kabat-Zinn 2003), determining which PPIs are optimized as a result of specific levels of mindfulness seems a worthwhile task. This means that individual's mindfulness levels can be improved to suit the task, or PPIs can be selected to suit individuals based on whether or not they possess high levels of mindfulness. Higher levels of mindfulness practice have been associated with increased levels of positive affect and decreased levels of negative affect (Jha et al. 2010) and increased psychological well-being (Huppert and Johnson 2010). However, how mindfulness levels influence the efficacy of PPIs has not been the focus of research to date.

Socioeconomic Status and Demographics

Typically, research studies have relied on participants from high socioeconomic and westernized backgrounds. This middle class, white bias may impact significantly on the outcomes obtained on the efficacy of PPIs. It has been found that higher education and income levels are related to higher SWB (Cummins 2000). Hence, PPIs may not be as effective for individuals with lower levels of education and income or from different cultural backgrounds. Moreover, PPIs appear to be more effective for older people (Sin and Lyubomirsky 2009). These findings suggest that some consideration of the interaction effects of individuals' socioeconomic status and demographic details is warranted when selecting PPIs, and greater effort is needed to recruit more diverse and representative samples in future research studies on PPIs so that more about the influence of individual difference and cultural factors on the efficacy of PPIs can be learned.

Nature of the PPI

Frequency of Undertaking the PPI

The specific components and qualities of PPIs, such as the response format, frequency of completion, delivery mode, and content coverage and depth, may impact the success of the intervention for specific individuals. Some of these factors will now be examined in more detail.

The frequency with which PPIs are undertaken appears to be an important factor. Huppert and Johnson (2010), in their RCT of the efficacy of mindfulness training to improve well-being in 155 adolescent boys, found that there was no significant difference in mindfulness, resilience, and psychological well-being between the mindfulness and control groups. There was, however, a positive relationship between the amount of practice undertaken by the adolescents and improvements in psychological well-being and mindfulness. Jha et al. (2010) also found similar results in their study on mindfulness, with improvements evident only for those participants with higher levels of mindfulness training. Therefore, there is escalating evidence to suggest that the number of times a PPI is undertaken is important. However, it is not known what the optimal frequency rate is for each activity and whether there is a saturation point whereby the activity no longer remains effective due to, for example, hedonic adaptation. For instance, Sheldon and Lyubomirsky (2004) found that individuals who counted their blessings once a week, as opposed to those who counted their blessings three times per week, reported more significant gains in well-being. This demonstrates that the relationship between frequency of PPI and well-being is not always a linear one. Hence, PPIs will need to be adapted into several different versions to ensure there is sufficient variety to mitigate boredom and adaptation (e.g., count blessings relating to a different life domain each week for a month).

Writing-Based PPIs

Many PPIs require participants to write. This raises the question about whether those individuals who are more proficient in or comfortable with writing are more likely to derive greater benefits from PPIs. Interestingly, placebo control groups which involve writing about early memories or daily events have been shown to be equally effective in increasing well-being as the PPI conditions in some studies (e.g., Seligman et al. 2005, at the immediate post-intervention time point). Therefore, it can be deduced from these findings that the writing task may be the active ingredient rather than the positive nature of the intervention per se. Subsequently, more extensive exploration of the content and length of the writing activity, as well as the individual's preferred response style (e.g., writing versus verbal), seems relevant.

In terms of content, it has been found that when individuals are asked to write about intensely positive events, positive affect is significantly improved (Burton and King 2004). However, writing and journaling have been used as deliberate psychosocial strategies which promote emotional expression and disclosure of stressful events (Nazarian and Smyth 2008). For example, it has been shown that when participants who have experienced a relationship dissolution are asked to write about what the relationship was like prior to the break-up, the factors that may have triggered the break-up, and the consequences of the break-up, they experienced fewer adverse health symptoms in comparison to control participants (Lewandowski 2009). Research findings relating to this area of investigation have been mixed, but it seems that the use of positively oriented words is related to better health outcomes, whereas the use of words reflecting negative emotions results in negative health outcomes (see Lewandowski 2009). Less is known about the ideal length of the writing activity in relation to PPIs or about the individual's preferred response mode, and research directed at understanding more about these factors is needed.

Combination Interventions

Some PPIs, such as PPT or Cheavens et al.'s (2006) hope intervention, involve a combination of positive activities rather than a single activity, thus making it difficult to identify what the active ingredients associated with the successful or unsuccessful outcomes are. If a positive outcome is achieved, it is not possible to know whether all aspects of the combined interventions were effective or whether it was just one or two of the activities which generated the desired outcome. Hence, identifying the unique contributions each activity makes to specific outcome variables is difficult with these combination interventions, and more tightly designed studies are needed to first identify the unique contributions of specific interventions and then to examine the effects of various combinations of activities.

Preliminary findings suggest that combination activities may be less effective for enhancing well-being than are interventions which focus exclusively on one activity. For example, Giannopoulos and Vella-Brodrick (2011), in their study comparing four activity groups asking participants to write daily about (1) three pleasurable things; (2) three engaging things; (3) three meaningful things; and (4) a combination group of one pleasurable, one engaging, and one meaningful thing, found that the combination activity group was the least effective group. One explanation for this finding is that by attempting to cover a greater breadth of topics, depth is sacrificed, and this may have detrimental effects on the efficacy of PPIs in enhancing well-being. Given the time and commitment restrictions many individuals face, insight into the right balance of breadth and depth is needed.

Delivery Mode

PPIs can be delivered via a variety of mediums and settings. One medium that is gaining increasing attention is the Internet. Mitchell et al. (2009) conducted an RCT comparing the well-being effects of an online strengths intervention with a problem-solving intervention and a problem-solving information-only placebo control condition. In this study the measurement of well-being included domain-specific indices, cognitive and emotional well-being, and the pleasure, engagement, and meaning orientations to happiness. Results were mixed and tended to favor improvement of the cognitive component of well-being relative to the affective component. Although the study demonstrated that it is possible to improve specific aspects of well-being using self-guided Internet PPIs, this was not the case for many of the study outcome variables. This raises the question of whether different delivery modes impact the efficacy of interventions.

Although online, self-guided PPIs are currently scarce, they will become more prevalent given the large network of people that can be reached using the Internet and the convenience associated with responding via the Internet. However, one major challenge for scholars utilizing online interventions concerns the high attrition rates which, in the case of Mitchell et al.'s study, were 83% at the 3-month follow-up. The inclusion of methods which provide human support, such as e-coaching or regular reminders and follow-up, may increase the likelihood that participants will be (1) more fully engaged in online interventions, (2) comply with instructions, and (3) commit to completing online programs. Research exploring these propositions is critical to the advancement of practical online methods for enhancing well-being.

Contextual Factors

Contextual factors appear to be the least emphasized of the three broad categories of factors which may influence the success of PPIs. The importance of contextual aspects relating to lifestyle (e.g., time availability) and support from significant others should not be ignored. These will now be discussed briefly.

Time Availability

PPIs need to suit the lifestyles of the users. Quick and simple interventions are likely to be more readily adopted by individuals. This is clearly an advantage of PPIs, which tend to be self-administering, easy to do, enjoyable, and quick to complete. More specific information on how individuals embed these PPIs into their lifestyle and how much time they take to complete using a variety of different samples is needed to guide the development of future PPIs and ensure they remain practical for the end user.

Support from Significant Others

It has been shown that the support structure of individuals is important for any change process (Williams et al. 2006). For example, if an adolescent was involved in a PPI, the support and encouragement of peers, parents, and teachers may be helpful in completing the activity. Health initiatives in work settings have also demonstrated the beneficial effects of supportive workplace supervisors (Della et al. 2008). Hence, it appears that for PPIs to have maximal impact, a support network comprised of individuals and systems that will facilitate and encourage the practice of the PPI is likely to lead to better well-being outcomes; however, this has not been tested explicitly with PPIs.

Progressing PPI Research and Applications: Issues to Consider

Monitoring PPIs

Studies on PPIs, to date, have raised a number of important issues which need to be considered in future research so that the study of PPIs can continue to progress and deliver practical and effective outcomes for those in pursuit of optimal psychological health. Some of these issues pertain to the administration of the PPI, the selection of comparison and control groups, and the selection and types of measures employed.

Many PPIs are self-regulated and self-administered, which means that they are not required to be completed under standardized conditions with the researchers present to oversee program integrity. Therefore, it is not known whether participants have completed the PPIs in accordance with the specified instructions. Most studies do not monitor the extent to which participants have followed instructions, although some studies do ask participants for self-reports, for example, on the frequency of completing the activity. However, these responses are likely to be overinflated due to a range of response biases. For PPIs that involve writing, one possible solution is to ask participants to submit their journals detailing the frequency and content of their activities, to researchers, so this information can also be analyzed. While access to this level of information would provide valuable insight, it may make participants apprehensive about disclosing personal information to researchers. In many studies, however, participants remain anonymous; hence, privacy may not always be an issue. Unless information about the adherence of the intervention is monitored, it is not possible to know exactly what participants are doing as part of the positive intervention. In some recent studies undertaken by the author, participants were asked to complete the assigned intervention online, and these activity responses were recorded as part of the research study. It was found that the quality of the responses varied considerably, with participants assigned to an active intervention group not completing the activity. Others who did complete their assigned activity varied tremendously with regard to the quality and quantity of the responses. Therefore, researchers should not presume that all participants have adhered to the researchers' instructions. Instead, researchers should collect data to verify, within reason, that PPI activities have indeed been undertaken and completed as instructed, by participants.

More standardized instructions around the duration that one should spend on the activity (e.g., 20 min of writing or listing three things that happened today), or the quantity of responses expected (e.g., one pleasurable thing, one engaging thing, and one meaningful thing), may also provide more guidance and encourage greater compliance by participants. The key challenge will be to gain verification of completion of self-guided and self-administered activities as instructed and to promote adherence to instructions, without compromising participant autonomy and privacy.

Placebo Control and Control Conditions

Careful selection and monitoring of placebo control activities is needed. It is common for studies investigating PPIs to use daily events or early childhood memories placebo control groups which, on the whole, are believed to be fairly neutral conditions. It is possible, however, that participants in these conditions, particularly those with an optimistic outlook, can be selecting and writing about positive life events, thus transforming this neutral condition into a positive one. This may explain why some studies (e.g., Seligman et al. 2005) have found that their placebo control conditions have also been effective in increasing well-being in some post-intervention measures. Consequently, the content of placebo control activities should also be monitored and accounted for in the interpretation of study findings.

Research participants who have been assigned to a no-activity control group may have decided to adopt their own well-being strategy independent of the study. Although research participants of RCTs are informed that they have an equal chance of being in an intervention or control group, participants of PPI studies often sign up because they have an interest in improving their own well-being. This implies that they may wish to be proactive in meeting this goal during the course of the study. Therefore, asking participants questions about significant life events or lifestyle changes can provide valuable information, which can then be factored into the analysis.

What Are the Desirable Outcomes Resulting from PPIs?

One point for further discussion concerns how the success of PPIs should be evaluated. The majority of research undertaken on PPIs has focused primarily on increased positive affect and satisfaction with life and decreased negative affect and depression, as the target outcome variables. Less focus on short-term, hedonic outcomes, to instead include a wider range of well-being outcomes related to eudaimonia, is desirable. Target outcomes that benefit the community and include long-term growth and other-oriented benefits should be utilized more frequently and extensively in future studies. This will align more closely with contemporary conceptualizations of well-being and help to refine the specific well-being outcomes likely to be attained by various PPIs.

Measurement of Well-Being Change

Measures of well-being most commonly used in PPI studies are limited. Most are self-report measures, which may not be sufficiently sensitive to change. Others focus on narrow conceptualizations of well-being (e.g., high activation emotions). Greater use of a broader range of existing measurement methods is needed. For example, experience sampling and day reconstruction methods may provide greater insights than the exclusive use of standard well-being questionnaires commonly employed in well-being research. Physiological and neurological measures may also help confirm the accuracy of emotional reports. Ideally, more of an *assessment* approach rather than a *testing* approach employing both quantitative and qualitative methods would be valuable.

Multidisciplinary Interventions

It is important that well-being and positive psychology scholars draw on the expertise and knowledge currently available. Incorporating other interventions outside of positive psychology may provide valuable insight and may encourage the development of more diverse and potentially powerful interventions. For example, emotion regulation strategies or music therapy may provide some fruitful avenues for PPIs. Moreover, multidisciplinary collaborations would promote this multifaceted approach to the study and measurement of well-being.

Conclusion

In sum, it appears that positive interventions are generally effective at increasing well-being and decreasing depression for the middle class individual who is motivated to achieve positive changes. However, not all PPIs have been shown to produce all the desired or predicted outcomes, and not all individuals benefit from specific PPIs. Moreover, there are particular groups of people who have not been sufficiently examined in relation to PPIs, resulting in speculation over whether positive interventions are helpful with individuals across the full life span (e.g., for adolescents and older samples) and with specific populations such as those with particular illnesses or learning difficulties. Nevertheless, many studies supporting the efficacy of PPIs are of a high quality (RCTs and meta-analyses). This means that the evidence for PPIs is steadily increasing. Additional appealing features of PPIs are that most are simple, cost-effective, and self-administered, implying that they have real world applicability. Most PPIs appear to have met the two fundamental criteria of being evidence-based and demonstrating ecological validity. What is currently lacking, however, are insights into the optimal conditions for PPIs to achieve the greatest benefits. Given the infancy of PPIs, and the rapid developments gained in the field thus far, it is expected that this knowledge will continue to emerge over time and that robust interventions to suit most individual needs will be developed.

References

Aspinwall, L. G. (1998). Rethinking the role of positive affect in self-regulation. *Motivation and Emotion, 22*, 1–32.

Brickman, P., & Campbell, D. T. (1971). Hedonic relativism and planning the good society. In M. H. Appley (Ed.), *Adaptation-level theory: A symposium* (pp. 287–302). New York: Academic.

Brickman, P., Coates, D., & Janoff-Bulman, R. (1978). Lottery winners and accident victims: Is happiness relative? *Journal of Personality and Social Psychology, 36*, 917–927.

Brown, K. W., & Ryan, M. (2003). The benefits of being present: Mindfulness and its role in psychological well-being. *Journal of Personality and Social Psychology, 84*, 822–848.

Burton, C. M., & King, L. A. (2004). The health benefits of writing about intensely positive experiences. *Journal of Research in Personality, 38*, 150–163.

Cheavens, J. S., Feldman, D. B., Gum, A., Scott, T. M., & Snyder, C. R. (2006). Hope therapy in a community sample: A pilot investigation. *Social Indicators Research, 77*, 61–86.

Cummins, R. A. (2003). Normative life satisfaction: Measurement issues and a homeostatic model. *Social Indicators Research, 64*, 225–256.

Danner, D. D., Snowdon, D. A., & Friesen, W. V. (2001). Positive emotions in early life and longevity: Findings from the nun study. *Journal of Personality and Social Psychology, 80*, 804–813.

Davidson, R. J., Kabat-Zinn, J., Schumacker, J., Rosenkranz, M., Muller, D., Sontorelli, S. F., et al. (2003). Alterations in brain and immune function produced by mindfulness meditation. *Psychosomatic Medicine, 65*, 564–570.

Della, L. J., DeJoy, D. M., Goetzel, R. Z., Ozminkowski, R. J., & Wilson, M. G. (2008). Assessing management support for worksite health promotion: Psychometric analysis of the leading by example (LBE) instrument. *American Journal of Health Promotion, 22*, 359–367.

Delle Fave, A., Brdar, I., Freire, T., Vella-Brodrick, D. A., & Wissing, M. P. (2011). The eudaimonic and hedonic components of happiness: Qualitative and quantitative findings. *Social Indicators Research, 100*, 185–207. Accessible online at: http://www.deepdyve.com/lp/springer-journals/the-eudaimonic-and-hedonic-components-of-happiness-qualitative-and-Dx1x5gb4Gx

Diener, E. (1994). Assessing SWB: Progress and opportunities. *Social Indicators Research, 31*, 103–157.

Diener, E., Suh, E. M., Lucas, R. E., & Smith, H. L. (1999). SWB: Three decades of progress. *Psychological Bulletin, 125*, 276–302.

Diener, E., Lucas, R. E., & Scollon, C. N. (2006). Beyond the hedonic treadmill: Revising the adaptation theory of well-being. *American Psychologist, 61*, 305–314.

Emmons, R. A., & McCullough, M. E. (2003). Counting blessings versus burdens: An experimental investigation of gratitude and SWB in daily life. *Journal of Personality and Social Psychology, 84*, 377–389.

Estrada, C., Isen, A. M., & Young, M. J. (1994). Positive affect influences creative problem solving and reported source of practice satisfaction in physicians. *Motivation and Emotion, 18*, 285–299.

Fava, G. A., Rafanelli, C., Cazzaro, M., Conti, S., & Grandi, S. (1998). Well-being therapy: A novel psychotherapeutic model for residual symptoms of affective disorders. *Psychological Medicine, 28*, 475–480.
Fordyce, M. W. (1977). Development of a program to increase happiness. *Journal of Counseling Psychology, 24*, 511–521.
Fordyce, M. W. (1983). A program to increase happiness: Further studies. *Journal of Counseling Psychology, 4*, 483–498.
Fredrickson, B. L. (2001). The role of positive emotions in positive psychology: The broaden-and-build theory of positive emotions. *American Psychologist, 56*, 218–226.
Fredrickson, B. L., & Levenson, R. W. (1998). Positive emotions speed recovery from the cardiovascular sequelae of negative emotions. *Cognition and Emotion, 12*, 191–220.
Freedman, S. R., & Enright, R. D. (1986). Forgiveness as an intervention goal with incest survivors. *Journal of Consulting and Clinical Psychology, 64*, 983–992.
Froh, J. J., Kashdan, T. B., Ozimkowsk, K. M., & Miller, N. (2009). Who benefits the most from a gratitude intervention in children and adolescents? Examining positive affect as a moderator. *The Journal of Positive Psychology, 4*, 408–422.
Giannopoulos, V. L., & Vella-Brodrick, D. A. (2011). Effects of positive interventions and orientations to happiness on subjective well-being. *Journal of Positive Psychology, 6*, 95–105.
Harker, L., & Keltner, D. (2001). Expressions of positive emotions in women's college yearbook pictures and their relationship to personality and life outcomes across adulthood. *Journal of Personality and Social Psychology, 80*, 112–124.
Headey, B. (2006). Life goals matter to happiness: A revision of set-point theory. *Social Indicators Research, 86*, 213–231.
Holmes, E. A., & Mathews, A. (2010). Mental imagery in emotion and emotional disorders. *Clinical Psychology Review, 30*, 349–362.
Holmes, E. A., Mathews, A., Mackintosh, B., & Dalgleish, T. (2008). The causal effect of mental imagery on emotion assessed using picture-word cues. *Emotion, 8*, 395–409.
Huppert, F. A., & Johnson, D. M. (2010). A controlled trial of mindfulness training in schools: The importance of practice for an impact on well-being. *The Journal of Positive Psychology, 5*, 264–274.
Jha, A. P., Stanley, E. A., Kiyonaga, A., Wong, L., & Gelfand, L. (2010). Examining the protective effects of mindfulness training on working capacity and affective experience. *Emotion, 10*, 54–64.
Kabat-Zinn, J. (2003). Mindfulness-based interventions in context: Past, present, and future. *Clinical Psychology: Science and Practice, 10*, 144–156.
Kashdan, T. B., Biswas-Diener, R., & King, L. A. (2008). Reconsidering happiness: The cost of distinguishing between hedonics and eudaimonia. *The Journal of Positive Psychology, 3*, 219–233.
Keyes, C. L. M. (2002). The mental health continuum: From languishing to flourishing in life. *Journal of Health and Social Research, 43*, 207–222.
Keyes, C. L. M. (2005). Mental illness and/or mental health? Investigating axioms of the complete state model of health. *Journal of Consulting and Clinical Psychology, 73*(3), 539–548.
Keyes, C. L. M. (2007). Promoting and protecting mental health as flourishing: A complementary strategy for improving national mental health. *American Psychologist, 62*(2), 95–108.
Keyes, C. L. M., Shmotkin, D., & Ryff, C. D. (2002). Optimizing well-being: The empirical encounter of two traditions. *Journal of Personality and Social Psychology, 82*, 1007–1022.
King, L. A. (2001). The health benefits of writing about life goals. *Personality and Social Psychology Bulletin, 27*, 798–807.
Lewandowski, G. (2009). Promoting positive emotions following relationship dissolution through writing. *The Journal of Positive Psychology, 4*, 21–31.
Lykken, D., & Tellegen, A. (1996). Happiness is a stochastic phenomenon. *Psychological Science, 7*, 186–189.
Lyubomirsky, S. (2008). *The how of happiness: A scientific approach to getting the life you want.* New York: Penguin Press.
Lyubomirsky, S., King, L., & Diener, E. (2005a). The benefits of frequent positive affect: Does happiness lead to success? *Psychological Bulletin, 131*, 803–855.

Lyubomirsky, S., Sheldon, K. M., & Schkade, D. (2005b). Pursuing happiness: The architecture of sustainable change. *Review of General Psychology, 9*, 111–131.
Martin, K. A., Moritz, S. E., & Hall, C. R. (1999). Imagery use in sport: A literature review and applied mode. *The Sport Psychologist, 13*, 245–268.
Mitchell, J., Stanimirovic, R., Klein, B., & Vella-Brodrick, D. (2009). A randomised controlled trial of a self-guided internet intervention promoting well-being. *Computers in Human Behavior, 25*, 749–760.
Nazarian, D., & Smyth, J. (2008). Expressive writing. In W. O'Donohue & N. Cummings (Eds.), *Evidence-based adjunctive treatments* (pp. 221–241). New York: Elsevier Inc.
Odou, N., & Vella-Brodrick, D. A. (2011). The efficacy of positive psychology interventions to increase well-being and the role of mental imagery ability. *Social Indicators Research* (published on-line 20 August, 2011).
Otake, K., Shimai, S., Tanaka-Matsumi, J., Otsui, K., & Fredrickson, B. L. (2006). Happy people become happier through kindness: A counting kindness intervention. *Journal of Happiness Studies, 7*, 361–375.
Peters, M. L., Flink, I. K., Boersma, K., & Linton, S. J. (2010). Manipulating optimism: Can imagining a best possible self be used to increase positive future expectancies? *The Journal of Positive Psychology, 5*, 204–211.
Peterson, C., Park, N., & Seligman, M. E. (2005). Orientations to happiness and life satisfaction: The full life versus the empty life. *Journal of Happiness Studies, 6*, 25–41.
Pressman, S. D., & Cohen, S. (2005). Does positive affect influence health? *Psychological Bulletin, 131*, 925–971.
Reed, G. L., & Enright, R. D. (2006). The effects of forgiveness therapy on depression, anxiety and, post-traumatic stress for women after spousal emotional abuse. *Journal of Consulting and Clinical Psychology, 74*, 920–929.
Richardson, A. (1969). *Mental imagery*. London: Routledge & Kegan Paul.
Ryan, R. M., & Deci, E. L. (2001). On happiness and human potentials: A review of the research on hedonic and eudaimonic well-being. *Annual Review of Psychology, 52*, 141–166.
Ryff, C. D. (1989). Happiness is everything, or is it? Explorations on the meaning of psychological well-being. *Journal of Personality and Social Psychology, 57*, 1069–1081.
Schueller, S. M. (2010). Preferences for positive psychology exercises. *The Journal of Positive Psychology, 5*, 192–203.
Schueller, S. M. (2011). To each his own well-being boosting intervention: Using preference to guide selection. *The Journal of Positive Psychology, 6*, 300–313.
Seligman, M. E. P. (2011). Flourish: A Visionary New Understanding of Happiness and Well-being. New York: Free Press.
Seligman, M. E. P. (2002). *Authentic happiness*. New York: Free Press.
Seligman, M. E. P., & Csikszentmihalyi, M. (2000). Positive psychology. An introduction. *American Psychologist, 55*, 5.
Seligman, M. E. P., Steen, T. A., Park, N. P., & Peterson, C. (2005). Positive psychology progress: Empirical validation of interventions. *American Psychologist, 60*, 410–421.
Seligman, M. E. P., Rashid, T., & Parks, A. C. (2006). Positive psychology progress: Empirical validation of interventions. *American Psychologist, 60*, 410–421.
Sergeant, S., & Mongrain, M. (2011). Are positive psychology exercises helpful for people with depressive personality styles? *The Journal of Positive Psychology, 6*, 260–272.
Sheldon, K. M., & Lyubomirsky, S. (2004). Achieving sustainable new happiness: Prospects, practices, and prescriptions. In A. Linley & S. Joseph (Eds.), *Positive psychology in practice* (pp. 127–145). Hoboken: Wiley.
Sheldon, K. M., & Lyubomirsky, S. (2006). How to increase and sustain positive emotion: The effect of expressing gratitude and visualizing best possible selves. *The Journal of Positive Psychology, 1*, 73–82.
Silberman, J. (2007). Positive intervention self-selection: Developing models of what works for whom. *International Coaching Psychology Review, 2*, 70–77.

Sin, N. L., & Lyubomirsky, S. (2009). Enhancing well-being and alleviating depressive symptoms with positive psychology interventions: A practice-friendly meta-analysis. *Journal of Clinical Psychology, 65*, 467–487.

Tennant, R., Hiller, L., Fishwick, R., Platt, S., Joseph, S., Weich, S., et al. (2007). The Warwick-Edinburgh Mental Well-being Scale (WEMWBS): Development and UK validation. *Health and Quality of Life Outcomes, 5*(63).

Thomas, D. C. (2006). Domain and development of cultural intelligence: The importance of mindfulness. *Group and Organization Management, 31*, 78–79.

Vella-Brodrick, D. A., Park, N., & Peterson, C. (2009). Three ways to be happy: Pleasure, engagement, and meaning—findings from Australian and US samples. *Social Indicators Research, 90*, 165–179.

Waterman, A. S. (2008). Reconsidering happiness: A eudaimonist's perspective. *The Journal of Positive Psychology, 3*, 234–252.

Waterman, A. S., Schwartz, S. J., Zamboanga, B. L., Ravert, R. D., Williams, M. K., Bede Agocha, V., et al. (2010). The questionnaire for eudaimonic well-being: Psychometric properties, demographic comparisons, and evidence of validity. *The Journal of Positive Psychology, 5*, 41–61.

Waugh, C. E., & Fredrickson, B. L. (2006). Nice to know you: Positive emotions, self-other overlap, and complex understanding in the formation of a new relationship. *The Journal of Positive Psychology, 1*, 93–106.

Williams, S., & Shiaw, W. T. (1999). Mood and organizational citizenship behavior: The effects of positive affect on employee organizational citizenship behavior intentions. *Journal of Psychology, 133*, 656–668.

Williams, G. C., Lynch, M. F., McGregor, H. A., Ryan, R. M., Sharp, D., & Deci, E. (2006). Validation of the "important other" climate questionnaire: Assessing autonomy support for health-related change. *Families, Systems and Health, 24*, 179–194.

Chapter 16
Promoting Positive Mental Health and Well-Being: Practice and Policy

Margaret M. Barry

Promoting positive mental health and well-being is an integral part of improving the overall health of a population. Positive mental health is fundamental to good health and is a resource which enables people to manage their lives successfully and thereby contributes to the functioning of individuals, families, communities, and society. The concept of mental health cannot be separated from that of overall health, which was defined in the World Health Organization Constitution of 1946 as a state of complete physical, mental, and social well-being, and not merely the absence of disease or injury. More recent definitions have gone on to describe health as a resource for living and as a positive concept, emphasizing social and personal resources as well as physical capacities (WHO 1986). Positive mental health is conceptualized as encompassing the dimensions of both subjective emotional well-being and positive psychological and social functioning (Keyes 2007; Kovess-Masfety et al. 2005). Empirical findings support the independence of positive and negative mental health, showing that the absence of mental disorder does not equal the presence of mental health (Keyes 2005, 2007; Huppert 2005). As a positive resource, mental health contributes to the social, human, and economic capital of society (Lehtinen et al. 2005). The promotion of positive mental health is, therefore, important in its own right.

There is increased global recognition of the importance of promoting mental health, as reflected in a number of key international publications and policy documents. The WHO (2001) World Health Report advocated a comprehensive public health approach to mental health, including mental health promotion and prevention, in order to reduce the burden of mental health problems at a population level. The Prevention and Promotion in Mental Health report (WHO 2002) further prioritized the role of promotion and prevention, acknowledging that policies focused on curing

M.M. Barry (✉)
WHO Collaborating Centre for Health Promotion Research,
School of Health Sciences, National University of Ireland Galway,
Galway, Ireland
e-mail: margaret.barry@nuigalway.ie

C.L.M. Keyes (ed.), *Mental Well-Being: International Contributions to the Study of Positive Mental Health*, DOI 10.1007/978-94-007-5195-8_16,

or preventing mental ill-health alone will not necessarily deliver on improved mental health at a population level.

A population approach to mental health underscores the universal relevance of mental health for the general population and identifies the need for strategies that can be applied across population groups. These strategies range from building resilience and promoting mental health for healthy populations to reducing risk for those at higher risk of developing mental health problems and promoting recovery and well-being for people with mental disorders. A population approach to mental health improvement requires the development of policy and program interventions, which extend beyond the clinical, and treatment, focus of current mental health service delivery, in order to address the influence of broader social and environmental determinants of mental health.

The WHO reports on Promoting Mental Health: Concepts, Emerging Evidence, Practice (WHO 2004a; Herrman et al. 2005) and the International Union for Health Promotion and Education special issue on the evidence of mental health promotion effectiveness (Jané-Llopis et al. 2005) clearly outline the concepts relating to the promotion of mental health, emerging evidence for the effectiveness of interventions, and public health policy and practice implications. A separate WHO report on the Prevention of Mental Disorders was also published in tandem (WHO 2004b). Through these landmark publications, the rationale for mental health promotion, its conceptual and research base, and its distinctive approach to mental health improvement have become more clearly established internationally. The feasibility of implementing effective strategies that promote mental health has also been demonstrated through increased focus on evidence-based practice (Herrman et al. 2005; Barry and Jenkins 2007). In keeping with this international momentum, mental health promotion policy and practice have been introduced and strengthened in a number of countries.

Much progress has been made over the last 20 years in establishing an evidence base for the promotion of mental health. There is consensus that there are clusters of known risk and protective factors for mental health (Mrazek and Haggerty 1994). There is also a growing body of evidence that interventions exist which can modify these factors. A number of intervention programs evaluated in efficacy and effectiveness trials have been established and disseminated (Hosman and Jané-Llopis 1999; Jané-Llopis et al. 2005; Herrman et al. 2005; Keleher and Armstrong 2005; Barry and Jenkins 2007). There is compelling evidence from high-quality studies that interventions promoting mental health, when implemented effectively, can lead to lasting positive effects on a range of health and social outcomes (Friedli 2003; Keleher and Armstrong 2005; Herrman et al. 2005; Barry and Jenkins 2007; Barry et al. 2009a). The accumulating evidence demonstrates the feasibility of implementing effective mental health promotion programs across a range of diverse population groups and settings (Jané-Llopis and Barry 2005; Barry and Jenkins 2007). Findings from systematic reviews indicate that there is sufficient knowledge to guide effective practice and policy in this field (Jané-Llopis et al. 2005).

There is also increasing recognition of the wider policy and economic case for investing in promoting mental health and well-being at a population level

(Marshall-Williams et al. 2005). Good mental health is recognized as a key asset and resource for population well-being and for the long-term social and economic prosperity of society (WHO 2002, 2005a; Lehtinen et al. 2005; Foresight Project on Mental Capital and Wellbeing 2008). There is a growing realization that interventions promoting mental health and well-being, which can be implemented and sustained at a reasonable cost, will generate clear health and social gains for the general population and, therefore, represent a strong case for policy investment (WHO 2002, 2005a; Friedli and Parsonage 2007; Zechmeister et al. 2008; Barry and Friedli 2008).

This chapter provides an overview of international developments concerning the policy and practice of promoting positive mental health. The key concepts and principles of mental health promotion are outlined, and the implications of embracing a health promotion perspective and a socioecological model of mental health are discussed. The distinction between the conceptual frameworks for the practice of mental health promotion, which aims to enhance positive mental health, and the prevention of mental disorders, which aims to reduce mental ill-health, is outlined. The adoption of a competence-enhancement model of mental health promotion, as opposed to a risk reduction model for mental disorders, is explained. The evidence of effective interventions that promote positive mental health across life stages from the early years through adulthood in key settings such as the home, school, workplace, and community is examined. Policy developments on mental health promotion in a number of countries are presented, including policies which embrace a positive well-being focus and advocate for a flourishing society based on promoting population mental health and well-being. The importance of mainstreaming and sustaining policy and practice developments for maximizing population impact is considered. The need to build capacity, including workforce development for the implementation of effective mental health promotion interventions, is discussed.

Promoting Positive Mental Health and Well-Being: A Framework for Action

Positive mental health is a broad concept, and as outlined elsewhere in this book, there are a range of constructs and theories relevant to its understanding. The emerging literature conceptualizes positive mental health as encompassing aspects of emotional (affect/feeling), psychological (positive functioning), social (relations with others and society), physical (physical health and fitness), and spiritual (sense of meaning and purpose in life) well-being (Keyes 2002, 2007; Huppert 2005; Kovess-Masfety et al. 2005; Zubrick and Kovess-Masfety 2005; Ryff et al. 2006). A number of key constructs have been used to inform the development of indicators of positive mental health, including concepts such as resilience, self-esteem, self-efficacy, optimism, life satisfaction, hopefulness, sense of control, meaning in life, fulfillment, and social integration (Keyes 2005; Stewart-Brown 2005; Zubrick and Kovess-Masfety 2005; Ryff and Singer 1996). Indicators of positive mental health, which include both general measures and validated scales, have been found to be associated with indicators of better physical health, fewer limitations in daily living, higher educational attainment, better employment and earnings, better quality of life, supportive social relationships, and positive health behaviors (Lehtinen et al. 2005; Lyubomirsky et al. 2005; Dolan et al. 2006; Barry et al. 2009b; Friedli 2009). Conceptualized as such, positive mental health is an integral component of general health and well-being. The challenge is, therefore, to understand the factors that build and enhance positive mental health and create the conditions and environments that support the development of psychological strengths, resilience, and positive relations with others and society. The development of this knowledge is key to realizing the potential of this new focus on positive aspects of mental health and well-being.

Promoting and enhancing positive mental health requires an understanding of appropriate frameworks for practice at a population level. Positioning its core focus on the *health* end of the mental health–disease continuum, mental health promotion provides a distinct framework for action informed by a multidisciplinary base of theory, research, and values. Many of the constructs that constitute positive mental health have already been incorporated into the practice of mental health promotion and have informed interventions designed to enhance the psychological strengths, competencies, and resources of individuals, families, and communities (Herrman et al. 2005; Jané-Llopis et al. 2005; Barry and Jenkins 2007). A framework for implementing mental health promotion interventions is presented in this chapter, along with the evidence that demonstrates the capacity of these interventions to have an impact on positive mental health and well-being.

Adopting a Health Promotion Approach to Promoting Positive Mental Health

A health promotion framework locates mental health within a holistic definition of health and builds on the basic tenets of health promotion, as outlined in the Ottawa Charter (WHO 1986) and subsequent WHO directives (WHO 2005b, 2009). Health promotion is understood to be the process of enabling people to increase control over, and to improve, their health. The Ottawa Charter embraces a positive definition of health and shifts the focus from an individual, disease prevention approach toward the health actions and wider social determinants that keep people healthy. Health promotion, therefore, embraces actions directed at strengthening the skills and capabilities of individuals, together with actions on changing the social, environmental, and economic conditions which have an impact on health. The principles of health promotion practice, as articulated in the Ottawa Charter for Health Promotion (WHO 1986), are based on an empowering, participative, and collaborative process which aims to improve health and reduce health inequities.

Health promotion is driven by a socioecological model of health, as it seeks to improve the everyday contexts (home, schools, communities, and workplaces) where people live and where health is created. Health promotion addresses the broader social, physical, and economic environments that determine the health of populations and individuals (Mittelmark et al. 2005). Applying this socioecological model to mental health, mental health is viewed as being embedded in, and influenced by, a wider social, economic, and cultural ecology (Zubrick and Kovess-Masfety 2005). This perspective stresses the interdependence of the individual, family, community, and society and moves the concept of mental health beyond an individualistic focus to consider the broader social, economic, cultural, political, and environmental determinants. Mental health promotion emphasizes that mental health is created and promoted within the everyday contexts or settings, such as the home, school, workplace, and community. Mental health promotion interventions address the broader social determinants of the mental health of populations and individuals.

Mental health promotion is, therefore, conceptualized as an empowering, participative, and collaborative process, which enables people to increase control over their mental health and its determinants. An emphasis on *enabling positive mental health* focuses attention on both the process of implementing mental health promotion (i.e., it should be an enabling process) and on the impact on positive mental health outcomes, as opposed to reductions in mental ill-health.

The Ottawa Charter for Health Promotion (WHO 1986) outlined five key areas for action to promote health, each of which can be applied to mental health promotion. *Building healthy public policy* puts mental health promotion on the agenda of all policy makers and calls for coordinated action across health, economic, and social policies for improved mental health. *Creating supportive environments* moves mental health beyond an individualistic focus to consider the influence of broader social, physical, cultural, and economic environments and highlights the importance of mediating structures such as the home, school, workplace, and community as key contexts or settings for creating and promoting positive mental health. *Strengthening community action* focuses on the empowerment of communities through their active engagement and participation in identifying their needs, setting priorities, planning, and implementing action to achieve better mental health at the community level. *Developing personal skills* involves enabling personal and social development through providing information, education, and enhancing life skills for improving mental health. *Reorienting health services* requires that health services embrace the importance of mental health to overall health and well-being and that mental health services embrace promotion and prevention strategies as well as treatment and rehabilitation.

The health promotion framework has been applied to the promotion of mental health, underscoring the need for integrated action at the level of the individual, community, supportive environments, and policies, in order to bring about sustainable change that will create and promote positive mental health (Health Education Authority 1997; Victorian Health Promotion Foundation 2005; Commonwealth Department of Health and Aged Care 2000; Barry 2001; Lahtinen et al. 2005; Ministry of Health New Zealand 2005; Herrman et al. 2005; Barry and Jenkins 2007). The Melbourne Charter for Promoting Mental Health and Preventing Mental and Behavioural Disorders (VicHealth 2009) endorses the health promotion approach to promoting mental health and outlines the principles and actions that can be taken by governments, communities, and organizations to influence the interconnecting social, economic, cultural, environmental, and personal factors that influence mental health and well-being. A number of current international policies have also embraced the Ottawa Charter as a basis for mental health promotion. The health promotion framework usefully informs the conceptualization and principles of promoting mental health, which have been articulated as follows (Barry 2007):

- Mental health promotion involves the population as a whole in the context of everyday life, rather than focusing exclusively on people at risk from specific mental disorders.
- Focuses on protective factors for enhancing well-being and quality of life.
- Addresses the social, physical, and socioeconomic environments that determine the mental health of populations and individuals.
- Adopts complementary approaches and integrated strategies, operating from the individual to socioenvironmental levels.
- Involves intersectoral action extending beyond the health sector.
- Is based on public participation, engagement, and empowerment.

The inextricable link between people and their environments forms the basis of the socioecological approach to mental health promotion and provides a distinctive conceptual framework for practice. This framework embraces a systems approach to mental health promotion, spanning individual, social, and environmental factors, and underlines the importance of multisectoral involvement and synergistic action from the micro- to the macrolevel, to bring about tangible and enduring change.

Conceptual Frameworks for Practice

The practice of mental health promotion is underpinned by multidisciplinary concepts, theories, and research, which provide integrated models for designing, conducting, and evaluating interventions. In considering frameworks for practice, it is useful to make a distinction between the practice of mental health promotion and the prevention of mental disorders. These two areas, while clearly related and overlapping, tend to operate within different conceptual frameworks. Mental health promotion focuses on positive mental health, and its aim is to enhance psychosocial strengths, competencies, and resources. In contrast, the area of prevention primarily concerns specific mental disorders and aims to reduce the incidence and prevalence, or seriousness, of targeted problems, that is, mortality, morbidity, and risk behavior outcomes. Articulated as such, these two fields have different starting points; one is concerned with competence enhancement and the other with risk reduction. They also seek to impact different outcomes, one is focused on the promotion of positive mental health and the other on the prevention of mental health disorders. In practice, however, there is some common ground between the two areas, particularly with regard to primary prevention and mental health promotion interventions.

The most widely used prevention framework in mental health was put forward by Mrazek and Haggerty (1994). Depicted as a half circle, this framework places prevention activities in the wider mental health intervention spectrum of treatment, maintenance, and rehabilitation. Three main categories of prevention activities are identified: universal prevention (targeting the general population), selected prevention (targeting high-risk groups), and indicated prevention (targeting high-risk individuals or groups with minimal, but detectable, signs or symptoms of mental disorder). While clearly articulating the different types of prevention, this framework does not include interventions that focus on promoting positive mental health. However, it would appear that, at least conceptually, there is quite an overlap between universal prevention activities as outlined in the framework and those of mental health promotion. The 2009 report by the US Committee on Prevention of Mental Disorders and Substance Abuse of Children, Youth, and Young Adults (O'Connell et al. 2009) strongly recommends the inclusion of mental health promotion in the spectrum of mental health interventions. This report endorses the view that mental health is more than the absence of disorder and that a focus on wellness and the promotion of mental health will have far-reaching benefits that extend beyond a specific disorder. Barry (2001) adapted the Mrazek and Haggerty (1994) prevention framework to include mental health promotion, which depicts mental health promotion as the largest part of the circle, given its universal relevance, and indicates the unifying central area between the different interventions as being strategies for promoting well-being and quality of life. An amended version of this figure, first published in 2001, is presented in Fig. 16.1.

Within the mental health promotion framework, recognition of the broader determinants of mental health has led to a growing emphasis on models of mental health promotion that seek to intervene in strengthening individuals and communities and removing the structural barriers to mental health through initiatives to reduce poverty, discrimination, and inequalities (Barry and Friedli 2008; Barry 2009; Herrman et al. 2005; Lahtinen et al. 2005). The existence of review-level evidence of the effectiveness of mental health promotion across these multiple levels strengthens the case for action (WHO 2004a; Jané-Llopis et al. 2005; Keleher and Armstrong 2005; Barry et al. 2009a).

The Evidence Base for Mental Health Promotion Practice

Systematic reviews and effectiveness studies have been published that show many examples of effective interventions which promote and enhance mental health and lead to wider social and health gains. The evidence supports the value of programs promoting positive mental health, demonstrating that many of these initiatives have a positive impact on mental health and have the dual effect of reducing risks of mental disorders (Durlak and Wells 1997; Hosman and Jané-Llopis 1999;

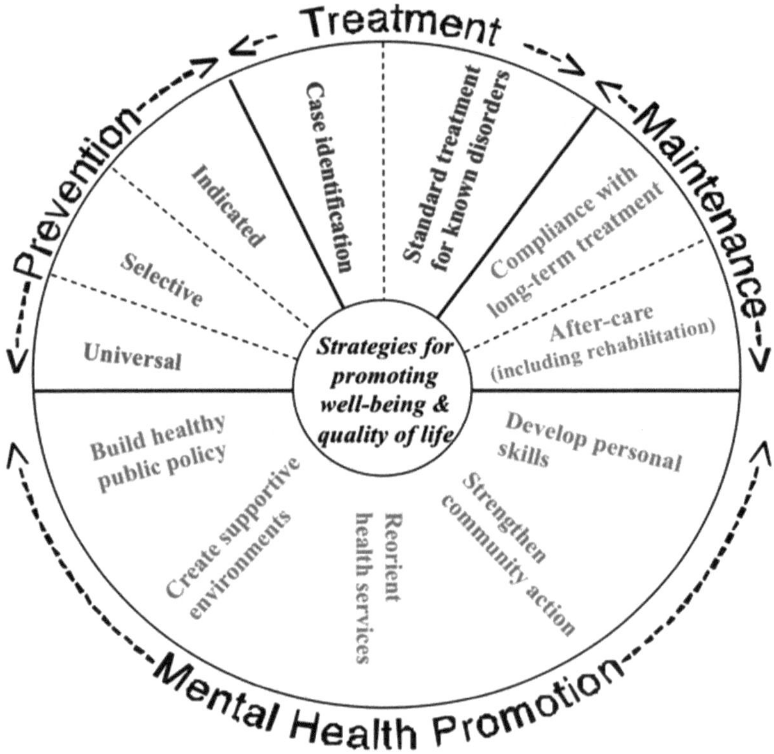

Fig. 16.1 Depicting mental health promotion within the spectrum of mental health interventions

Friedli 2003; Herrman et al. 2005; Jané-Llopis et al. 2005; Keleher and Armstrong 2005; Barry 2009). The available evidence supports the view that competence-enhancing programs carried out in collaboration with families, schools, and wider communities have the potential to have an impact on multiple positive outcomes across social and personal health domains (Jané-Llopis and Barry 2005; Barry 2009). This section reviews the evidence across life stages from the early years through adulthood and considers the findings in terms of effective interventions that promote positive mental health in the early years, in school, at the workplace, and in the community and broader society.

Promoting Positive Mental Health in the Early Years

A number of interventions have been developed which promote positive mental health in the early years of life, through empowering parents and enhancing resilience and competence in both children and parents (Kendrick et al. 2000, 2007; Barlow et al. 2003; Elkan et al. 2000; Ciliska et al. 1999; Olds et al. 1997). Systematic reviews indicate that interventions that provide quality family support programs, including parenting support, home visiting, and quality preschool programs, have the potential to achieve long-term mental health benefits for both children and their parents (Barry et al. 2009a). The value of these interventions lies not only on their ability to reduce the risk factors for negative developmental outcomes, such as delinquency, substance misuse, teenage pregnancy, violence, and school failure, but also in their potential to enhance positive child and family functioning through promoting competence, positive relationships, and supportive environments for development (Barry and Jenkins 2007; Jané-Llopis et al. 2005).

Home Visiting Programs

Systematic reviews of home visiting programs for parents of children in the first 2 years of life show robust evidence of improved parenting skills, improved child development, reduced behavioral problems, and improved maternal health and social functioning (Ciliska et al. 1999; Elkan et al. 2000; Kendrick et al. 2000, 2007; Bull et al. 2004; Tennant et al. 2007). Positive findings with medium to strong effect sizes are particularly evident for programs which start antenatally, are of high intensity, are of medium to long duration (up to at least 12 months), and are designed for parents considered to be at higher risk, for example, low-income parents, teenage parents, single parents, and mothers coping with postnatal depression (Tennant et al. 2007; Waddell et al. 2007).

Intensive and comprehensive programs, such as the Prenatal and Infancy Home Visitation by Nurses program (Olds et al. 1997, 1998, 2004), have established strong evidence over 30 years of their cost-effectiveness in terms of long-term positive health, social, and economic gains for pregnant women and their children up to 15 years postintervention. Findings from a number of randomized controlled trials with participants from diverse backgrounds (Olds et al. 2006) not only support the program's impact on reducing negative outcomes, such as child abuse, behavioral problems, and substance misuse, but also report a number of positive outcomes including improved prenatal health, enhanced child development, and mothers' personal development. A report from the Rand Corporation estimated that the cost savings on this intervention, due to reduced welfare, health care, crime costs, and increased taxes, are four times the original investment by the time a child reaches the age of 15 years (Karoly et al. 1998). Alongside such structured programs, which are delivered by trained nurse home visitors, there is also some convincing evidence concerning the effectiveness of peer-led interventions involving trained volunteer visitors, such as the Community Mothers Program (Johnson et al. 1993, 2000).

Parenting Programs

Parenting interventions have also been found to have a significant impact on positive mental health, including improving maternal psychosocial health (Barlow et al. 2002) and the emotional and behavioral adjustment of children (Barlow and Parson 2003;

Tennant et al. 2007). Based on a meta-analysis of 213 programs, Barlow et al. (2003) concluded that there is clear evidence of the impact of parenting programs in improving psychosocial outcomes for mothers of children aged 3–10 years, including; improved self-esteem, reduced anxiety, stress, and depression, and improved relationship with spouse and marital adjustment. Programs such as the Triple P Positive Parenting Program have been successfully incorporated into service delivery in a range of health and community services. Findings from a number of randomized controlled trials (Sanders 1999; Sanders et al. 2000; Dean et al. 2003) and a meta-analysis (De Graaf et al. 2008) have demonstrated that the Triple P Program results in increased positive parenting practices, which in turn result in improved children's behavior, lower levels of dysfunctional parenting, reduced parental conflict, and gains in parental mental health.

Preschool Programs

Systematic reviews demonstrate the effectiveness of early childhood and preschool education programs in enhancing the cognitive and social skills of children under 5 years of age, improved academic achievement, school readiness, and mental and social development (Anderson et al. 2003; Nelson et al. 2003; Karoly et al. 2005; Schweinhart et al. 2005; Sylva et al. 2007). Impressive long-term results have been achieved by programs, such as the High Scope Perry Preschool Project, that address preschool development, including enhancing language, cognitive, and social skills in children aged 3–4 years from disadvantaged backgrounds (Schweinhart et al. 2005). With follow-ups over 40 years, the High Scope Perry Preschool Project has been found to positively impact school success, improve employment rates and earnings, increase social responsibility (including fewer criminal arrests), reduce the need for social service benefits, and improve family functioning. The majority of preschool programs are designed for children from disadvantaged backgrounds, and the duration and intensity of the interventions are related to outcomes (Nelson et al. 2003). With regard to positive mental health impact, it is interesting to note that relatively large effect sizes are reported for social–emotional impacts (ES = 0.27–0.33) and cognitive outcomes (ES = 0.30) (Tennant et al. 2007).

Longitudinal studies not only show that the benefits from early years interventions can be long-lasting in multiple domains, but they also show that the savings the programs generate can be substantial. Economic analyses of several early childhood interventions demonstrate that effective programs, particularly those with long-term outcomes, can repay the initial investment with savings to governments and benefits to society, with those at most risk making the greatest gains (Karoly et al. 2005; Galinsky 2006; Friedli and Parsonage 2007).

The roll-out of multicomponent support interventions, such as the Sure Start programs for young children and their families living in deprived communities in England (Melhuish et al. 2008), has also reported improved social development outcomes for children, improved parenting, better home-learning environments, and greater use of support services. These findings are encouraging because they support the feasibility of scaling-up such interventions on a national scale.

Early interventions have an important role to play in addressing child health inequities. As home visiting and parenting programs often deal with the most vulnerable families, such as those living in socially and economically disadvantaged communities, these interventions are viewed as having the potential to break cycles of disadvantage and social exclusion. However, the effectiveness of these interventions needs to be viewed in the context of wider policy initiatives, addressing poverty and the wider structural determinants of child health inequities.

Promoting Positive Mental Health in Schools

Schools are one of the most important settings for promoting the mental health of young people. Schools have an important function in nurturing children's social and emotional development as well as their academic and cognitive development. Enhancing children's mental health will improve their ability to learn and to achieve academically as well as their capacity to become responsible adults and citizens (Weissberg et al. 1991; Zins et al. 2004; Payton et al. 2008).

There is a growing body of evidence that mental health promotion in schools, when implemented effectively, can produce long-term benefits for young people, including emotional and social functioning and improved academic performance (Tilford et al. 1997; Durlak and Wells 1997; Lister-Sharp et al. 1999; Greenberg et al. 2001; Harden et al. 2001; Wells et al. 2003; Payton et al. 2008). Reviews of the evidence show that comprehensive programs that are implemented continuously for more than one year, are aimed at the promotion of mental health as opposed to the prevention of mental disorder, and that target multiple health outcomes in the context of a coordinated whole-school approach, offer the most consistently effective strategies (Wells et al. 2003; Jané-Llopis et al. 2005). The evidence indicates that long-term interventions promoting the positive mental health of all pupils, and involving changes to the school environment, are likely to be more successful than brief class-based prevention programs.

Social and Emotional Learning Programs

A number of successful universal school-based programs targeting all pupils have employed cognitive skills training in promoting social and emotional competencies (Shure and Spivack 1988; Kellam et al. 1994; Bruene-Butler et al. 1997; Greenberg et al. 1995, 2001; Aber et al. 1998; Mishara and Ystgaard 2006; Clarke and Barry 2010). Many of these programs have been evaluated using randomized controlled trials and have been replicated with a wide range of children in different school settings across countries. Three large-scale meta-analyses of research on the impact of social and emotional learning (SEL) programs on children in the United States aged 5–13 years were conducted by Payton et al. (2008).

These reviews confirm that SEL improves students' social–emotional skills, attitudes about self and others, connection to school, positive social behavior, and students' academic performance by 11 percentage points. SEL programs were also found to reduce students' conduct problems and emotional distress and to be effective in both school and after-school settings, for racially and ethnically diverse students and for students with and without behavioral and emotional problems.

Whole-School Approaches

Programs adopting a whole-school approach seek to enhance the social and emotional well-being and positive life skills of pupils and work to create supportive environments that foster positive youth development and a sense of connectedness with the family, community, and broader social context of young people's lives (Rowling et al. 2002). Review evidence supports the effectiveness of mental health promotion programs in schools that take a whole-school approach (Wells et al. 2003; Lister-Sharp et al. 1999). Examples of whole-school programs that have been implemented at a national level include the Australian MindMatters program (Wynn et al. 2000) and the Social and Emotional Aspects of Learning (SEAL) initiative in England (Department for Education and Skills 2005). While evidence relating to programs that adopt a *truly* whole-school approach (i.e., include all elements) is quite limited, those that have been identified provide indication of a positive impact, with small to medium effect sizes being reported on outcome measures (Adi et al. 2007). Interventions employing a whole-school approach are more likely to be effective in decreasing bullying than curriculum-only programs. The Olweus Bullying Prevention Program (Olweus et al. 1998) is one such example of a comprehensive whole-school intervention designed to reduce bullying at the level of the individual pupil, the classroom, and the school as a whole.

A review of the cost-effectiveness of whole-school approaches by McCabe (2007) suggests that interventions of this type can lead to health, academic, and social gains, which lead to savings for health and social services and for the criminal justice system. Lack of investment in mental health promotion in schools is likely to lead to significant costs for society as children who experience emotional and social problems are more likely, at some point, to misuse drugs and alcohol, to have lower educational attainment, and to be untrained, unemployed, and involved in crime.

To date, there has been comparatively little research on mental health promotion in schools outside of the USA. There is a need for high-quality studies with longitudinal designs to assess the impact of school-based interventions across education systems, cultures, and structures. While there is still much to learn regarding how best to implement and support the effective implementation of school-based mental health promotion programs, the current evidence clearly demonstrates their value in promoting the mental health and well-being of young people.

Promoting Positive Mental Health in the Workplace

The workplace is a key environment that affects the mental health and well-being of working adults (WHO 2000). The importance of work in terms of role fulfillment, self-identity, sense of purpose, and participation in society is well recognized. Traditionally, many workplace health initiatives have placed more emphasis on physical health and safety issues in the workplace than on mental health. The promotion of positive mental health is relevant to many aspects of employment, including health and safety, equal opportunities, bullying and harassment, and work–life balance initiatives. Creating a healthy workplace entails creating an environment that is supportive of the psychosocial aspects of work, recognizing the potential of the workplace to promote workers' mental health and well-being and to reduce the negative impacts of work-related stress. Many of the factors that influence the positive health and well-being of workers relate to the social environment at work, such as style of management, working culture, the psychological demands of work, work overload, levels of social support, and job security.

Effective workplace interventions address the physical, environmental, and psychosocial factors influencing mental health. They strengthen modifying factors such as social support, control over decision making, and effort–reward balance, and they provide skills and competences for addressing short-term and long-term responses to work-related stress. Additionally, they enhance role clarity, staff involvement, and policies designed to tackle bullying and harassment (Stansfeld et al. 1999; Van Der Klink et al. 2001; Michie and Williams 2003). A poor work environment characterized by features such as high demand/low control (Karasek 1990; Karasek and Theorell 1990) and effort–reward imbalance (Siegrist 1996) is one of the main factors explaining the higher prevalence of depressive symptoms among participants in lower employment grades (Stansfeld et al. 1999).

Promoting workers' well-being and mental health requires change at the organizational level as well as more individual-focused approaches (Giga et al. 2003; Bambara et al. 2007). A systematic review by Bambra et al. (2007) reports that while microlevel interventions that change the psychosocial work environment and enhance employee's level of control have a positive impact on self-reported mental and physical health, the interventions that had more positive effects were those in which the macroenvironment was also supportive of employee control and participation. A comprehensive policy of mental health at work includes addressing the mental health of the organization itself as well as that of the individual employees (WHO 2000). The gain to both employees and the organization is reflected in reduced absenteeism, improved well-being, and productivity.

The macroeconomic labor market conditions and employment policies, including issues of salaries, career opportunities, and job security, also have a significant influence on employee well-being, and interventions addressing these structural factors need to be considered (Marmot et al. 1999). Policy initiatives, legislation, and regulatory mechanisms are required to safeguard the rights of workers against the negative impact of effort–reward imbalance, especially among vulnerable groups, such as migrant and contract workers.

The mental health impact of unemployment is well documented, including a higher risk of suicide, higher levels of anxiety, depression, uncertainty about the future, anger, shame, and loss of self-esteem (Murphy and Athanasou 1999; Jané-Llopis and Barry 2005, 2005; Paul and Moser 2009). Interventions, such as the JOBS program (Caplan et al. 1989; Vinokur et al. 2000), that combat the negative impact of unemployment on mental health and facilitate reemployment, are the most effective way of promoting the mental health of the unemployed. The JOBS program, which promotes the mental health of unemployed people and is cost-effective in terms of increased economic benefits for participants and the state, has been applied successfully in a number of countries (Vinokur et al. 2000; Vuori and Silvonen 2005; Barry et al. 2006; Reynolds et al. 2010).

The evidence for interventions promoting mental health in the workplace is only partial, and many authors comment on the poor-quality implementation of the interventions in many of the studies, with lack of management commitment being frequently cited as a specific problem. In particular, there is a paucity of studies that assess organizational-level approaches and organizational-level outcomes (Graveling et al. 2008). There is need for more evaluation of the impact of changes in employment practices and management style and of the inclusion of longer-term follow-ups and economic evaluations (Michie and Williams 2003). While acknowledging that the evidence needs to be strengthened, it can be concluded from the current evidence that a comprehensive and integrated approach to mental health promotion, which combines both individual- and organizational-level interventions, will be more effective in improving and maintaining positive mental health at work.

Promoting Positive Mental Health in the Community

The community setting offers important opportunities to work with diverse population groups in strengthening social networks and in addressing systems of socialization, social support, participation, and socioenvironmental influences on mental health and well-being. Interventions addressing community-level determinants of mental health aim to improve people's sense of social belonging, strengthen community networks, build social capital, improve neighborhood environments and community safety, and promote services and support networks to promote mental well-being.

Communities with high levels of social capital, including trust, reciprocity, participation, and cohesion, have important benefits for mental health (Morgan and Swann 2004; Whiteford et al. 2005; Friedli 2009; Wilkinson and Pickett 2009). Social support and social inclusion play a significant role in maintaining positive mental health (Lehtinen et al. 2005; Wilkinson and Marmot 2003). There are a number of review studies of social support interventions for older people which demonstrate their positive impact on mental health (Cattan et al. 2005). Research findings also support the effectiveness of peer-support programs for diverse groups delivered by trained community volunteers, including bereavement support

(Vachon et al. 1980), self-help groups, and care for older people (Cattan et al. 2005; Wheeler et al. 1998).

A culture of cooperation and tolerance, a sense of belonging, and strong social relationships are protective of positive mental health (Moodie and Jenkins 2005). Stigma and discrimination are identified as one of the most important barriers to well-being and quality of life in the community for people who experience mental health problems (WHO 2001). Tackling stigma in public attitudes to mental health and raising public awareness of the importance of positive mental health require focused interventions approaches, ranging from sophisticated mass media campaigns to more local initiatives involving community models of participation. Campaigns or social marketing interventions, particularly if they are supported by local community action, have been shown to have a significant impact on public knowledge, attitudes, and behavioral intentions (Wyllie et al. 2008; Myers et al. 2009) and are cost-effective (Vaithianathan and Pram 2010). Such interventions can increase understanding and tolerance, reduce stigma, and increase knowledge of sources of support. They also have the potential to positively impact on mental health literacy at the wider community level.

Community development programs, based on the participation and empowerment of local community members, including those who are socially marginalized, provide a useful model for promoting mental health in disadvantaged community settings (Arole et al. 2005). Community empowerment initiatives entail individuals and organizations working together to gain increased control over the quality of life in their community. Effective interventions include economic empowerment initiatives, such as microcredit schemes and community banks, literacy promotion, policies that promote gender and racial equality, violence prevention, and crime reduction in marginalized communities (Patel et al. 2005; Barry et al. 2007).

Environmental factors including access to open spaces and the quality of buildings and other structures have a beneficial impact on mental health (Dalgard and Tambs 1997; Ellaway et al. 2001; Weich et al. 2002; Whitley et al. 2005). Neighborhood disorder, mistrust, and powerlessness have negative impacts on mental health and serve to amplify a sense of hopelessness and alienation (Friedli 2009). Urban regeneration projects, which address the psychosocial aspects of deprivation, can have a significant mental health impact. A systematic review by Thomson et al. (2001), and a number of subsequent studies (Thomson et al. 2003, 2006), reports evidence that improving housing can lead to positive mental health impacts. Further mental health impact assessment of community-level initiatives, such as urban regeneration, which typically may not assess the impacts on health and well-being, is required if the potential of such initiatives to improve mental health and well-being is to be demonstrated.

Although the evidence is quite limited in terms of the documented impact of interventions on positive mental health, community initiatives aimed at building social capital, strengthening community networks, and increasing participation by excluded groups have an important contribution to make in promoting community mental health and well-being.

Promoting Positive Mental Health at the Societal Level

At the societal level, mental health promotion entails addressing the structural determinants of mental health. This includes reducing the structural barriers to mental health through initiatives to reduce poverty, discrimination, and social inequities and to promote access to education, meaningful employment, housing, and services and support for those who are most vulnerable. Poor mental health is consistently associated with poverty, unemployment, low levels of education, low-income or material standard of living, poor physical health, and adverse life events (Melzer et al. 2004; Patel et al. 2005; Kessler 2007; Prince et al. 2007). Recent studies across a number of countries also report that higher levels of positive mental health are associated with higher levels of education, paid employment, and higher social and economic position in society (Keyes 2002; Lehtinen et al. 2005; Barry et al. 2009b). Higher national levels of income inequality have also been found to be associated with a higher prevalence of mental disorders (Pickett et al. 2006). The experience of inequity is corrosive of good social relations and has a negative impact on people's mental health and their sense of emotional and social well-being. The experience of racial harassment and perceptions of racial discrimination have also been found to contribute to poor mental health outcomes (Chakraborty and McKenzie 2002; Aspinal and Jacobson 2004).

Responsibility for promoting mental health at the societal level extends across sectors and all government departments and encompasses a concern with the impact of economic and social policies on population well-being and the quality of people's lives. The evidence indicates that higher levels of education, improved standards of living, freedom from discrimination, fewer adverse life events, and good physical health enhance positive mental health (Barry and Friedli 2008). An integrated policy approach is required to address these structural factors and underlines the need for cross-sectoral policy implementation. The WHO Commission on the Social Determinants of Health report (World Health Organization 2008) concluded that the impact of daily living conditions on health, and the impact of inequitable distribution of power, money, and resources in particular, acts as structural drivers of inequity. Friedli (2009) argues that mental health is directly and indirectly related, at every level, to human responses to inequity, influencing people's sense of agency, self-esteem, efficacy, and connectedness, and their ability to deal with chronic stress and adversity. Wilkinson and Pickett (2009) posit that as inequity is an aspect of the broad structure of society, the powerful mechanisms that make people sensitive to inequity cannot be understood in terms of either social structure or individual psychology alone. Therefore, understanding the effects of inequity means understanding how individuals are affected by social structure, and this may produce useful policy insights into the well-being of whole societies. The impact of inequity on mental health and the role of psychosocial mechanisms in mediating the impact of inequity are under-researched and require further investigation.

International Policy Developments in Mental Health Promotion

The growing emphasis on the need for mental health promotion is both explicit and implicit in a wide range of policies on population health and mental health. There is also a growing interest in how a well-being focus could influence the future direction of public policy in areas such as education, employment, culture, and sustainable development (Marks and Shah 2005; Layard 2005; Dolan et al. 2006; Pickett et al. 2006; Eckersley 2006; Marks et al. 2006; Carlisle 2007; Friedli 2009). Greater integration of social, economic, and ecological policies is being advocated in order to maximize population well-being (New Economics Foundation 2003). The increasing focus on well-being is also reflected in the development of national well-being indicators, which seek to capture people's sense of well-being and how their lives are progressing, alongside indicators of economic growth (e.g., the National Accounts of Well-being by the New Economics Foundation 2008). A number of countries have developed national well-being indices, including countries as diverse as Bhutan and Canada. Such measures serve as national indicators of social progress, which can usefully inform policy making, and are designed to go beyond a traditional "silo approach" to public policy decisions.

Mental health policies, which embrace a positive well-being focus and advocate for a flourishing society based on promoting population mental health and well-being, have been introduced and are being strengthened in a number of countries (see, e.g., Towards a Mentally Flourishing Scotland, Scottish Government 2009). A review of international policy developments in mental promotion (GermAnn and Ardiles 2009) outlines the different types of policy models that have been adopted across a number of high-income countries (including Australia, Ireland, New Zealand, Scotland, and England) when incorporating the promotion of mental health into population health and mental health policies. Across all of these jurisdictions, there has been a focus on developing a population-based approach to mental health improvement, whether this be through a stand-alone mental health promotion policy as in Scotland (Scottish Government 2009) and Northern Ireland (Northern Ireland Association for Mental Health 2009) or as part of a more comprehensive mental health policy as in Australia (Council of Australian Governments 2006), New Zealand (Ministry of Health 2005), England (NIMHE 2005), and Ireland (Department of Health and Children 2006). It is noteworthy that in Australia (Commonwealth Department of Health and Aged 2000) and New Zealand (Ministry of Health 2002), specific policies for mental health promotion have also been developed in order to strengthen mental health promotion action. In a number of countries, there is also a stated aim to integrate mental health promotion into public health policy. In England, the New Horizons initiative (Department of Health 2009) presents a cross-government vision for mental health and well-being in England from 2010 onward. As part of the New Horizons initiative, a public mental health framework for developing well-being and resilience, and reducing inequalities, is presented. Based on a vision to create flourishing connected communities, a framework for promoting well-being is outlined which includes ensuring a positive start to life; building resilience and a safe, secure base; integrating physical and mental health and well-being; developing sustainable connected communities; and promoting meaning and purpose.

A number of national population health policies also include a focus on promoting positive mental health, underscoring the critical contribution of good mental health to population health and well-being. The relevance of the mental health improvement agenda to the broader policy context of addressing health inequities and the social determinants of health is also evident in a number of policies, recognizing that mental health is both a contributor and a consequence of social inequity. In such policy models, a whole-government approach is advocated, with responsibility for promoting mental health extending across government departments and encompassing a concern with the impact of economic and social policies on population mental health and well-being.

An overview of international policies clearly shows that, in almost all countries, the effective implementation of policy is identified as a key challenge (GermAnn and Ardiles 2009). While well-designed policies and plans give a mandate for action at a national level, implementation can be variable, particularly at the regional and local levels. A number of key influencing factors are identified, which include the need for sustained leadership for the implementation process, sufficient financial and human resources to support delivery, effective engagement across sectors, and the need for coordination of actions at multiple levels (national/state/local), especially across the service delivery and public health fields of practice. Building and strengthening an infrastructure for policy implementation is required, including sustained leadership and cross-sectoral partnerships, investment in research and evaluation to guide the implementation of policy and best practice, and building workforce capacity for quality implementation across sectors.

Building Capacity for the Effective Implementation of Mental Health Promotion

There is a growing body of knowledge from research and practice which shows that high-quality comprehensive programs promoting mental health, carried out in collaboration with individuals, families, and communities, can produce lasting positive benefits for mental health and social well-being. When these interventions are implemented effectively, they lead to improvements not only in mental health but also to improved social functioning, academic and work performance, and general health behaviors. The effects are especially evident in relation to the early years and for families from disadvantaged backgrounds, indicating that investment in such initiatives is cost-effective. The critical issue is ensuring that these interventions can be effectively implemented and sustained. It is, therefore, important to consider what is needed to ensure that effective policy and practice is at a scale, scope, and intensity to make a critical difference for population mental health.

Implementing programs in complex multilevel systems, such as schools, workplaces, and communities, requires a focus on the complex interaction of characteristics of the intervention, the implementer, the participants, the organizational capacity, and support of the delivery system (both general and intervention-specific capacity) and the specific contexts in which the intervention is being implemented (Chen 1998). The recognition of implementation complexity and the importance of relevance to the local context and community are critical considerations (Fixsen et al. 2005; Clarke et al. 2010). Current research indicates that implementation is often variable and imperfect in field settings and that the level of implementation influences outcomes (Durlak and DuPre 2008; Durlak 1998; Domitrovich and Greenberg 2000). The importance of a supportive implementation system in ensuring successful program implementation and replication is underscored by the literature (Mihalic et al. 2002; Barry et al. 2005). Influencing factors include; the quality of training and support, facilitatory and inhibitory factors in the local context such as readiness, mobilization of support, ecological fit of the program, cultural sensitivity, and the extent of participation and collaboration with key stakeholders. The level and extent of all these aspects of the implementation system need to be carefully planned and documented in order to ensure the quality and sustainability of program delivery. The generic processes underpinning the effective implementation of mental health promotion interventions are identified by Barry and Jenkins (2007) through examining a number of model programs and case studies to determine how effective implementation can be ensured through the use of research-based, theoretically grounded, and culturally appropriate interventions.

Translating from research into effective policy and practice requires not only scientific research evidence but also the skills of effective implementation. Program implementation involves working creatively with local resources, engaging participation, mobilizing support, and successfully navigating the process of collaboration and partnership-building with different stakeholders. Developing sustainable initiatives requires the ability to foster collaboration that will bring about system transformation for endurable change. The resources and skills required for effective implementation tend to be underestimated, and the leadership required for effective translation of plans into action needs to permeate all the way from the level of macro policy to local implementation. While public mental health is, indeed, everybody's business—as we all have mental health needs—dedicated resources and capacities are required for the effective implementation of policy and practice. A skilled and trained workforce with the necessary competencies to work at the level of population groups, communities, and individuals is recognized as being critical to effective implementation. Partnerships and cross-sectoral strategies that call for high-level expertise are needed in order to engage and facilitate the participation of diverse sectors. Building the capacity of workforce in developing and implementing mental health promotion programs is fundamental to mainstreaming and sustaining action in this area. Workforce development and training range from increasing awareness and training about the promotion of mental health for the wider workforce, to skills development needed to support and implement specific initiatives, through to dedicated mental health promotion specialists who facilitate and support the development and implementation of policy and practice across a range of settings. Continuing professional development and training is required to enhance the quality of practice and update the skill set required to work within changing social and political contexts. International developments in identifying core competencies for health promotion (Allegrante et al. 2009; Barry et al. 2009c) could usefully inform frameworks for workforce development and training in mental health promotion.

Conclusions

Positive mental health is an integral component of good health and quality of life and is critical to population well-being and the social and economic prosperity of society. There is a growing body of knowledge on the effective implementation of mental health promotion policy and practice in a number of countries around the world. Mental health promotion offers a distinctive framework for promoting positive mental health, through embracing an empowering, participatory approach based on the underpinning principles of health promotion and collaborative multisectoral action that addresses the structural determinants of mental health. This approach, which is being tried and tested in a number of countries, is based on a body of evidence that demonstrates its capacity to have a positive impact on the mental health and well-being of individuals, families, and communities. The wider health and social benefits that will accrue from promoting positive mental health are already apparent in the evidence base. Indeed, in many respects, demonstrating an impact on positive mental health is methodologically more feasible than demonstrating the successful prevention of mental disorders. However, for this potential to be fully realized, indicators of positive mental health, including standard measures in population health surveys, need to be further developed and refined so that they may be employed in determining the impact and outcomes of mental health promotion practice and policy.

Mental health promotion has an important role to play in empowering individuals, families, and communities in shaping the future direction and quality of their lives, and enhancing well-being in the face of challenges, such as changing family and work structures, economic crises, growing health inequities, and increasing globalization. The positive orientation of mental health promotion, in terms of its competence-enhancement approach, provides an appealing and practical framework for practice and policy. Broad engagement across society is needed to ensure that public policies and services are oriented toward the promotion of mental health and population well-being.

The promotion of mental health and well-being cannot be undertaken by any one sector, or any single profession or discipline on its own. Effective policy and practice requires different sectors and organizations to work together. The socioenvironmental nature of the determinants of mental health demands a cross-sectoral approach, involving the building of partnerships and collaboration across a range of sectors, agencies, organizations, and community groups. Collaboration across government departments and different sectors is key to effectively influencing the determinants of mental health. In keeping with the basic principles of health promotion, a multisectoral, integrated approach is needed that will ensure that mental health promotion is embedded firmly in policy across a range of sectors such as education, employment, housing, environment, social inclusion, and equality. These efforts need to be coordinated across the various sectors so that the impact of all public and social policies on population level mental health can be assessed and monitored.

Advocacy and active engagement across sectors is needed to promote a greater understanding of the concept of positive mental health and its importance for overall health and quality of life. To increase the visibility of positive mental health and its promotion at a societal level, it is necessary to remove the stigma surrounding mental ill-health and to promote greater public and professional understanding of the importance of promoting positive mental health as a resource for everyday life, good health, and societal well-being. This means effectively mobilizing a public demand for a greater focus on positive mental health and engaging the participation of the wider community in securing the conditions needed for a mentally healthy society.

References

Aber, J. L., Jones, S. M., Brown, J. L., Chaudry, N., & Samples, F. (1998). Resolving conflict creatively: Evaluating the developmental effects of a school-based violence prevention program in neighborhood and classroom context. *Development and Psychopathology, 10*, 187–213.

Adi, Y., Killoran, A., Janmohamed, K., & Stewart-Brown, S. (2007). *Systematic review of the effectiveness of interventions to promote mental wellbeing in children in primary education: Report 1: Universal approaches. Non-violence related outcomes*. London: NICE (National Institute for Health and Clinical Excellence). [online]. Available: http://guidance.nice.org.uk/page.aspx?o=441001 [July, 2007].

Allegrante, J. P., Barry, M. M., Airhihenbuwa, C. O., Auld, E., Collins, J. L., Lamarre, M.-C., Magnusson, M., McQueen, D., & Mittelmark, M. (2009). Domains of core competency, standards, and quality assurance for building global capacity in health promotion: The Galway Consensus Conference Statement. *Health Education & Behavior, 36*(3), 476–482.

Anderson, L. M., Shinn, C., Fullilove, M. T., Scrimshaw, S. C., Fielding, J. E., Normand, J., Carande-Kulis, V. G., & the Task Force on Community Preventive Services. (2003). The effectiveness of early childhood development programs: A systematic review. *American Journal of Preventive Medicine, 24*(3S), 32–46.

Arole, R., Fuller, B., & Deutschman, P. (2005). Community development as a strategy for mental health promotion: Lessons from a low income country. In H. Herman, S. Saxena, & R. Moodie (Eds.), *Promoting mental health: Concepts, emerging evidence, practice.* A WHO Report in collaboration with the Victorian Health Promotion Foundation and the University of Melbourne. Geneva: World Health Organization.

Aspinall, P. J., & Jacobson, B. (2004). *Ethnic disparities in health and health care: A focused review of the evidence and selected examples of good practice*. London: London Health Observatory.

Bambara, C., Egan, M., Thomas, S., Petticrew, M., & Whitehead, M. (2007). The psychosocial and health effects of workplace reorganisation: A systematic review of task restructuring interventions. *Journal of Epidemiology and Community Health, 61*, 1028–1037.

Barlow, J., & Parsons, J. (2003). Group-based parent-training programmes for improving emotional and behavioural adjustment in 0–3 year old children. *Cochrane Database of Systematic Reviews* 2003, Issue 2. Art. No.: CD003680. doi:10.1002/14651858.CD003680

Barlow, J., Parsons, J., & Stewart-Brown, S. (2002). *Systematic review of parenting programmes in the primary and secondary prevention of mental health problems*. Oxford: University of Oxford Health Services Research Unit.

Barlow, J., Coren, E., & Stewart-Brown, S. (2003). Parent-training programmes for improving maternal psychosocial health. *Cochrane Database of Systematic Reviews* 2003, Issue 4. Art. No.:CD002020. doi:10.1002/14651858.CD002020.pub2

Barry, M. M. (2001). Promoting positive mental health: Theoretical frameworks for practice. *International Journal of Mental Health Promotion, 3*(1), 25–34.

Barry, M. M. (2007). Generic principles of effective mental health promotion. *International Journal of Mental Health Promotion, 9*(2), 4–16.

Barry, M. M. (2009). Addressing the determinants of positive mental health: Concepts, evidence and practice. *International Journal of Mental Health Promotion, 11*(3), 4–17.

Barry, M. M., & Friedli, L. (2008). The influence of social, demographic and physical factors on positive mental health in children, adults and older people. *Foresight Mental Capital and Wellbeing Project. State-of-Science Review: SR-B3*. London: Government Office of Science and Innovation, UK.

Barry, M. M., & Jenkins, R. (2007). *Implementing mental health promotion*. Oxford: Churchill Livingstone Elsevier.

Barry, M. M., Domitrovich, C., & Lara, A. (2005). The implementation of mental health promotion programs. In E. Jané-Llopis, M. M. Barry, C. Hosman and V. Patel (Eds.). The Evidence of Mental Health Promotion Effectiveness: Strategies for Action. *Promotion and Education IUHPE Special Issue, Supplement 2*, 30–35.

Barry, M. M., Reynolds, C., Sheridan, A., & Egenton, R. (2006). Implementation of the jobs programme in Ireland. *Journal of Public Mental Health, 5*(4), 10–25.

Barry, M. M., Patel, V., Jané-Llopis, E., Raeburn, J., & Mittlemark, M. (2007). Strengthening the evidence base for mental health promotion. In D. C. McQueen & C. M. Jones (Eds.), *Global perspectives on health promotion* (pp. 67–86). New York: Springer.

Barry, M. M., Canavan, R., Clarke, A., Dempsey, C., & O'Sullivan, M. (2009a). *Review of evidence-based mental health promotion and primary/secondary prevention*. Report prepared for the Department of Health, London. Health Promotion Research Centre, National University of Ireland Galway. Accessible at: http: www.nuigalway.ie/hprc

Barry, M. M., van Lente, E., Molcho, M., Morgan, K., McGee, H., Conroy, R., Watson, D., Shelley, E., & Perry, I. (2009b). *SLÁN 2007: Survey of lifestyle, attitudes and nutrition in Ireland: Mental health and social well-being report*. Department of Health and Children. Dublin: The Stationery Office. Accessible at: www.slan07.ie

Barry, M. M., Allegrante, J. P., Lamarre, M.-C., Auld, E., & Taub, A. (2009c). The Galway Consensus Conference: International collaboration on the development of core competencies for health promotion and health education. *Global Health Promotion, 16*(2), 5–11.

Bruene-Butler, L., Hampson, J., Elias, M. J., Clabby, J., & Schuyler, T. (1997). The 'improving social awareness-social problem solving' project. In G. W. Albee & T. P. Gullotta (Eds.), *Primary prevention works, Vol 6: Issues in children's and families' lives*. Thousand Oaks: Sage.

Bull, J., McCormick, G., Swann, C., & Mulvihill, C. (2004). *Ante-and post-natal home-visiting programmes: A review of reviews*. NHS Health Development Agency. [online]. Available: http://www.nice.org.uk/niceMedia/documents/home_visiting.pdf

Caplan, R. D., Vinokur, A. D., Price, R. H., & Van Ryn, M. (1989). Job seeking, reemployment, and mental health: A randomized field experiment in coping with job loss. *Journal of Applied Psychology, 74*(5), 759–769.

Carlisle, S. (2007). *Series of papers on cultural influences on mental health and well-being in Scotland*. Available: http://www.wellscotland.info/publications/consultations4.html. Accessed Apr 2009.

Cattan, M., White, M., Bond, J., & Learmouth, A. (2005). Preventing social isolation and loneliness among older people: A systematic review of health promotion interventions. *Ageing & Society, 25*, 41–67.

Chakraborty, A., & McKenzie, K. (2002). Does racism cause mental illness? *The British Journal of Psychiatry, 180*, 475–477.

Chen, H. (1998). Theory-driven evaluations. *Advances in Educational Productivity, 7*, 15–34.

Ciliska, D., Mastrilli, P., Ploeg, J., Hayward, S., Brunton, G., & Underwood, J. (1999). *The effectiveness of home visiting as a delivery strategy for public health nursing interventions to clients in the prenatal and postnatal period: A systematic review*. Hamilton: Effective Public Health Practice Project (EPHPP).

Clarke, A. M., & Barry, M. M. (2010). *An evaluation of the Zippy's friends emotional wellbeing programme for primary schools in Ireland*. Health Promotion Research Centre, National University of Ireland Galway. Accessible at www.nuigalway.ie/hprc

Clarke, A. M., O'Sullivan, M., & Barry, M. M. (2010). Context matters in programme implementation. *Health Education, 110*(4), 273–293.

Commonwealth Department of Health and Aged Care. (2000). *National action plan for promotion, prevention and early intervention for mental health 2000*. Canberra: Mental Health and Special Programs Branch, Cw. Department of Health and Aged Care. Accessible online at: www.health.gov.au/internet/main/publishing.nsf/Content/mental-pubs-n-promote

Council of Australian Governments. (2006). *National Action Plan on Mental Health 2006–2011*. Accessible: www.coag.gov.au/reports/docs/AHMC_COAG_mental_health.doc

Dalgard, O. S., & Tambs, K. (1997). Urban environment and mental health: A longitudinal study. *The British Journal of Psychiatry, 171*, 530–536.

De Graaf, I., Speetjents, P., Smit, F., de Wolff, M., & Tavecchio, L. (2008). Effectiveness of The Triple P Parenting Program on behavioral problems in children: A meta-analysis. *Behavior Modification, 32*(5), 714–735.

Dean, C., Myors, K., & Evans, E. (2003). Community-wide implementation of a parenting programme: The south east Sydney positive parenting project. *Australian e-Journal for the Advancement of Mental Health, 2*(3), 1–12.

Department for Education and Skills DfES. (2005). Primary national strategy. Excellence and enjoyment. Social and emotional aspects of learning. Guidance Booklet (Ref 1378–2005). London: The Stationery Office.

Department of Health. (2009). *New horizons: A shared vision for mental health*. London: HM Government.

Department of Health and Children. (2006). *A vision for change: Report of the expert group on mental health policy*. Dublin: The Stationery Office.

Dolan, P., Peasgood, T., &White, M. (2006). *Review of research on the influences on personal well-being and application to policy making*. London: DEFRA (Department of the Environment, Food and Rural Affairs). Accessible online at: http://www.defra.gov.uk/science/project_data/DocumentLibrary/SD12005/SD12005_4017_FRP.pdf

Domitrovich, C. E., & Greenberg, M. T. (2000). The study of implementation: Current findings from effective programs that prevent mental disorders in school-aged children. *Journal of Educational and Psychological Consultation, 11*(2), 193–221.

Durlak, J. A. (1998). Why program implementation is important. *Journal of Prevention & Intervention in the Community, 17*(2), 5–18.

Durlak, J. A., & DuPre, E. P. (2008). Implementation matters: A review of research on the influence of implementation on program outcomes and the factors affecting implementation. *American Journal of Community Psychology, 41*(3–4), 327–350.

Durlak, J. A., & Wells, A. M. (1997). Primary prevention mental health programs for children and adolescents: A meta-analytic review. *American Journal of Community Psychology, 25*(2), 115–152.

Eckersley, R. (2006). Is modern western culture a health hazard? *International Journal of Epidemiology, 35*, 252–258. PDF: http://ije.oxfordjournals.org/cgi/content/full/35/2/252?etoc

Elkan, R., Kendrick, D., Hewitt, M., Robinson, J. J. A., Tolley, K., Blair, M., Dewey, M., Williams, D., & Brummell, K. (2000). The effectiveness of domiciliary health visiting: A systematic review of international studies and a selective review of the British literature. *Health Technology Assessment, 4*(13).

Ellaway, A., Macintyre, S., & Kearns, A. (2001). Perceptions of place and health in socially contrasting neighbourhoods. *Urban Studies, 38*(12), 2299–2316.

Fixsen, D. L., Naoom, S. F., Blasé, K. A., Friedman, R. M., & Wallace, F. (2005). *Implementation research: A synthesis of the literature*. Tampa: Louis de la Parte Florida Mental Health Institute, The National Implementation Research Network, University of South Florida.

Foresight Project on Mental Capital and Wellbeing. (2008). *Final project report*. London: Government Office for Science, London. Accessible online at: www.foresight.gov.uk

Friedli, L. (2003). *Making it effective: A guide to evidence based mental health promotion*. London: Mentality, London.

Friedli, L. (2009). *Mental health, resilience and inequalities*. Copenhagen: WHO Regional Office for Europe.

Friedli, L., & Parsonage, M. (2007). *Mental health promotion: Building an economic case*. Belfast: Northern Ireland Association for Mental Health.

Galinsky, E. (2006). *The economic benefits of high-quality early childhood programs: What makes the difference?* Washington, DC: CED (Committee for Economic Development).

GermAnn, K., & Ardiles, P. (2009). Toward flourishing for all: Mental health promotion and mental illness prevention policy background paper. Commissioned by the Pan-Canadian Steering Committee for Mental Health Promotion and Mental Illness Prevention. Accessible at: http://www.utoronto.ca/chp/mentalhealthpdffinal/Toward%20Flourishing%20for%20All%20Companion%20Document%20%20Final%20Version%20April%202009.pdf

Giga, S. I., Noblet, A. J., Faragher, B., & Cooper, C. L. (2003). The UK perspective: A review of research on organisational stress management interventions. *Australian Psychologist, 39*(2), 158–164.

Graveling, R. A., Crawford, J. O., Cowie, H., Amati, C., & Vohra, S. (2008). *A review of workplace interventions that promote mental wellbeing in the workplace -Draft report*. London: Institute of Occupational Medicine. [online]. Available: http://www.nice.org.uk/nicemedia/pdf/MentalWellbeingWorkFinalReport.pdf

Greenberg, M. T., Kusche, C. A., Cook, E. T., & Quamma, J. P. (1995). Promoting emotional competence in school-aged children: The effects of the PATHS curriculum. *Development and Psychopathology, 7*, 117–136.

Greenberg, M. T., Domitrovich, C. E., & Bumbarger, B. (2001). The prevention of mental disorders in school-aged children: current state of the field. *Prevention and Treatment, 4*(1). [online]. Available: http://journals.apa.org/prevention/volume4/pre0040001a.html. Accessed June 2009.

Harden, A., Rees, R., Shepherd, J., Brunton, G., Oliver, S., & Oakley, A. (2001). *Young people and mental health: A systematic review on barriers and facilitators*. England: EPPI-Centre. [Online]. Available: http://eppi.ioe.ac.uk

Health Education Authority. (1997). *Mental health promotion: A quality framework*. London: Health Education Authority.

Herrman, H., Saxena, S., & Moodie, R. (Eds.) (2005). *Promoting mental health: Concepts, emerging evidence, practice*. A report of the World Health Organization, Department of Mental Health and Substance Abuse in collaboration with the Victorian Health Promotion Foundation and University of Melbourne. Geneva: World Health Organization. [online]. Available: www.who.int/mental_health/evicence/MH_Promotion_Book.pdf

Hosman, C., & Jané-Llopis, E. (1999). Political challenges 2: Mental health. In *The evidence of health promotion effectiveness: Shaping public health in a New Europe*. Chapter 3: 29–41, A Report for the European Commission. International Union for Health Promotion and Education. Paris: Jouve Composition & Impression.

Huppert, F. A. (2005). Positive mental health in individuals and populations. In F. Huppert, N. Bayliss, & B. Keverne (Eds.), *The science of well-being*. Oxford: Oxford University Press.

Jané-Llopis, E., & Barry, M. M. (2005). What makes mental health promotion effective? In E. Jané-Llopis, M. M. Barry, C. Hosman and V. Patel (Eds.). The Evidence of Mental Health Promotion Effectiveness: Strategies for Action. *Promotion and Education IUHPE Special Issue, Suppl 2*, 47–55.

Jané-Llopis, E., Barry, M. M., Hosman, C., & Patel, V. (2005). Mental health promotion works: A review. In E. Jané-Llopis, M.M. Barry, C. Hosman and V. Patel (Eds.). The Evidence of Mental Health Promotion Effectiveness: Strategies for Action. *Promotion and Education IUHPE Special Issue, Suppl 2*, 9–25.

Johnson, Z., Howell, F., & Molloy, B. (1993). Community mothers programme: Randomised controlled trial of non-professional intervention in parenting. *British Medical Journal, 306*, 1449–1452.

Johnson, Z., Molloy, B., Scallon, E., Fitzpatrick, P., Rooney, B., Keegan, T., & Byrne, P. (2000). Community Mothers Programme: Seven year follow-up of a randomised controlled trial of non-professional intervention in parenting. *Journal of Public Health Medicine, 22*(3), 337–342.

Karasek, R. A. (1990). Lower health risk with increased job control among white collar workers. *Journal of Organizational Behaviour, 11*, 171–185.

Karasek, R. A., & Theorell, T. (1990). *Healthy work: Stress, productivity and the reconstruction of working life*. New York: Basic Books.

Karoly, L. A., Greenwood, P. W., Everingham, S. S., Houbé, J., Kilburn, M. R., Rydell, C. P., Sanders, M., & Chiesa, J. (1998). *Investing in our children: What we know and don't know about the costs and benefits of early childhood interventions*. Santa Monica: Rand Publications.

Karoly, L. A., Kilburn, R. A., & Cannon, J. S. (2005). *Early childhood interventions: Proven results, future promises*. [online]. Available: http://www.rand.org/pubs/monographs/MG341

Keleher, H., & Armstrong, R. (2005). *Evidence-based mental health promotion resource*. Melbourne: Department of Human Services.

Kellam, S. G., Rebok, G. W., Ialongo, N., & Mayer, L. S. (1994). The course and malleability of aggressive behaviour from early first grade into middle school: Results of a developmental epidemiologically based preventive trial. *Journal of Child Psychology and Psychiatry, 35*, 259–281.

Kendrick, D., Elkan, R., Hewitt, M., Dewey, M., Blair, M., Robinson, J., Williams, D., & Brummell, K. (2000). Does home visiting improve parenting and the quality of the home environment? A systematic review and meta-analysis. [Electronic Version] *Arch. Dis. Child.* 2000; 82, 443–451. doi:10.1136/adc.82.6.443

Kendrick, D., Barlow, J., Hampshire, A., Polnay, L., & Stewart-Brown, S. (2007). Parenting interventions for the prevention of unintentional injuries in childhood. *Cochrane Database of Systematic Reviews* 2007, Issue 4. Art. No.: CD006020. doi:10.1002/14651858.CD006020.pub2

Kessler, R. C. (2007). The global burden of anxiety and mood disorders: Putting the European study of the epidemiology of mental disorders (ESEMeD) findings into perspective. *The Journal of Clinical Psychiatry, 68*(Suppl 2), 10–19.

Keyes, C. L. M. (2002). The mental health continuum: From languishing to flourishing in life. *Journal of Health and Social Research, 43*, 207–222.

Keyes, C. L. M. (2005). Mental illness and/or mental health? Investigating axioms of the complete state model of health. *Journal of Consulting and Clinical Psychology, 73*, 539–548.

Keyes, C. L. M. (2007). Promoting and protecting mental health as flourishing. *American Psychologist, 62*(2), 1–14.

Kovess-Masfety, M., Murray, M., &, Gureje, O, (2005). Positive mental health. In H. Herrman, S. Saxena, & R. Moodie (Eds.), *Promoting mental health: Concepts, emerging evidence, practice* (pp. 35–45). A report of the World Health Organization, Department of Mental Health and Substance Abuse in collaboration with the Victorian Health Promotion Foundation and University of Melbourne. Geneva: World Health Organization.

Lahtinen, E., Joubert, N., Raeburn, J., & Jenkins, R. (2005). Strategies for promoting the mental health of populations. In H. Herrman, S. Saxena, & R. Moodie (Eds.), *Promoting mental health: Concepts, emerging evidence, practice* (pp. 226–242). A report of the World Health Organization, Department of Mental Health and Substance Abuse in collaboration with the Victorian Health Promotion Foundation and University of Melbourne. Geneva: World Health Organization.

Layard, R. (2005). *Happiness: Lessons from a new science*. London: Allen Lane.
Lehtinen, V., Ozamiz, A., Underwood, L., & Weiss, M. (2005). The intrinsic value of mental health. In H. Herrman, S. Saxena, & R. Moodie (Eds.), *Promoting mental health: Concepts, emerging evidence, practice* (pp. 46–58). A report of the World Health Organization, Department of Mental Health and Substance Abuse in collaboration with the Victorian Health Promotion Foundation and University of Melbourne. Geneva: WHO.
Lister-Sharp, D., Chapman, S., Stewart-Brown, S., & Sowden, A. (1999). Health promoting schools and health promotion in schools: Two systematic reviews. *Health Technology Assessment, 3*(22), 1–207.
Lyubomirsky, S., King, L., & Diener, E. (2005). The benefits of frequent positive affect: Does happiness lead to success? *Psychological Bulletin*. http://www.apa.org/journals/releases/bul1316803.pdf
Marks, N., & Shah, H. (2005). A well-being manifesto for a flourishing society. *Journal of Mental Health Promotion, 3*(4), 9–15.
Marks, N., Thompson, S., Eckersley, R., Jackson, T., & Kasser, T. (2006). *Sustainable development and well-being: Relationships, challenges and policy implications. A report by the centre for well-being, nef (the New Economics Foundation) for DEFRA (Department of the Environment, Food and Rural Affairs),* London. Accessible at: http://www.defra.gov.uk/science/project_data/DocumentLibrary/SD12007/SD12007_4606_FRP.pdf
Marmot, M., Siegrist, J., Therorell, T., … NOW LIST LAST AUTHOR. (1999). Health and the psychosocial environment at work. In M. Marmot, & R. Wilkinson (Eds.), *Social determinants of health*. Oxford: Oxford University Press.
Marshall-Williams, S., Saxena, S., & McQueen, D. V. (2005). The momentum for mental health promotion. *Promotion and Education, 2*, 6–9.
McCabe, C. (2007). *A systematic review of cost-effectiveness analyses of whole school interventions to promote children's mental health*. Leeds: Leeds Institute of Health Sciences, University of Leeds. [online] Available: http://www.nice.org.uk/nicemedia/pdf/MentalWellbeingChildrenCostEffectiveness.pdf
McKee-Ryan, F. M., Song, Z., Wanberg, C. R., & Kinicki, A. J. (2005). Psychological and physical well-being during unemployment: A meta-analytic study. *Journal of Applied Psychology, 90*, 53–76.
Melhuish, E. Belsky, J., Leyland, A. H., & NESS Research Team. (2008). *The impact of sure start local programmes on three year olds and their families* (The National Evaluation of Sure Start Research Report 027). London: University of London.
Melzer, D., Fryers, T., & Jenkins, R. (2004). *Social inequalities and the distribution of common mental disorders* (Maudsley Monographs). Hove: Psychology Press.
Michie, S., & Williams, S. (2003). Reducing work related psychological ill health and sickness absence: A systematic literature review. *Occupational and Environmental Medicine, 60*, 3–9.
Mihalic, S., Fagan, A., Irwin, K., Ballard, D., & Elliott, D. (2002). *Blueprints for violence prevention replications: Factors for implementation success*. Boulder: Center for the Study of Prevention of Violence, Institute of Behavioral Science, University of Colorado.
Ministry of Health (New Zealand). (2002). *Building on strengths: A new approach to promoting mental health in New Zealand/Aotearoa*. Accessible: www.moh.govt.nz/moh.nsf/f872666357c511eb4c25666d000c8888/7083a9302c12c0f9cc256e7f00056967?OpenDocument
Ministry of Health, New Zealand. (2005). *Te Tahuhu: Improving mental health 2005–2015*. Wellington: Ministry of Health. Accessible online at: www.moh.govt.nz/moh.nsf/0/F2907744575A9DA9CC25702C007E8411/$File/tetahuhu-improvingmentalhealth.pdf
Mishara, B. L., & Ystgaard, M. (2006). Effectiveness of a mental health promotion program to improve coping skills in young children: Zippy's Friends. *Early Childhood Quarterly, 21*, 110–123.
Mittelmark, M., Puska, P., O'Byrne, D., & Tang, K. -C. (2005). Health promotion: A sketch of the landscape. In H. Herrman, S. Saxena, & R. Moodie (Eds.), *Promoting mental health: Concepts, emerging evidence, practice* (pp. 18–34). A WHO Report in collaboration with the Victorian Health Promotion Foundation and the University of Melbourne. Geneva: World Health Organization.

Moodie, R., & Jenkins, R. (2005). I'm from the government and you want me to invest in mental health promotion: Well why should I? *Promotion and Education, Suppl 2*, 37.

Morgan, A., & Swann, C. (Eds.). (2004). *Social capital for health: Issues of definition, measurement and links to health*. London: Health Development Agency.

Mrazek, P. J., & Haggerty, R. J. (Eds.). (1994). *Reducing risks for mental disorders: Frontiers for preventive intervention research*. Washington, DC: National Academy Press.

Murphy, G. C., & Athanasou, J. A. (1999). The effect of unemployment on mental health. *Journal of Occupational and Organizational Psychology, 72*, 83–99.

Myers, F., Woodhouse, A., Whitehead, I., McCollam, A., McBryde, L., Pinfold, V., Thornicroft, G., McBrierty, R., & Wilson, L. (2009). *Evaluation of 'see me'. The national campaign against the stigma and discrimination associated with mental ill-health* (Research Report for the Scottish Government). Accessible at: www.scotland.gov.uk/socialresearch

Nelson, G., Westhues, A., & MacLeod, J. (2003). A meta-analysis of longitudinal research on preschool prevention programs for children. *Prevention and Treatment 6*. Available at: http://journals.apa.org/prevention/volume6/toc-dec18-03.html; http://www.hm-treasury.gov.uk/d/cypreview2006_cphva7.pdf

New Economics Foundation. (2003). *A well-being manifesto for a flourishing society*. London: nef. Available: www.neweconomicsfoundation.org

New Economics Foundation. (2008). *National accounts of well-being: Bringing real wealth on the balance sheet*. London: nef. Available: www.nationalaccountsofwellbeing.org

NIMHE – National Institute for Mental Health in England. (2005). Making it possible: Improving mental health and well-being in England. Accessible: http://kc.nimhe.org.uk/upload/making%20it%20possible%20Final%20pdf.pdf

Northern Ireland Association for Mental Health. (2009). *A flourishing society: Aspirations for emotional health and wellbeing in Northern Ireland*. Belfast: Northern Ireland Association for Mental Health.

O'Connell, M. A., Boat, T., & Warner, K. (2009). *Preventing mental, emotional and behavioral disorders among young people: Progress and possibilities*. Washington, DC: National Academies Press.

Olds, D. L., Eckenrode, J. J., Henderson, C. R., Kitzman, H., Powers, J., Cole, R., Sidora, K., Morris, P., Pettitt, L. M., & Luckey, D. (1997). Long term effects of home visitation on maternal life course and child abuse and neglect: Fifteen year follow up of a randomised trial. *Journal of the American Medical Association, 278*(8), 637–643.

Olds, D. L., Henderson, C. R., Kitzman, H. H., Eckenrode, J., Cole, R., & Tatelbaum, R. (1998). The promise of home visitation: Results of two randomised trials. *Journal of Community Psychology, 26*(1), 5–21.

Olds, D. L., Kitzman, J., Cole, R., Robinson, J., Sidora, K., Luckey, D. W., Henderson, C. R., Hanks, C., Bondy, J., & Holmberg, J. (2004). Effects of nurse-home-visiting on maternal life course and child development: Age 6 follow-up results of a randomised trial. *Pediatrics, 114*(6), 1550–1559.

Olds, D. L., Sadler, L., & Kitzman, H. J. (2006). Programs for parents of infants and toddlers: Recent evidence from randomized trials. *Journal of Child Psychology and Psychiatry, 48*(3/4), 355–391. doi:10.1111/j.1469-7610.2006.01702.x.

Olweus, D., Limber, S., & Mihalic, S. (1998). *Blueprints for violence prevention. Book Nine: Bullying Prevention Program*. Boulder: Center for the Study and Prevention of Violence, Institute of Behavioral Science.

Patel, V., Swartz, L., & Cohen, A. (2005). The evidence for mental health promotion in developing countries. In H. Herman, S. Saxena, & R. Moodie (Eds.), *Promoting mental health: Concepts, emerging evidence, practice*. A WHO Report in collaboration with the Victorian Health Promotion Foundation and the University of Melbourne. Geneva: World Health Organization.

Paul, K. I., & Moser, K. (2009). Unemployment impairs mental health: Meta-analyses. *Journal of Vocational Behavior, 55*(2), 188–220.

Payton, J., Weissberg, R. P., Durlak, J. A., Dymnicki, A. B., Taylor, R. D., Schellinger, K. B., & Pachan, M. (2008). *The positive impact of social and emotional learning for kindergarten to eight-grade students: Findings from three scientific reviews*. Chicago: Collaborative for Academic, Social, and Emotional Learning.

Pickett, K. E., James, O. W., & Wilkinson, R. G. (2006). Income inequality and the prevalence of mental illness: A preliminary international analysis. *Journal of Epidemiology and Community Health, 60*, 646–647.
Prince, M., Patel, V., Saxena, S., Maj, M., Maselko, J., Phillips, M. R., & Rahman, A. (2007). No health without mental health. *Lancet, 370*, 859–877.
Reynolds, C., Barry, M. M., & NicGabhainn, S. (2010). Evaluating the impact of the winning new jobs programme on the re-employment and mental health of a mixed profile of unemployed people. *International Journal of Mental Health Promotion, 12*(2), 32–41.
Rowling, L., Martin, G., & Walker, L. (2002). *Mental health promotion and young people: Concepts and practice*. Sydney: McGraw-Hill.
Ryff, C. D., & Singer, B. (1996). Psychological well-being: Meaning, measurement, and implications for psychotherapy research. *Psychotherapy and Psychosomatics, 65*, 14–23.
Ryff, C., Love, G., Urry, H., Muller, D., Rosenkranz, M., Friedman, E., Davidson, R., & Singer, B. (2006). Psychological well-being and ill-being: Do they have distinct or mirrored biological correlates? *Psychotherapy and Psychosomatics, 75*, 85–95.
Sanders, M. R. (1999). The Triple P-positive parenting programme: Towards an empirically validated multilevel parenting and family support strategy for the prevention of behaviour and emotional problems in children. *Clinical Child and Family Psychology Review, 2*(2), 71–90.
Sanders, M. R., Markie-Dadds, C., Tully, L., & Bor, W. (2000). The Triple P-positive parenting programme: A comparison of enhanced, standard and self-directed behavioural family intervention from parents of children with early onset conduct problems. *Journal of Consulting and Clinical Psychology, 68*(4), 624–640.
Schweinhart, L. J., Montie, J., Xiang, Z., Barnett, W. S., Belfield, C. R., & Nores, M.(2005). *Lifetime effects: The high/scope Perry pre-school study through age 40. Monographs of the High/Scope Educational Research Foundation, 14*. Ypsilanti, Michigan: High/Scope Press. [Online]. Available: http://www.highscope.org/Research/PerryProject/PerryAge40SumWeb.pdf
Scottish Government. (2009). *Toward a mentally flourishing Scotland: Policy and action plan 2009–2011*. Accessible: www.scotland.gov.uk/Publications/2009/05/06154655/
Shure, M. B., & Spivack, G. (1988). Interpersonal cognitive problem solving. In R. H. Price, E. L. Cowen, R. P. Lorion, et al. (Eds.), *Fourteen ounces of prevention: A casebook for practitioners*. Washington, DC: American Psychological Association.
Siegrist, J. (1996). Adverse health effects of high-effort/low-reward conditions. *Journal of Occupational Health Psychology, 1*, 27–41.
Stansfeld, S. A., Fuhrer, R., Shipley, M. J., & Marmot, M. G. (1999). Work characteristics predict psychiatric disorder: Prospective results from the Whitehall II study. *Occupational and Environmental Medicine, 56*, 302–307.
Stewart-Brown, S. (2005). Interpersonal relationships and the origins of mental health. *Journal of Public Mental Health, 4*(1), 24–29.
Sylva, K., Melhuish, E., Sammons, P., Siraj-Blatchford, I., & Taggart, B. (2007). *Effective pre- school and primary education 3–11 project (EPPE 3–11) a longitudinal study funded by the DfES (2003–2008) Promoting Equality in the Early Years: Report to the Equalities Review*. London: Institute of Education. http://archive.cabinetoffice.gov.uk/equalitiesreview/upload/assets/www.theequalitiesreview.org.uk/promoting_equality_in_the_early_years.pdf
Tennant, R., Goens, C., Barlow, J., Day, C., & Stewart-Brown, S. (2007). A systematic review of reviews of interventions to promote mental health and prevent mental health problems in children and young people. *Journal of Public Mental Health, 6*(1), 25–32.
Thompson, E. A., Eggert, L. L., Randell, B. P., & Pike, K. C. (2001). Evaluation of indicated suicide risk prevention approaches for potential high school dropouts. *American Journal of Public Health, 91*(5), 742–752.
Thomson, H., Petticrew, M., & Douglas, M. (2003). Health impact assessment of housing improvements: Incorporating research evidence. *Journal of Epidemiology and Community Health, 57*, 11–16.

Thomson, H., Atkinson, R., Petticrew, M., & Kearns, A. (2006). Do urban regeneration programmes improve public health and reduce health inequalities? A synthesis of the evidence from UK policy and practice (1980–2004). *Journal of Epidemiology and Community Health, 60*(2), 108–115.

Tilford, S., Delaney, F., & Vogels, M. (1997). *Effectiveness of mental health promotion interventions: A review*. London: Health Education Authority.

Vachon, M. L., Lyall, W. A., Rodgers, J., Freedman-Letofsky, K., & Freeman, S. J. J. (1980). A controlled study of self-help interventions for widows. *The American Journal of Psychiatry, 137*, 1380–1384.

Vaithianathan, R., & Pram, K. (2010). *Cost benefit analysis of the New Zealand National Mental Health Destigmatisation Programme ("Like-Minds programme")*. Prepared for Phoenix Research, Ministry of Health, New Zealand.

Van Der Klink, J. J. L., Blonk, R. W. B., Schene, A. H., & Van Dijk, F. J. H. (2001). The benefits of interventions for work-related stress. *American Journal of Public Health, 91*(2), 270–276.

VicHealth. (2009). *The Melbourne charter for promoting mental health and preventing mental and behavioral disorders*. Accessible online at: http://www.vichealth.vic.gov.au/en/Resource-Centre/Publications-and-Resources/Mental-health-promotion/Melbourne-Charter.aspx

Victorian Health Promotion Foundation. (2005). *A plan for action 2005–2007: Promoting mental health and well-being*. Accessible online at: www.vichealth.vic.gov.au/assets/contentFiles/VH%20action%20plan-web.pdf

Vinokur, A. D., Schul, Y., Vuori, J., & Price, R. H. (2000). Two years after a job loss: Long-term impact of the JOBS program on reemployment and mental health. *Journal of Occupational Health Psychology, 5*(1), 32–47.

Vuori, J., & Silvonen, J. (2005). The benefits of a preventive job search program on re- employment and mental health at two years follow-up. *Journal of Occupational and Organizational Psychology, 78*, 43–52.

Waddell, C., Hua, J. M., Garland, O., Peters, R., De, V. & McEwan, K., (2007). Preventing mental disorders in children: A systematic review to inform policy-making. *Canadian Journal of Public Health, 98*(3), 166–173.

Weich, S., Blanchard, M., Prince, M., & Burton, E. (2002). Mental health and the built environments: Cross-sectional survey of individual and contextual risk factors for depression. *The British Journal of Psychiatry, 180*, 428–433.

Weissberg, R. P., Caplan, M., & Harwood, L. (1991). Promoting competent young people in competence-enhancing environments: A systems-based perspective on primary prevention. *Journal of Consulting and Clinical Psychology, 59*(6), 830–841.

Wells, J., Barlow, J., & Stewart-Brown, S. (2003). A systematic review of universal approaches to mental health promotion in schools. *Health Education, 103*(4), 197–220.

Wheeler, J., Gorey, K., & Greenblatt, B. (1998). The beneficial effects of volunteering for older volunteers and the people they serve: A meta-analysis. *International Journal of Aging & Human Development, 47*(1), 69–79.

Whiteford, H., Cullen, M., & Baingana, F. (2005). Social capital and mental health. In H. Herman, S. Saxena, & R. Moodie (Eds.), *Promoting mental health: Concepts, emerging evidence, practice*. A WHO Report in collaboration with the Victorian Health Promotion Foundation and the University of Melbourne. Geneva: World Health Organization. [online]. Available: www.who.int/mental_health/evicence/MH_Promotion_Book.pdf

Whitley, R., Prince, M., & Cargo, M. (2005). Thinking inside the bubble: Evidence for a new contextual unit in urban mental health. *Journal of Epidemiology and Community Health, 59*(10), 893–897.

Wilkinson, R. G., & Marmot, M. (2003). *Social determinants of health: The solid facts* (2nd ed.). Copenhagen: World Health Organization Regional Office for Europe.

Wilkinson, R. G., & Pickett, K. (2009). *The spirit level: Why equality is better for everyone*. London: Penguin.

World Health Organization. (1986). *Ottawa charter for health promotion*. Geneva: World Health Organization.

World Health Organization. (2001). *Mental health: New understanding, new hope. The World Health Report*. Geneva: World Health Organization.
World Health Organization. (2002). *Prevention and promotion in mental health*. Geneva: World Health Organization.
World Health Organization. (2004a). *Promoting mental health: Concepts, emerging evidence, and practice* (Summary Report. A report of the World Health Organization, Department of Mental Health and Substance Abuse in collaboration with the Victorian Health Promotion Foundation and the University of Melbourne). Geneva: World Health Organization. Accessible online at: www.who.int/mental_health/evidence/en/promoting_mhh.pdf
World Health Organization. (2004b). *Prevention of mental disorders: Effective interventions and policy options* (Summary Report. A report of the World Health Organization Department of Mental Health and Substance Abuse in collaboration with the Prevention Research Centre of the Universities of Nijmegen and Maastricht). Geneva: WHO. Accessible: http://www.who.int/mental_health/evidence/en/prevention_of_mental_disorders_sr.pdf
World Health Organization. (2005a). *Mental health action plan for Europe: Facing the challenges, building solutions*. Accessible online at: www.euro.who.int/document/mnh/edoc07.pdf
World Health Organization. (2005b). *The Bangkok charter for health promotion in a globalized world*. Geneva: World Health Organization.
World Health Organization Commission on the Social Determinants of Health. (2008). *Closing the gap in a generation: Health equity through action on the social determinants of health. Final Report of the Commission on the Social Determinants of Health*. Geneva: World Health Organization.
World Health Organization. (2009). *Nairobi call to action for closing the implementation gap in health promotion. 7th Global Conference on Health Promotion*. World Health Organization, Geneva. Accessible online at: http://www.gesundheitsfoerderung.ch/pdf_doc_xls/e/GFPstaerken/Netzwerke/Nairobi-Call-to-Action-Nov09.pdf
World Health Organization. (Harnois, G., Gabriel, P. (Eds.)) (2000). *Mental health and work: Impact, issues and good practices*. Geneva: A joint publication of the World Health Organization and the International Labour Organization.
Wyllie, A., Cameron, A., & Howearth, J. (2008). *Impacts of national media campaigns to counter stigma and discrimination associated with mental illness*. Survey 9 Results for Campaign 4. Research Report for Ministry of Health, New Zealand.
Wynn, J., Cahill, H., Holdsworth, R., Rowling, L., & Carson, S. (2000). MindMatters, a whole school approach to promoting mental health and well-being. *Australia and New Zealand Journal of Psychiatry, 34*, 594–601.
Zechmeister, I., Kilian, R., McDaid, D., & the MHEEN Group. (2008). Is it worth investing in mental health promotion and prevention of mental illness? A systematic review of the evidence from economic evaluations. *BMC Public Health, 8*, 20. Accessed online at: http://www.ncbi.nlm.nih.gov/pmc/articles/PMC2245925/
Zins, J. E., Weissberg, R. P., Wang, M. C., & Walberg, H. J. (Eds.). (2004). *Building academic success on social and motivational learning: What does the research say?* New York: Teachers College Press.
Zubrick, S., & Kovess-Masfety, M. (2005). Indicators of mental health. In H. Herrman, S. Saxena, & R. Moodie (Eds.), *Promoting mental health: Concepts, emerging evidence, practice* (pp. 148–168). A report of the World Health Organization, Department of Mental Health and Substance Abuse in collaboration with the Victorian Health Promotion Foundation and University of Melbourne. Geneva: World Health Organization.

Index

C.L.M. Keyes (ed.), *Mental Well-Being: International Contributions to the Study of Positive Mental Health*, DOI 10.1007/978-94-007-5195-8,

MIX
Papier aus verantwortungsvollen Quellen
Paper from responsible sources
FSC® C105338

If you have any concerns about our products,
you can contact us on
ProductSafety@springernature.com

In case Publisher is established outside the EU,
the EU authorized representative is:
Springer Nature Customer Service Center GmbH
Europaplatz 3, 69115 Heidelberg, Germany

Printed by Libri Plureos GmbH
in Hamburg, Germany